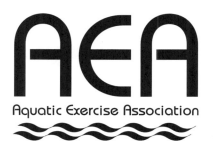

Aquatic Exercise Association

Aquatic Fitness
Professional Manual

5th Edition

Distributed by Human Kinetics

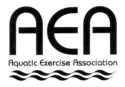

AEA
Aquatic Exercise Association

Published by:
Aquatic Exercise Association
201 S. Tamiami Trail, Suite 3
Nokomis, FL 34275
Phone: (941) 486-8600
Fax: (941) 486-8820
E-mail: info@aeawave.com
Website: www.aeawave.com

Distributed by:
Human Kinetics
Web site: www.HumanKinetics.com

United States: Human Kinetics
P.O. Box 5076
Champaign, IL 61825-5076
800-747-4457
e-mail: humank@hkusa.com

Canada: Human Kinetics
475 Devonshire Road Unit 100
Windsor, ON N8Y 2L5
800-465-7301 (in Canada only)
e-mail: orders@hkcanada.com

Europe: Human Kinetics
107 Bradford Road
Stanningley
Leeds LS28 6AT, United Kingdom
+44 (0) 113 255 5665
e-mail: hk@hkeurope.com

Australia: Human Kinetics
57A Price Avenue
Lower Mitcham, South Australia 5062
08 8277 1555
e-mail: liaw@hkaustralia.com

New Zealand: Human Kinetics
Division of Sports Distributors NZ Ltd.
P.O. Box 300 226 Albany
North Shore City
Auckland
0064 9 448 1207
e-mail: info@humankinetics.co.nz

Editorial Team:
Managing Editor – June Lindle, MS
Assistant Editors – Paul Baran and Julie See
Production Editor – Angie Proctor
Layout and Design – Carolyn Mac Millan
Photographer – Troy Nelson
Models – Ashley Acton, Heather Acton, Monique Acton,
   Greg Peterson, Norma Proctor and Kenroy Simmons

Illustrations and Graphics provided by:

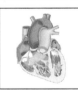
LifeART®;
Lippincott, Williams and Wilkins,
2005
To view all products, visit
www.lifeart.com

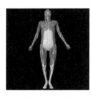
Primal Pictures ©
3D Images Copyright Primal Pictures
Ltd. 2005
To see the full range of this interactive
3D software please visit
www.primalpictures.com
2nd Floor, Tennyson House, 159-165 Great Portland
Street, London, W1W 5PA, UK

AEA thanks Speedo for the financial assistance and
support in the production of this Manual.

speedo

ISBN-10: 0-9760021-0-8
ISBN-13: 978-0-9760021-0-9

Acknowledgement

The Aquatic Exercise Association acknowledges that education is a never-ending process.

This manual is in recognition of over 40,000 aquatic fitness professionals worldwide who have dedicated their time, energy, motivation, leadership and expertise to promote global health and longevity for all people.

AEA thanks all supporters of aquatic fitness and the many industry leaders who have donated both time and experience to accomplishing this educational manual.

Mission Statement

The Aquatic Exercise Association is a not-for-profit educational organization dedicated to the growth and development of the aquatic fitness industry and the public served.

Table of Contents

Introduction

This manual is intended as a resource for students and fitness professionals seeking knowledge in aquatic fitness application, education and training. It contains both condensed and simplified information as well as in-depth knowledge in many subject areas relevant to aquatic fitness theory and application. AEA hopes that this manual will help all fitness professionals to study, review, learn and update skills necessary to effectively lead aquatic fitness programming. May all utilizing this manual continue to learn and grow in the pursuit of a healthier and more fit planet.

Chapter 1: Exercise Anatomy

INTRODUCTION

Chapter one gives you an overview of the organization of the human body, with a more in-depth look at the five bodily systems most closely related to exercise. You will take a surface look at how the skeletal, muscular, nervous, respiratory, and cardiovascular systems function within the body. At the end of the chapter, you will learn how all five of these systems work together on an "organismic" level to initiate, perpetuate, and regulate exercise within the human organism.

Unit Objectives

After completing Chapter 1, you should be able to:
1. Name the 11 systems of the human body.
2. Define the anatomical reference terms and use them in an example.
3. Identify the major bones in the human skeleton.
4. Describe the four classifications of bone, the structural composition of bone, and how bones grow.
5. Understand the characteristics of human muscle tissue.
6. Define the terms agonist and antagonist and use them in an example.
7. Identify the major muscle groups in the body, their location, the joint(s) moved, and basic movements.
8. Understand the basic organization of the nervous system.
9. Describe the flow of oxygen in the respiratory system.
10. Understand the basic anatomy of the heart muscle. Be able to trace the pathway of blood in the cardiovascular system.
11. Define general cardiovascular terms.

Key Questions:
1. How are body parts referenced to one another in the body?
2. How many bones are in the human skeleton?
3. How do bones grow?
4. How do muscles attach to bones?
5. Which muscles move the major joints in the body?
6. What is the difference between the afferent and efferent systems?
7. How is oxygen and carbon dioxide exchanged in the lungs?
8. What role does the cardiovascular system play in exercise?

Structural Organization of the Human Body

It is often overwhelming for an entry-level fitness professional to start studying the structures and systems of the body. This chapter strives to present a very basic overview of human anatomy relevant to the entry-level aquatic fitness professional.

To begin your study of human anatomy, think of your body as consisting of several layers of structural organization. These levels become more and more complex, and are associated with each other in several ways. The first level, called the "chemical" level, consists of all of the chemical substances found within the body that are essential to maintaining life. The next level is called the "cellular" level. As it implies, this level consists of the basic structural and functional unit of the body called the cell. The body is composed of numerous different kinds of cells including muscle cells, blood cells, mucous cells, etc. These cells are organized into similar groups called tissues, which make up the next level of structural organization called the "tissue" level. Cells grouped together to form tissues have similar functions and structures. Often these various types of tissues are combined to make organs. Organs comprise an even higher level of organization called the "organ" level. Organs have definite shapes and functions. Examples would include the heart, liver, stomach, brain, etc. The next level of organization is called the "system" level. In a body system, several associated organs are grouped together to perform a particular function such as digestion, hormone secretions, or supplying the body with blood or oxygen. We will primarily be discussing systems of the body in this chapter and how they work together to form the highest level of structural organization called the "organismic" level. This level represents all of the systems of the body working together to constitute an organism- a living person.

Systems of the Human Body

The human body is divided into 11 systems or parts. These systems interrelate and work together in several ways to allow humans to function as a whole person. One example of systems working together at this level, which would be of particular interest to fitness instructors, would be the skeletal, muscular, and nervous systems working together to cause gross and fine motor movement.

The 11 systems of the body are organized as follows:

1. Integumentary, (in teg′ yə men′ tə rē), which includes skin and all of the structures derived from it (hair, nails, etc.).
2. Skeletal, which includes all of the bones of the body, associated cartilage and joints.
3. Muscular, which includes all of the skeletal muscles, visceral muscles, cardiac muscle, tendons, and ligaments.
4. Nervous, which includes the brain, spinal cord, nerves, and sensory organs (eyes and ears).
5. Endocrine, which includes all the glands that produce hormones.
6. Cardiovascular, which includes blood, the heart, and blood vessels.
7. Lymphatic, which includes lymph, lymph nodes, lymph vessels, and lymph glands.
8. Respiratory, which includes the lungs and the passageways leading into and out of them.
9. Digestive, which includes a long tube and associated organs (liver, gallbladder, pancreas, etc.).
10. Urinary, which includes organs that produce, collect, and eliminate urine.
11. Reproductive, which includes organs that produce reproductive cells and organs that store and transport reproductive cells.

Not all of these systems are directly related to exercise. The systems of particular interest to fitness instructors would include the skeletal, muscular, nervous, cardiovascular, and respiratory systems. This chapter fosters a very basic understanding of the function and role that these five particular bodily systems play in the process of movement and exercise. The endocrine system and the hormones it produces play an important role in regulating many exercise processes but will not be discussed in depth in the scope of this manual.

Anatomical Reference Terms

There are several anatomical descriptive terms which refer to body parts, areas, location, and position. Medical terminology is very complicated and can be a college course in itself. In exercise, we are primarily interested in some of the anatomical terms that describe location and position. These terms are more specifically used in exercise to describe one body part's position in relation to another. These terms include:

- **superior**, which means "above"
- **inferior**, which means "below"
- **anterior**, which means "in front of"
- **posterior**, which means "behind"
- **medial**, which means "toward the midline of the body"
- **lateral**, which means "away from the midline of the body"

These terms can be used when the position of one body part is described in relation to another. For example, the quadriceps muscles, which are located in the front of the thigh, could be described as being "anterior" or "in front of" the hamstring muscles, which are located in the back of the thigh. The pectoralis muscle in the chest would be considered "superior" to the rectus abdominis muscle located in the abdomen. The adductor muscle in the inner thigh would be considered "medial" in comparison to the abductor muscles in the outer thigh. The humerus bone in the upper arm would be considered "lateral" to the ribs. The tibia bone in the lower leg would be considered "inferior" to the femur bone in the upper leg. You can see how these anatomical terms are used to describe one part's location in the body as compared to another.

The next two terms describe a positioning of the body in spatial terms. The term **supine** refers to the body lying in a "face-up" position. The term **prone** refers to the body lying in a "face-down" position. These terms are often used to describe the body's position when starting, performing, or finishing a particular exercise. The next three terms describe a surface of the body independent of its positioning in space. The term **ventral** describes the front surface of the body. The term **dorsal** describes the back surface of the body. Dorsal also refers to the top part of the foot or the instep. **Plantar** refers to the bottom surface or the sole of the foot.

The Skeletal System

The skeletal system is composed of all the bones in the body as well as their associated cartilage and joints. We will focus on the primary or major bones in the body associated with gross movements. Joints or articulations will be discussed in Chapter 3.

The function of the skeletal system is to give rigidity and form to the body. Your basic body shape is genetically determined in large part by your bone structure. If we had no bones we would be a mass of flesh and organs resembling a jellyfish. The skeletal system provides our bodies with support, protection, and shape. The rib cage and scapula protect vital organs like the lungs, kidneys, and liver found in the thoracic cavity of the body. The skull bones in the head surround and house the brain. Bones also provide the body with leverage, something essential to movement. The bones manufacture red blood cells and store minerals.

Types of Bones

Bones are divided into four basic types or classifications. (see figures 1-1a and 1-1b) Bone classification is based primarily on the shape of the bone. **Long bones** are longer than they are wide and are primarily found in the appendages (arms and legs). Long bones would include the femur, tibia, fibula, radius, ulna, and humerus. Long bones are slightly curved for strength and designed to absorb stress at several points. They consist of a long, thin part called the diaphysis or shaft, and two bulbous-type ends called the epiphysis.

Short bones are basically cube shaped and are about as wide as they are long. Examples of this bone would be the bones found in the wrist and ankle.

Flat bones are thin and generally flat as the term implies. Flat bones offer considerable protection and a great deal of surface area for muscles to attach. Examples of flat bones would be the cranial bones,

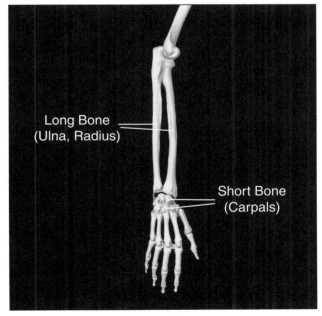

Long Bone
(Ulna, Radius)

Short Bone
(Carpals)

Figure 1-1a Types of Bones

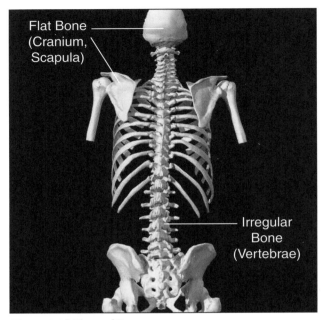

Figure 1-1b Types of Bones

which protect the brain, and the scapula or shoulder blade.

Irregular bones include many of the bones that do not fall into the other three categories. They have complex shapes and include bones like the vertebrae.

Structural Composition of Bone

A bone is made of many parts, with the proportions of each part being dependent upon the size and shape of the bone. For the most part, bones

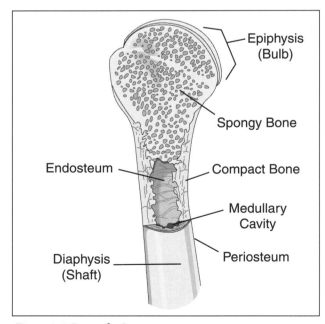

Figure 1-2 Parts of a Bone

are composed of spongy and compact bone, periosteum and endosteum, and a medullary cavity. (see figure 1-2) The periosteum is a dense, white, fibrous sheath that covers the surface of the bone and is where muscles and tendons attach. The medullary cavity of the bone is a cavity in the center of the bone filled with yellow, fatty marrow. The endosteum is the layer of cells that line the medullary cavity. The rigid part of the bone is made of spongy and compact bone. The spongy bone is less dense and contains spaces so blood vessels and other nutrients can be supplied to the bone. The compact part of the bone contains few spaces and provides protection and strength.

How Bones Grow

The process by which bone grows in the body is called **ossification**. Bones, in particular long bones, have cartilaginous growth plates located at either end called epiphyseal plates. Initially, these plates are not completely hardened and are where growth occurs in the bone. These fragile growth plates can be damaged in growing children or teens and affect bone growth. As a person matures, the epiphyseal plate hardens and growth stops between the ages of 21 and 25.

Children have large amounts of organic material in their bones, making their bones softer and more pliable. As we age, we have larger proportions of inorganic material, which causes bones to become brittle and more fragile. The structures in bones are in a continuous state of being built up and broken down. When exercise is combined with adequate rest and nutrition, it causes healthy bones to become thicker and stronger. Exercise helps build and promote healthy bone tissue and reduces the risk of bone disease such as osteoporosis.

The Human Skeleton

The human skeleton consists of 206 bones and is divided into two parts: the **axial skeleton** and the **appendicular skeleton**. (see figure 1-3) The axial skeleton consist of the bones found around the "axis" or imaginary midline of the body and includes the skull, vertebral column, sternum, and the ribs. The appendicular skeleton refers to the bones associated with the "appendages" and includes the bones in the arms, shoulders, legs, and hips.

An articulation or joint is the point of contact between bones or cartilage and bones. Joints are classified as immovable, slightly movable, or freely movable. The amount of movement possible at a joint

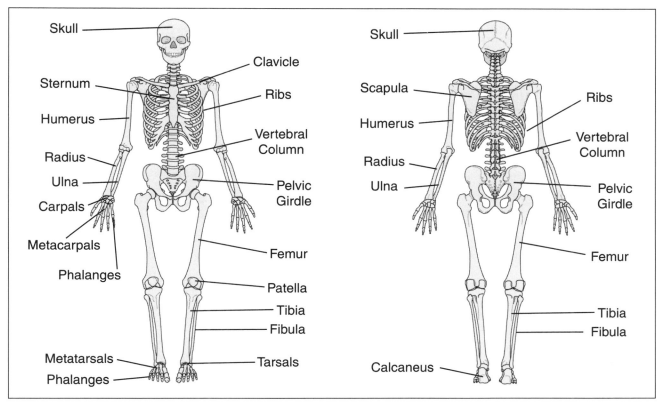

Figure 1-3 The Human Skeleton

depends upon the way in which the bones fit together, the tightness of the tissue that surround the joint, and the position of ligaments, muscles, and tendons. **Ligaments** are dense, regular, connective tissue that attach bone to bone at movable joints and help to protect the joint from dislocation.

The vertebral column, or backbone of the human skeleton, is typically made up of 26 bones called vertebrae. (see figure 1-4) These vertebrae are divided into five sections. The part of the vertebral column found in the neck is called the **cervical** spine and contains seven smaller vertebrae. The part of the vertebral column found behind the rib cage is called the **thoracic** spine and consists of 12 mid-sized vertebrae. The low back area of the vertebral column is called the **lumbar** spine and consists of five large vertebrae. Below the lumbar spine is the **sacrum** which is one bone made up of five fused sacral vertebrae. The **coccyx**, or tailbone, is made up of four vertebrae fused into one or two bones.

A fibro cartilaginous tissue, called an intervertebral disc, is found between each vertebra. This tissue is often injured due to trauma or overuse in the lumbar or weight bearing area of the spine or in the delicate

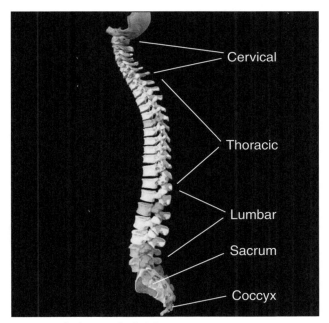

Figure 1-4 The Vertebral Column

cervical area of the spine. Disc problems are not as common in the thoracic area of the spine due to the support and stability the ribs give the vertebral column in this area.

The Muscular System

There are more than 600 muscles in the human body. The muscular system is comprised of skeletal, visceral, and cardiac muscle tissue. **Visceral muscle**, the "smooth" or "involuntary" muscle over which we have no conscious control, is found in the walls of organs such as the intestines and esophagus. **Cardiac muscle** is found in the heart. As a fitness professional, you will likely find **skeletal muscle** tissue to be of the most interest.

The skeletal system may give our bodies shape and support, but the bones alone cannot move our bodies. The skeletal muscles attach to and work with the bones in the skeletal system to create or allow movement to occur, much like the strings on a puppet. Skeletal muscle is often called "voluntary" or "striated" muscle because it is under our conscious control and looks like "bands" of tissue. When the skeletal and muscular systems work together to cause movement, they are often referred to collectively as the "musculoskeletal" system.

The muscular system has three basic functions: to work with other systems in the body to assist in causing movement, to maintain posture, and to create heat. Muscle performs these three functions through contraction, which is shortening the muscle tissue.

Characteristics of Muscle Tissue

All muscle tissue possesses four principle characteristics: **excitability**, **contractility**, **extensibility**, and **elasticity**. All four of these characteristics are necessary for muscles to function as they do. Imagine a muscle being unable to stretch, or if it did stretch, not being able to return to its original length.

Excitability allows the muscle to receive and respond to stimuli. A stimulus is some kind of change that occurs in the muscle itself, or a change that occurs in the external environment of the muscle tissue. This change must be strong enough to initiate a nerve impulse. The muscular system is very intricately associated with the nervous system.

Contractility is simply the ability of muscle tissue to shorten and thicken or to contract when it is stimulated to do so. Most muscle contractions actually result in the length of the muscle becoming shorter.

Extensibility is the characteristic that allows a muscle to stretch. Just as a muscle has the ability to shorten, it also has the ability to lengthen. The ability of muscles to contract or shorten and to extend or lengthen is what allows us to move.

Elasticity is a very important characteristic. If a muscle did not possess elasticity, it could not return to its original shape after it contracted or extended (much like putty). The property of elasticity allows the muscle to return to its original shape so it can contract or extend again to repeat the same movement or cause a different movement (somewhat like a rubber band).

Muscle Structure

Skeletal muscle is a grouping of very specialized cells working together to cause a muscle to contract. Because muscles are attached to bones, these bones move when the muscles contract. Structurally, muscles are bands of fibers anchored firmly to bones by **tendons**. Tendons are a very strong, fibrous, connective tissue which connects the **fascia**, a covering on the muscles, to the periosteum, which is the fibrous membrane covering the bones. Most muscles have at least two tendons, each one attaching to a different bone. One of these attachments tends to be more stationary or immobile and is referred to as the muscle's **origin**. The other attachment, which tends to be more mobile, is called the muscle's **insertion**.

The bands of muscle fibers that comprise a given muscle are bound firmly together by connective tissue. If you look at a cross section of muscle, you will see

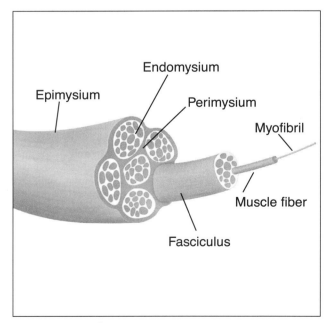

Figure 1-5 Muscle Tissue

that these bundles of fibers called **fasciculus** are actually bundles of muscle cells bound by connective tissue as well. (see figure 1-5) This deep connective tissue is innervated by blood vessels which supply oxygen and nutrients needed for contraction to the muscle cells. The anatomy of a muscle cell and how muscles contract is covered in Chapter 2.

Muscle Arrangements

Muscles are, for the most part, found in pairs in the body on either side of a joint allowing them to move bones in both directions. (see figure 1-6) Paired muscles have a relationship which allows one muscle to relax or stretch while the other muscle is shortening or contracting.

In a muscle pair, the muscle that is actively contracting at any given time is referred to as the **agonist** or prime mover. This contracting muscle is doing the "agony of the work." The other muscle of the muscle pair must relax or yield in order for the agonist to contract. This relaxed or stretched muscle is referred to as the **antagonist**. The agonist and antagonist in a muscle pair work together to contract and relax on either side of a joint so that movement can occur in different directions and at various angles. If both muscles would contract at the same time, movement at that joint would not be possible.

The biceps and triceps located in the upper arm would be an example of a muscle pair. The biceps muscle is located in the front of the upper arm, crosses

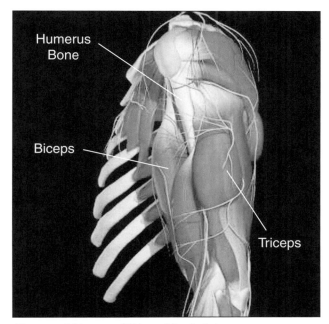

Figure 1-6 Biceps and Triceps Muscle Pair

the elbow joint, and attaches into the forearm. When the biceps muscle is contracted, the forearm raises toward the upper arm. The elbow would remain in this bent position if not for the triceps muscle located on the back of the upper arm. The triceps runs through the back of the elbow joint and attaches into the forearm as well. When the triceps contracts, it straightens the forearm. The arrangement of these "paired" muscle groups throughout the body is what allows us to perform a variety of movements. Muscle pairs will be discussed in more depth in Chapters 2 & 3.

It is important to consider the effects of gravity when looking at how the muscles work. In the standing arm curl mentioned above, gravity assists the downward movement (straightening of the arm) and greatly reduces the work required by the triceps muscle. On land in the presence of gravity, many of our "return" moves are assisted by gravity. The body has to be positioned so that the muscle can work against gravity in order to train a muscle on land. Thus one exercise would need to be performed for the biceps muscle, and a different exercise would need to be performed for the triceps muscle on land in the presence of gravity.

It is important for even the entry-level fitness instructor to have a general knowledge of the basic muscle groups and how they are involved in movement. In order to design and implement an effective program, you must be aware of what muscles are responsible for what movements. In this chapter, we will look at the location of these major muscles and the associated joint(s) involved. In Chapter 3, you will learn more about what muscles are responsible for what movement at any given joint. So your study of muscles will have two parts: where muscles are located and the joints they move, as well as which muscles are involved in a specific movement at a particular joint. This dual approach will allow you to design more effective programming to improve muscle tone and strength in all of the major muscles in the body as opposed to randomized, hit-or-miss type programming. You need to gain a basic knowledge of what each move in your choreography accomplishes from the muscle's viewpoint. This way you can design an effective, safe, balanced program.

(See figure 1-7a and 1-7b for a full view of the major muscles in the body.)

(See chart 1-1 for names of major muscles, their location in the body, the joints they move, and the movements they cause.)

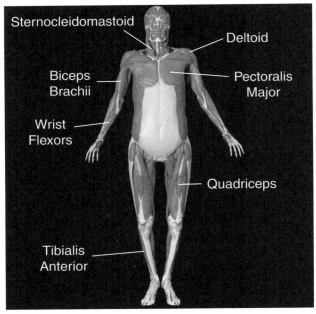

Figure 1-7a Muscles in the Body

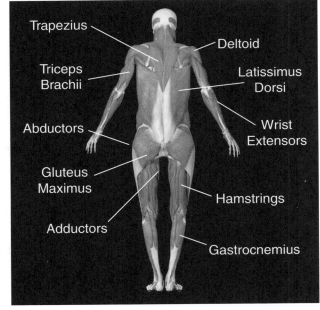

Figure 1-7b Muscles in the Body

Chart 1-1

The Major Muscles of the Body

Name of Muscle	Location	Joint(s) Moved	Movement(s)
Sternocleidomastoid	Front of the neck	Cervical spine	Flexion and rotation of the head
Pectoralis Major	Chest	Shoulder Sternoclavicular	Flexion and transverse adduction of the arm at the shoulder

Trapezius
  Upper (U)
  Middle (M)
  Lower (L)
	Upper back and neck	Scapula Sternoclavicular Cervical spine	(U) Scapular elevation and neck extension
			(M) Scapular retraction
			(L) Scapular depression

Latissimus Dorsi	Middle and low back	Shoulder	Extension and adduction of the arm at the shoulder

Deltoid
  Anterior (A)
  Medial (M)
  Posterior (P)
	Cap of shoulder	Shoulder	(A) Transverse adduction,
			(M) Abduction, and
			(P) Transverse abduction of the arm at the shoulder

Biceps Brachii	Front of upper arm	Elbow Shoulder	Flexion of the forearm at the elbow Flexion of the arm at the shoulder
Triceps Brachii	Back of upper arm	Elbow Shoulder	Extension of the forearm at the elbow Extension of the arm at the shoulder
Wrist Flexors	Front of the forearm	Wrist Phalanges	Flexion of the hand at the wrist Flexion of the phalanges

Wrist Extensors	Back of the forearm	Wrist Phalanges	Extension of the hand at the wrist Extension of the phalanges
Erector Spinae	Back, along spine	Intervertebral joints of spine	Extension of the trunk along the vertebral column
Quadratus Lumborum	Low back	Lumbar spine	Lateral flexion of the trunk
Rectus Abdominis	Abdomen	Lumbar spine	Flexion of the trunk
Internal and External Obliques	Abdomen	Lumbar spine	Flexion and rotation of the trunk
Transversus Abdominis	Abdomen	Lumbar spine	Abdominal compression and posterior pelvic tilt
Iliopsoas (psoas major and minor, iliacus)	Front of hip	Hip	Flexion of the leg at the hip
Gluteus Maximus	Buttocks	Hip	Extension of the leg at the hip
Hip Abductors (gluteus medius and minimus)	Outer thigh	Hip	Abduction of the leg at the hip
Hip Adductors	Inner thigh	Hip	Adduction of the leg at the hip
Quadriceps Femoris (rectus femoris, vastus medialis, vastus intermedius, vastus lateralis)	Front of thigh	Hip (rectus femoris) Knee	Flexion of the leg at the hip Extension of the lower leg at the knee
Hamstrings (biceps femoris, semimembranosus, semitendinosus)	Back of thigh	Hip Knee	Extension of the leg at the hip Flexion of the lower leg at the knee
Gastrocnemius	Calf	Ankle	Plantar flexion at the ankle
Soleus	Calf	Ankle	Plantar flexion at the ankle
Tibialis Anterior	Shin	Ankle	Dorsi flexion at the ankle

Muscles of the Upper Torso and Extremities

Major muscles of the upper torso include the sternocleidomastoid, pectoralis major, trapezius, latissimus dorsi, deltoids, biceps brachii, triceps brachii, wrist flexors and wrist extensors. There are several other muscles involved in movement in the upper torso. Once you learn the primary muscles, you are encouraged to learn additional muscles in the upper torso. To start, you should have a basic idea of the bones to which a particular muscle attaches as opposed to learning the name of every origin and insertion. This will aid in identifying the joint(s) each muscle moves. It will also give you valuable information about the movement each muscle produces.

The location of the muscle, where it attaches, the primary joint(s) moved, and the primary movements for that muscle are provided with the description of each muscle or muscle group in the following text. Although movement terms are not discussed until Chapter 3, the movements are listed with the description of the muscle to help when you come back to review muscle anatomy. The movement terminology may not make complete sense until you read Chapter 3. Use Chart 1 as a summary for the name, location, joint(s) moved, and primary movements for each muscle or group.

Sternocleidomastoid: (ster′-nō-klī-dō-MAS-toid) The sternocleidomastoid is found in the front of the neck. As its name implies, this muscle attaches from the sternum and clavicle up to the jaw area. The primary joints moved are the intervertebral spine in the cervical or neck area. Primary movements include flexion of the head at the cervical spine and rotation of the head at the cervical spine. (see figure 1-8)

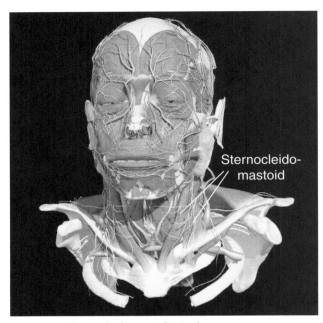

Figure 1-8 Sternocleidomastoid Muscle

Pectoralis Major: (pek´-tor-A-lis) The pectoralis major muscle is found in the chest. It originates at the sternum and ribs and attaches into the upper arm. The primary joint moved is the shoulder joint. The pectoralis muscle moves the sternoclavicular joint (where the sternum and clavicle meet) as well. Primary movements include flexion of the arm at the

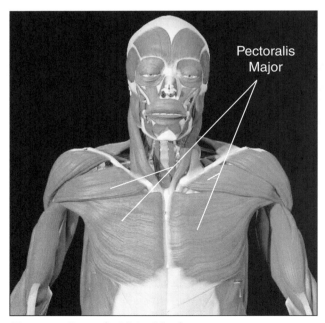

Figure 1-9 Pectoralis Major Muscle

shoulder and transverse adduction of the arm at the shoulder. (see figure 1-9)

Trapezius: (tra-PĒ-zē-us) The trapezius is a large, diamond-shaped muscle found in the upper back and up in to the back of the neck. The fibers in this muscle run primarily in three different directions. It is divided into three parts based on the direction the fibers run and the movements for which they are responsible. The fibers in the upper trapezius run at an angle down the neck and out toward the shoulder blade. The middle trapezius fibers run horizontally across the upper back. The lower trapezius fibers run at an angle from the spine up and out toward the shoulder blade. Surprisingly, the trapezius muscle does not cross the shoulder joint or attach into the humerus bone and therefore cannot be responsible for movements at the shoulder joint. The trapezius moves the scapulae and sternoclavicular joint and the upper trapezius extends the head. Primary movements include shoulder elevation (upper), neck extension (upper), shoulder retraction (middle), and shoulder depression (lower). (see figure 1-10)

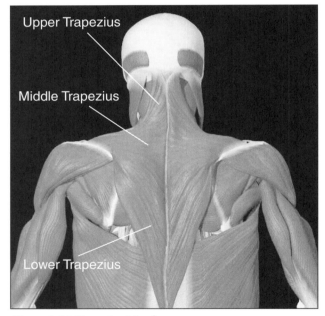

Figure 1-10 Trapezius Muscle

Latissimus dorsi: (la-TIS-i-mus DOR-sī) The latissimus dorsi muscle is located in the middle and low back. It is a large, flat muscle that attaches into the pelvic bone and vertebral column and runs up and out either side of the low back to attach in the upper arm or humerus bone. The primary joint this muscle moves is the shoulder joint. Primary movements include extension of the arm at the shoulder and adduction of the arm at the shoulder. (see figure 1-11)

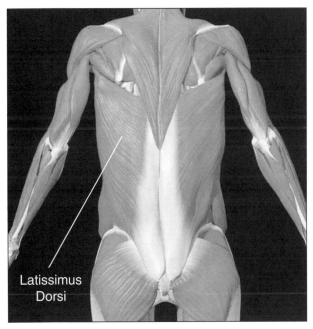

Figure 1-11 Latissimus Dorsi Muscle

Deltoid: (DEL-toyd) The deltoid is the muscle that caps the shoulder. Because it is attached on the front and back of the shoulder, the deltoid is involved in three ranges of motion and is divided into the anterior, middle, and posterior deltoid muscle fibers. The deltoid muscle runs over the top of the shoulder and attaches into the upper arm or humerus bone. It

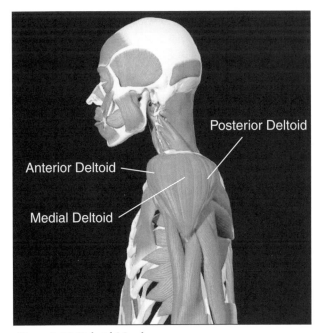

Figure 1-12 Deltoid Muscle

moves the shoulder joint. Primary movements include abduction of the arm at the shoulder and transverse adduction (anterior) and abduction (posterior) of the arm at the shoulder. (see figure 1-12)

Biceps brachii: (BĬ-ceps BRĀ-kē-ī) The biceps brachii muscle is so named because it has two (bi) origins. It is located on the front of the upper arm. The biceps brachii moves three joints. It originates above the shoulder and attaches into the forearm. We are primarily concerned with how it moves the elbow joint. It also crosses the shoulder joint and the radioulnar joint in the forearm. Primary movements include flexion of the arm at the shoulder and flexion of the forearm at the elbow. (see figure 1-13)

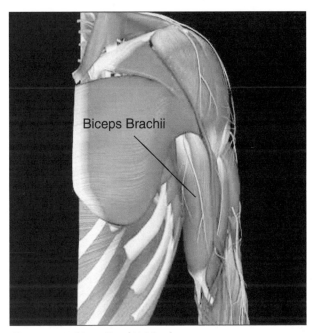

Figure 1-13 Biceps Brachii Muscle

Triceps brachii: (TRĬ-ceps BRĀ-kē-ī) The triceps brachii muscle is found in the back of the upper arm. It originates in three places, as its name implies. Like the biceps muscle, the triceps moves the elbow and shoulder joints and attaches into the forearm. Primary movements include extension of the arm at the shoulder and extension of the forearm at the elbow. (see figure 1-14)

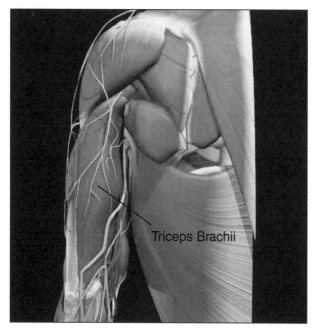

Figure 1-14 Triceps Brachii Muscle

Wrist flexors: The wrist flexors are a group of muscles found in the front of the forearm. They move the wrist and fingers. Their arrangement and attachment from the arm into the hand allows flexion of the wrist as well as movement in the hand and thumb. (see figure 1-15)

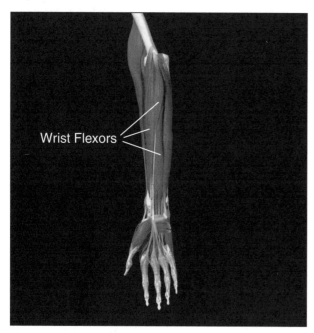

Figure 1-15 Wrist Flexor Muscles

Wrist extensors: The wrist extensors are a group of muscles found in the back of the forearm that work in opposition to the wrist flexors. They also move the wrist and fingers. Just as their name implies, their attachment from the arm into the hand allows extension of the wrist and movement in the hand and thumb. (see figure 1-16)

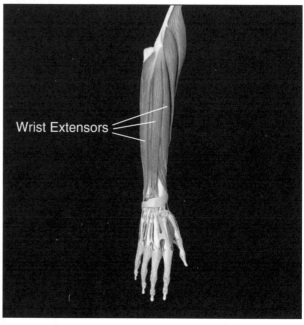

Figure 1-16 Wrist Extensor Muscles

Muscles of the Torso

Major muscles in the midsection of the body include the erector spinae, quadratus lumborum, rectus abdominis, internal and external obliques, and the transversus abdominis. These muscles provide support and stability for the lumbar or weight-bearing area of the vertebral column. Having adequate strength and flexibility in these muscles enhances postural alignment and reduces risk of low back problems.

Erector spinae: (e-REK-tor SPI-nē) The erector spinae muscle is located in the back, along the entire length of the vertebral column. This muscle is a large mass of tissue that splits and attaches in an overlapping fashion as it goes up the back. The erector spinae moves the intervertebral spine joints. Primary movement is extension of the trunk at the spine. (see figure 1-17)

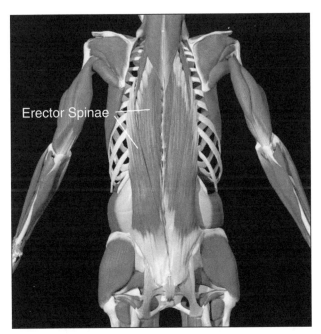

Figure 1-17 Erector Spinae Muscles

Quadratus lumborum: (kwod-RĂ-tus lum BOR-um) The quadratus lumborum muscle is located in the low back. It attaches from the pelvic bone up into the ribs and lumbar vertebrae. The fibers run at a slight angle and can flex the spine laterally if only one side is contracted. They also help with deep breathing. (see figure 1-18)

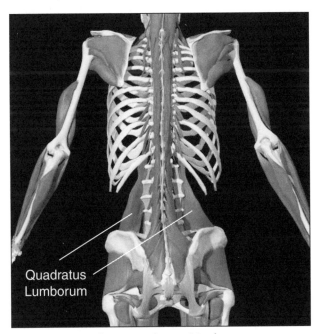

Figure 1-18 Quadratus Lumborum Muscle

Rectus abdominis: (REK-tus ab-DOM-in-is) This long, flat muscle runs from the pubic bone in the abdomen up into the sternum and ribs. Its fibers run

parallel to the midline; the term "rectus" refers to "straight." It is often referred to as the natural biological brace for the low back. Many people believe that exercises such as leg lifts, bicycles, or lifting your legs while hanging from the side of the pool, actively work the rectus abdominis muscle. These exercises, involving movement at the hip joint, do not actively involve the rectus abdominis because it does not cross the hip joint and attach into the femur. The rectus abdominis muscle is contracted to stabilize the pelvis and protect the low back when lifting the legs and moving from the hip. It is not actively doing the work. Like the erector spinae, it moves the joints of the intervertebral spine. Its primary movement is flexion of the trunk at the spine. (see figure 1-19)

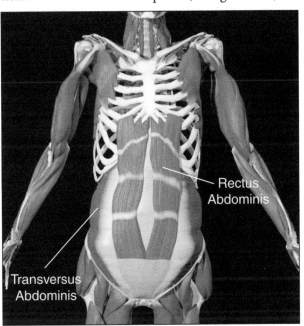

Figure 1-19
Rectus Abdominis and Transversus Abdominis Muscles

Transversus abdominis: (tranz-VER-sus ab-DOM-in-is) The transversus abdominis is much like a sling that runs horizontally across the front of the abdominal cavity. This muscle helps to hold the abdominal organs up and in place. After pregnancy, or as we age, these muscles can become weak and flaccid and need to be strengthened. Their action works to compress the abdomen and take the pelvis into a posterior tilt. Abdominal exercise is most effective when initiated by an abdominal compression or engagement of the transversus abdominis. (see figure 1-19)

Internal and external obliques: (ō-BLĒK) The internal and external obliques work with the rectus abdominis muscle in the abdomen. The term oblique refers to muscle fibers that run diagonal to midline. The first of these muscles, the internal oblique, lies beside the rectus abdominis muscle and below the external oblique in an inverted "V" pattern. (see figure 1-20) The external oblique lies over the internals in a "V" pattern, the opposite of the internal oblique. (see figure 1-21) Both the internal and external oblique muscles wrap around the waist and move the intervertebral joints of the spine. They help the rectus abdominis with flexion of the trunk at the spine, but also allow for rotation of the trunk at the lumbar spine.

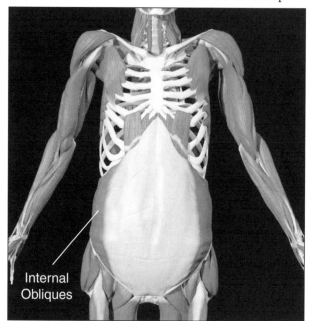

Figure 1-20 Internal Oblique Muscles

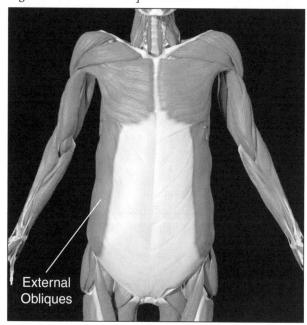

Figure 1-21 External Oblique Muscles

Muscles of the Lower Torso and Extremities

Muscles of the lower extremities include all of the major muscles in the hips and legs. Some of these muscles are the largest skeletal muscles in the body and are capable of powerful contractions to move the weight of the body. They are also capable of processing large amounts of fat and sugar to produce energy to fuel their contractions. These muscles include the iliopsoas, gluteus maximus, hip abductors and adductors, the quadriceps femoris, hamstrings, gastrocnemius, soleus, and the tibialis anterior.

Iliopsoas: (il'-ē-ō-SŌ-as) The iliopsoas is actually comprised of three muscles called the psoas major, psoas minor, and the iliacus. Better known as the hip flexors, these muscles originate on the lumbar vertebrae and pelvic bone and insert onto the upper leg or femur. These muscles are often confused with the abdominal muscles because they run through the lower abdomen. They actually move the hip joint and work independently of the abdominal muscles. The primary movement is flexion of the leg at the hip. (see figure 1-22)

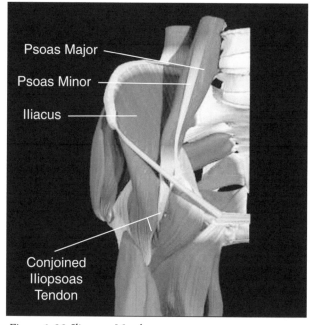

Figure 1-22 Iliopsoas Muscle

Gluteus maximus: (GLOO-tē-us MAK-si-mus) As the term maximus implies, this muscle is the larger of the three gluteal muscles. It is located in the buttocks. It originates along the lower vertebrae and along the pelvic bone and inserts on to the femur. It moves the hip joint. The primary movement is extension of the leg at the hip. (see figure 1-23)

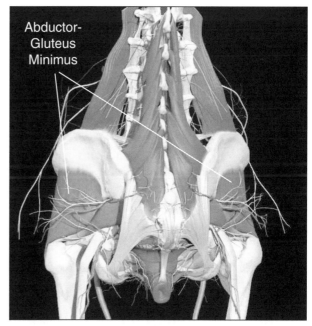

Figure 1-23 Gluteus Maximus Muscle

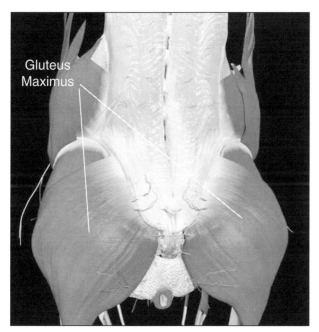

Figure 1-24b Gluteus Minimus Muscle

Hip abductors: These muscles, named after the movement they initiate, are located in the outer thigh. This group is composed of the **gluteus medius** and **gluteus minimus**. These muscles originate along the back crest of the pelvic bone and attach onto the femur. They move the hip joint. Primary movement is abduction of the leg at the hip. (see figure 1-24a and 1-24b)

Hip adductors: The hip adductors work in opposition to the hip abductors. This group is primarily made up of five smaller muscles located on the inside of the thigh. They originate for the most part on the low center part of the pelvic bone called the pubis and insert onto the femur. They also move the hip joint. Primary movement includes adduction of the leg at the hip. (see figure 1-25)

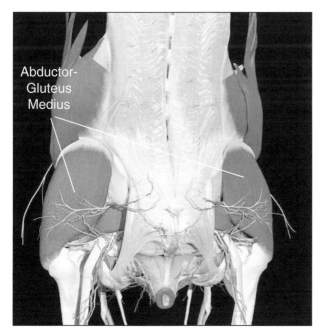

Figure 1-24a Gluteus Medius Muscle

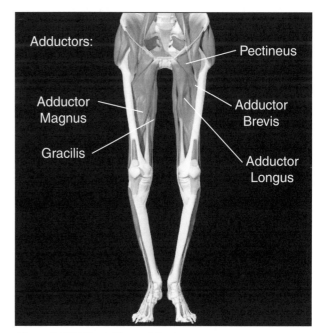

Figure 1-25 Hip Adductor Muscles

Quadriceps femoris: (KWOD-ri-ceps FEM-or-is) The term "quad" refers to "four" and there are four parts to the quadriceps femoris muscle group found in the front of the thigh. The **rectus femoris** (fibers running parallel to the midline of the femur) is a large, long muscle that originates above the hip. It is the only part of the quadriceps group that moves the hip. The three vastus muscles, the **vastus lateralis**, **vastus intermedius** and the **vastus medialis**, originate on the femur. All four parts of the quadriceps cross the knee joint and insert onto the lower leg. Primary movements include flexion of the leg at the hip (rectus femoris) and extension of the lower leg at the knee. (see figure 1-26)

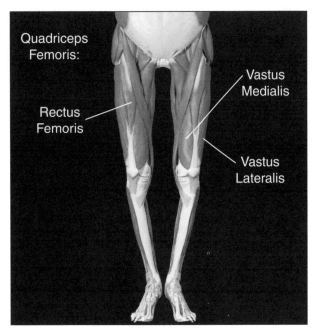

Figure 1-26 Quadriceps Femoris Muscles

Hamstrings: The hamstrings group, in the back of the thigh, is comprised of three muscles. The **biceps femoris** ("two heads of origin") has one head that originates above the hip and one that originates on the femur. The **semimembranosus** and the **semitendinosus** originate above the hip, and all three insert on to the lower leg. The hamstrings muscles move the hip and knee joints. Primary movements include extension of the leg at the hip and flexion of the lower leg at the knee. (see figure 1-27)

Gastrocnemius: (gas´-trok-NĒ-mē-us) The gastrocnemius muscle is the large muscle found in the calf. The gastrocnemius originates at the very lower end of the femur and the back of the knee and inserts onto the underside of the heel by way of the large

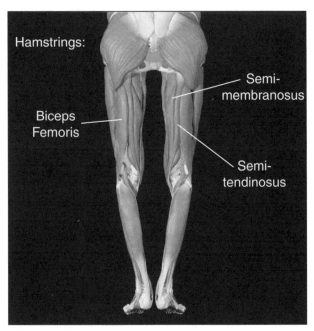

Figure 1-27 Hamstrings Muscles

Achilles tendon. The primary joint moved is the ankle joint. The primary movement is plantar flexion of the foot at the ankle. (see figure 1-28)

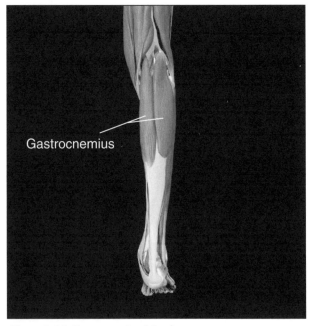

Figure 1-28 Gastrocnemius Muscle

Soleus: (SŌ-lē-us) The soleus is the muscle that lies right under and works with the gastrocnemius in the calf. The soleus muscle originates near the gastrocnemius on the tibia and fibula and inserts onto the underside of the heel by way of the large Achilles tendon. The primary joint moved is the ankle joint.

The primary movement is plantar flexion of the foot at the ankle. (see figure 1-29)

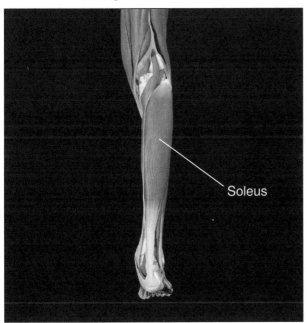

Figure 1-29 Soleus Muscle

Tibialis anterior: (tib´-ē-A-lis) As its name implies, the tibialis anterior is located in front of the tibia bone or in the shin. It originates on the front of the lower leg and inserts onto the top of the foot and therefore moves the ankle joint. The primary movement is dorsi flexion of the foot at the ankle. (see figure 1-30)

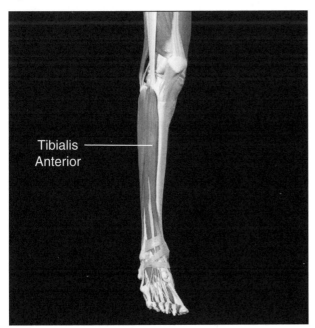

Figure 1-30 Tibialis Anterior Muscle

The Nervous System

The nervous system is comprised of the brain, spinal cord, nerves, and the sense organs. It serves as the control center and communication network within the body. (see figure 1-31) The split-second reactions determined by the nervous system and carried out by nerve impulses are instrumental in keeping the body functioning efficiently. The endocrine system shares the responsibility of maintaining homeostasis in the body with the nervous system through the secretion of hormones. Hormone induced adjustments made in the body are much slower than those made by the nervous system but are equally as important.

The nervous system has three primary functions. First, internal and external changes are sensed via a variety of sense organs and tissues. Next, the nervous system interprets these changes. And lastly, it responds to these interpretations through muscular contractions or glandular secretions. In this overview of the nervous system, focus will be on its relationship with skeletal muscles in the initiation of voluntary muscle contractions.

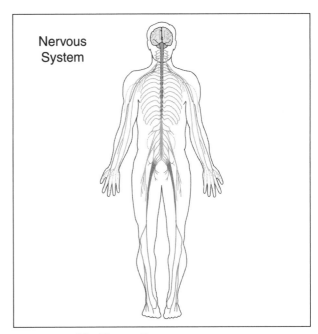

Figure 1-31 The Nervous System

Organization of the Nervous System

The nervous system somewhat resembles the cardiovascular system in how it innervates the body. The brain and spinal cord are the primary structures and are classified as the **central nervous system**

(CNS). In a sense, the central nervous system acts as the heart does in the cardiovascular system. The various nerve processes that branch off from the spinal cord and brain, much like the vascular system, constitute the **peripheral nervous system** (PNS). The peripheral nervous system connects the brain and spinal cord with receptors, muscles, and glands.

The peripheral nervous system can be broken down into the **afferent** and **efferent** systems. (see figure 1-32) The afferent system conveys information via neurons, or nerve cells, from sensors in the periphery of the body to the central nervous system. This system conveys "incoming" information about position, tone, etc., from the muscle to the central nervous system. The efferent neurons, also known as motor neurons, relay "outgoing" information from the central nervous system to the muscle cells.

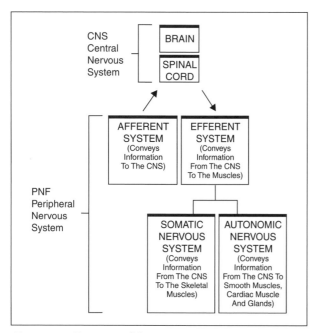

Figure 1-32 Divisions of the Nervous System

The efferent system is further divided into the **somatic** and **autonomic** nervous systems. The autonomic system consists of efferent neurons that transmit impulses to involuntary muscles and glands and is not of major concern to the fitness instructor. The somatic system consists of efferent neurons that transmit messages or impulses to voluntary skeletal muscle under our conscious control. The somatic nervous system is important to fitness instructors in that it serves as an important part of the link between the mind and the muscle to allow us to move, bend, twist, and stretch as we wish.

Figure 1- 33 depicts a typical efferent or motor neuron in the somatic nervous system and its connection to skeletal muscle tissue. How it causes the muscle to contract (the sliding filament theory) is discussed in Chapter 2.

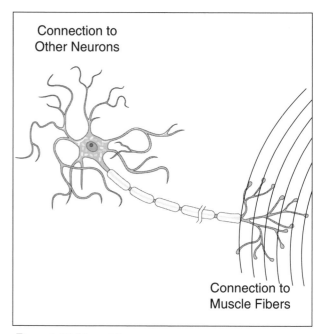

Figure 1-33 Motor Neuron

Figure 1- 34 shows how larger neurons from the brain and spinal cord branch to numerous neurons (one of which is shown in figure 1- 33) in a muscle fiber in what is called a "diverging circuit." A single motor neuron in the brain may stimulate several

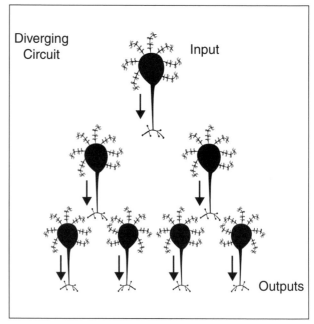

Figure 1-34 Diverging Circuit

neurons in the spinal cord, which in turn stimulate several fibers in the skeletal muscle. Thus, a single impulse from the brain will result in the contraction of several muscle fibers.

The Primary Peripheral Nerves

The entry-level fitness instructor need not know all of the nerve branches and nerves in the body. A general understanding of how the system is organized and knowledge of a few of the primary nerves would be beneficial. At times, a participant who suffers a musculoskeletal injury may have associated nerve damage as well. An example would be pain in the hip and leg associated with sciatic nerve damage when the lumbar area of the spine is injured.

There are four primary nerve branches along the spine originating from the central nervous system or the spinal cord. These four groupings are referred to as: the **cervical plexus**, originating from the cervical vertebrae; the **brachial plexus**, also originating from the cervical area and from a few of the thoracic vertebrae; the **lumbar plexus**, originating from the lumbar vertebrae; and the **sacral plexus**, originating from the lower lumbar vertebrae and sacrum. (see figures 1-35a and 1-35b) These large nerves branch from the spinal column and come out through openings between the vertebrae in pairs to service the right and left sides of the body.

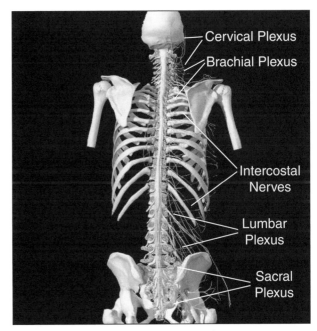
Figure 1-35b Major Spinal Nerve Branches

The nerves branching from the **cervical plexus** service the upper torso and extremities and are not primarily associated with motor movement. The nerves originating from the **brachial plexus** service the arms and shoulder area. Of particular concern would be three large motor nerves: the **median** nerve, the **ulnar** nerve, and the **radial** (largest in the brachial plexus) nerve. All of these supply motor fibers to several muscles in the upper arms, forearms, and hands.

The **lumbar plexus** nerves are the **femoral** nerve, the **saphenous** nerve, and the **obturator** nerve. The femoral nerve is the largest and supplies the skin of the leg and foot, and the obturator supplies motor fibers to the adductor muscles of the thigh. The **sacral plexus** contains the largest and longest nerve in the body, the **sciatic** nerve. The sciatic nerve supplies the hamstring muscle and divides into nerves that service the lower leg.

The Respiratory System

The respiratory system is made up of the lungs and a series of passageways leading into and out of the lungs. The respiratory system is important in exercise because it functions to supply oxygen to the body from the air we breathe. This oxygen is critical in the production of energy used for sustained muscular contraction. Another important function of the respiratory system is to rid the body of carbon dioxide,

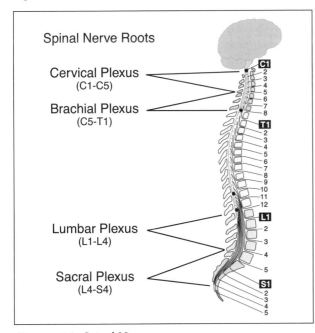

Figure 1-35a Spinal Nerves

a by-product of energy production, by "blowing it off" or exhaling it through the respiratory system in the opposite direction from which oxygen enters.

Organization of the Respiratory System

The respiratory system is divided into an upper and lower respiratory tract. (see figure 1-36) The upper respiratory tract consists of the parts which are located outside the chest cavity. These parts would include the nose and nasal cavities, as well as the upper **trachea** (the tube that connects the nasal passages to the lungs). The lower respiratory tract consists of the lower trachea and the lungs which include bronchial tubes and alveoli.

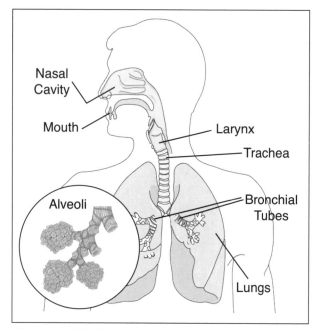

Figure 1-36 The Respiratory System & Figure 1-37 Alveoli

Oxygen Flow in the Respiratory System

Air enters and leaves the respiratory system through the nose and mouth. The nose is comprised of bone and cartilage covered by skin and contains little hairs, which block the entry of dust. Air passes through the nasal passage, past the soft palate and larynx (voice box), and into the upper trachea. The trachea is 4-5 inches long and contains several c-shaped cartilages, which hold it open. The trachea travels down into the chest cavity and splits into the right and left primary bronchi. These two bronchi enter the lungs and continue to split and branch into smaller and smaller **bronchial tubes**. The smallest bronchial tubes terminate into small balloon-like air sacs in the lungs call the **alveoli**. (see figure 1-37)

The alveoli are where oxygen and carbon dioxide are exchanged with the vascular system. The alveoli are surrounded by a rich supply of pulmonary capillaries. Oxygen crosses into the pulmonary capillaries from the alveoli to be transported by the bloodstream to the muscles. In the opposite direction, carbon dioxide is carried from the muscle tissue to the lungs via the bloodstream. At the alveoli, carbon dioxide crosses from the blood into the alveoli where it is ultimately exhaled through the respiratory tract.

Inhalation and exhalation are involuntary responses, controlled primarily by the autonomic nervous system. Involuntary nerve impulses to the diaphragm and intercostal muscles cause them to contract. The **diaphragm** moves downward, and the intercostal muscles contract to expand the rib cage. This expansion of the chest cavity creates pressure, which causes the lungs to expand and fill with air. When the pressure in the lungs and outside of the lungs equalizes, a normal inhalation is completed. A more forceful contraction of the diaphragm and intercostal muscles will further expand the lungs, allowing you to take an even deeper breath.

Exhalation is a much simpler process. When the nerve impulses are decreased, the diaphragm and intercostal muscles relax. The chest cavity becomes smaller and compresses the lungs and alveoli tissue, forcing air out through the respiratory tract.

Breathing properly during exercise is very important. If a participant holds his/her breath while straining, unequal pressure is created in the chest, blood pressure drops, and blood flow to the heart diminishes. When the participant starts breathing again and relaxes, blood surges to the heart causing a sharp increase in blood pressure. This is known as the **Valsalva maneuver**, and can create dangerous conditions for people with high blood pressure or cardiovascular disease. Breathing correctly during exercise is critical to proper oxygenation of the body as well as circulatory stability.

The Cardiovascular System

The cardiovascular system is named for the organs from which it is made: "cardio," which means heart, and "vascular," which represents the blood vessels and the blood they carry to all parts of the body.

The cardiovascular system has many important functions in the body. These functions include:
• distribution of oxygen and nutrients to the cells.

- removal of carbon dioxide and wastes from the cells.
- maintaining the acid-base balance of the body.
- helping the body regulate body heat.
- helping the body protect itself from disease.

Organization of the Cardiovascular System

As previously stated, the cardiovascular system is comprised of the heart, blood vessels, and blood. The heart is an organ found within the chest cavity that serves as the "pump" for the system. The blood vessels are the "pipes" which originate from the heart and eventually return to the heart. Blood is the oxygen and nutrient-rich "fluid" that the pump pushes through the pipes to all parts of the body. (see figures 1-38a and 1-38b)

The Heart:

Your heart is a hollow, fist-sized muscle found slightly to the left of your sternum in your chest cavity. (see figure 1-39) It is made up of four chambers- two receiving chambers called atria and two sending or pumping chambers called ventricles. Blood only flows in one direction through the heart. A wall or **septum** is found between the right and left sides of the heart, and several membranous folds called **valves** open to allow blood to flow into the heart's chambers then close to prevent backflow. Blood enters the **right atrium** of the heart through two large veins called the **superior vena cava** (carries blood from the upper body) and the **inferior vena cava** (carries blood from the lower body). Blood then flows through a valve into the **right ventricle**. The right ventricle contracts to force blood through the **pulmonary artery** to the capillaries at the alveoli in the lungs. Here the blood is oxygenated and sent back to the **left atrium** of the heart via the **pulmonary vein**. It then travels through a valve into the **left ventricle** where it is forcefully pumped out of the heart through a large artery called the **aorta** to the body.

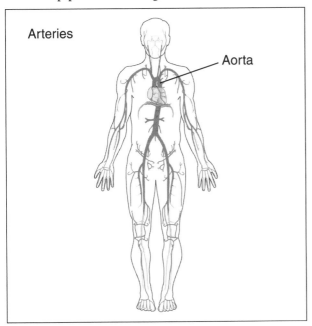

Figure 1-38a The Arteries of the Cardiovascular System

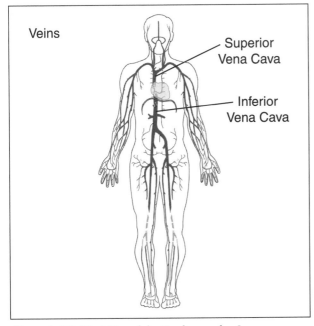

Figure 1-38b The Veins of the Cardiovascular System

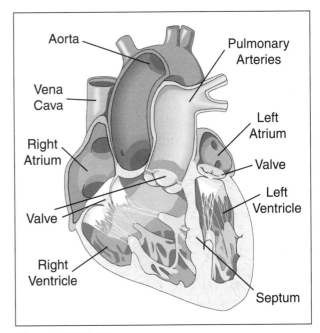

Figure 1-39 The Heart

Since the heart itself is made of cardiac muscle, it also must be supplied with the nutrients and oxygen found in blood. The heart has its own supply of blood vessels called the **coronary** arteries. If one of these coronary vessels becomes clogged or blocked, blood flow is restricted to the heart muscle. When the heart does not get enough oxygen and nutrients needed to contract due to blocked coronary vessels, a heart attack will result. Part of the heart muscle can actually "die" from lack of oxygen, damaging the heart and making it a much less efficient organ or pump. (see figure 1-40)

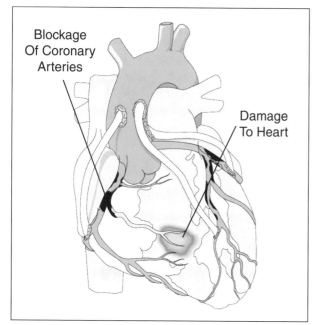

Figure 1-40 Heart Attack

The Vessels:

Three of the largest blood vessels in the body have already been mentioned along with their functions- the inferior vena cava, the superior vena cava, and the aorta. The vascular system is divided into **arteries**, **capillaries**, and **veins**. All arteries, except for the pulmonary arteries, carry oxygenated blood from the heart muscle to all parts of the body. The large aorta, stemming from the left ventricle of the heart, branches over and over into smaller and smaller arteries called **arterioles**. Arterioles are the smallest branches of the arteries found at the capillary beds. Capillaries are where the arteries and veins meet. (see figure 1-41) Capillaries have very thin membranes, which readily allow the exchange of oxygen and nutrients for carbon dioxide and waste products through their walls. This exchange actually occurs between the blood and tissue fluids. After the blood passes through the capillaries, exchanging its precious cargo for carbon dioxide and waste products, it then passes through the **venules**,

which are the smallest branches of the veins. All veins, except for the pulmonary veins, carry deoxygenated blood back through the body to the heart. These veins, many of which contain little valves to prevent the backflow of blood, connect with more and more veins, until they reach the inferior and superior vena cava at the heart. The blood vessels are like miles and miles of pipes carrying blood in a continuous loop from the heart, through the body, and back to the heart again.

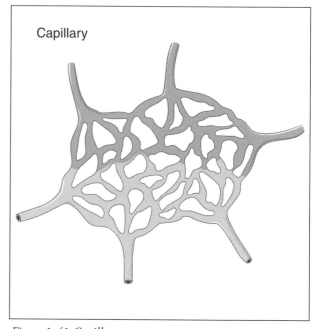

Figure 1-41 Capillary

The Blood:

Humans have between four and six liters of blood. Fifty-two to sixty-two percent of your blood is made of plasma, or the liquid portion. Thirty-eight to forty-eight percent is made up of the formed elements or various blood cells. General functions of the blood include transportation, regulation, and protection. The blood transports nutrients, gases, hormones, and waste products. The blood helps to regulate body temperature, fluid and electrolyte balance, and acid-base balance. Our blood protects us with white blood cells and by clotting when we are injured.

Blood can be visualized as a chunky soup with plasma being the broth and the various blood cells providing the "chunks." **Erythrocytes**, or red blood cells, are of particular interest to the fitness instructor. Erythrocytes contain the protein **hemoglobin**, which is the site where oxygen is carried in the blood. Iron is an essential component of hemoglobin, and it is the

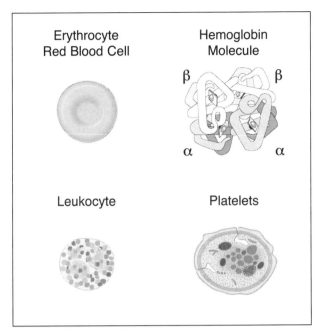

Figure 1-42 Blood Cells

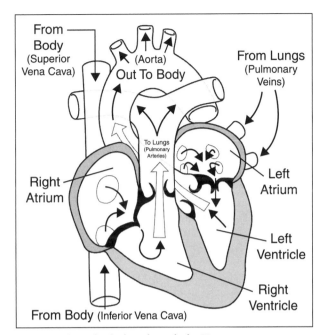

Figure 1-43a Blood Flow through the Heart

iron that actually bonds with oxygen. We inherit our blood type from our parents. Blood types are primarily determined by variations in the red blood cells.

Another important cell in blood is the white blood cell, also called a **leukocyte**. White blood cells are larger than red blood cells and function to protect the body from infectious diseases as well as provide immunity.

Platelets, or thrombocytes, are cells which function in several ways to prevent blood loss when we are injured, including the blood clotting mechanism.

Blood Flow and Oxygenation

This section will combine and review the path blood takes through the body and includes how blood is oxygenated. (see figures 1-43a, 1-43b, and 1-43c)

- Blood enters the heart through the inferior and superior vena cava and goes to the right atrium.
- It then passes into the right ventricle where it is sent through the pulmonary artery to the lungs.
- In the lungs, the arteries branch into smaller and smaller vessels called arterioles at the capillary beds.
- At the capillary beds, oxygen and carbon dioxide are exchanged through the alveoli of the lungs.
- At the alveoli, oxygen attaches to the iron in the hemoglobin of red blood cells.
- The oxygenated blood travels through the venules combining with other vessels to make the pulmonary vein.

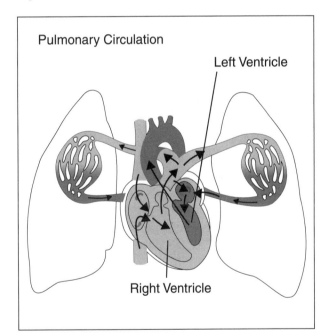

Figure 1-43b Pulmonary Circulation

- The pulmonary vein enters the left atrium of the heart and passes through to the left ventricle.
- The left ventricle contracts forcefully to pump blood through the aorta to the miles of other arteries of the body.
- The arteries branch into smaller and smaller units to arterioles located at the capillaries in various tissues of the body.
- At the capillaries, oxygen and nutrients from the

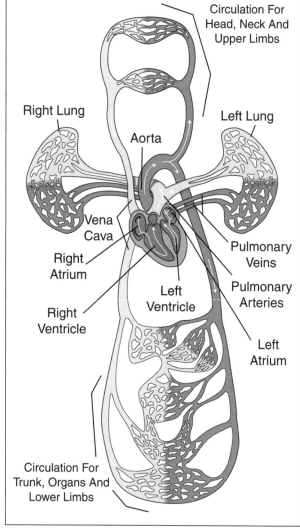

Figure 1-43c Blood Flow through the Body

blood are exchanged for carbon dioxide and waste products from tissue fluids.

- The blood passes into the <u>venules</u> which combine to end in the inferior and superior vena cava.
- There the process begins again in an unending cycle that brings life and vitality to the organism.

Cardiovascular Terms

1. Cardiac Cycle: Simultaneous contraction of the atria followed by simultaneous contraction of the ventricles. The sequence of events in one heartbeat.
2. Systole: The active contraction of the heart muscle. Ventricular contraction forces blood into the arteries.
3. Diastole: Relaxation of the heart muscle in the cardiac cycle.

4. Blood Pressure: The force the blood exerts against the blood vessel walls. Two numbers are obtained (the systolic blood pressure and the diastolic blood pressure) and are normally expressed as a fraction. Systolic blood pressure is the pressure exerted during the active contracting part of the cardiac cycle. This number is considered normal if between 90 and 135 when taken in the arm. Blood pressure is lower at the capillaries to permit filtration without rupturing the delicate membrane walls. A systolic blood pressure is the pressure in the vessels when the heart is relaxed in the cardiac cycle. Normal diastolic pressure is between 60 and 85 in the arm. A diastolic blood pressure in the arm of 90 is considered borderline high. A blood pressure of 120/80 would be considered normal, and blood pressure of 140/90 would be considered borderline high. High blood pressure can weaken the blood vessel walls and increase your risk of cardiovascular disease.
5. Cardiac Output: The volume of blood pumped by a ventricle in one minute. Usually expressed as CO = SV X HR, or cardiac output equals stroke volume times heart rate.
6. Stroke Volume: The amount of blood pumped by a ventricle in one heartbeat.
7. Heart Rate: The number of times the heart beats or completes a cardiac cycle in one minute. Heart rate is lower when at rest and increases as activity level increases.
8. Arrhythmia: An abnormal or irregular rhythm of the heart.
9. Tachycardia: An abnormally rapid or high heart rate.
10. Bradycardia: An abnormally slow or low heart rate.
11. Atherosclerosis: An abnormal collection of fat and other materials in the walls of arteries, narrowing the openings and increasing the risk of blockage.
12. Coronary Artery Disease: When atherosclerosis affects the arteries of the heart muscle.
13. Angina: Chest pain caused by lack of blood flow and consequently lack of oxygen to the heart muscle. Angina is a symptom of heart disease.
14. Heart Murmur: An abnormal or extra heart sound caused by the malfunctioning of a heart valve.

Summary-Exercise and the Bodily Systems

It was mentioned at the start of this chapter how all of the systems in the body work together to create the organism or individual. The five systems just discussed (the skeletal, muscular, nervous, respiratory, and cardiovascular systems) work together to allow us to move and sustain prolonged exercise. Each system contributes its special attributes, which allow us to initiate, perpetuate, and regulate exercise.

In exercise, the skeletal system provides the rigid structure to which our muscles attach. Without the leverage the skeletal system provides, human movement would not be possible.

The muscular system provides the power that moves the skeleton. Our muscles attach from bone to bone across joints and have the ability to contract. When our muscles contract, the bones move.

Coordinated, or voluntary movement of the musculoskeletal system, is made possible by the nervous system. The nervous system gives us the mind-to-muscle connection we need to be able to "will" our movement. Without the nervous system we would not be able to control the quality or quantity of our contractions.

The respiratory and cardiovascular systems provide the oxygen and nutrients the bones need to grow and the muscles need to contract. Without these two systems we would not be able to sustain contraction of the skeletal muscles - we would "run out of gas." The cardiovascular and respiratory systems also play a critical role in removing carbon dioxide and wastes from our bodies.

These five systems, aided by the other bodily systems, work together to make us the marvelous creatures we are - creatures capable of running, dancing, swimming and biking. The human body is truly a complicated but incredible machine.

Review Questions

1. The rib cage is _____ to the pelvic girdle. (Use an anatomical reference term.)
2. The humerus is classified as a _____ bone.
3. Which characteristic of muscle allows it to shorten and thicken?
4. The _____ muscle group flexes the leg at the knee.
5. What is a motor neuron?
6. Describe the Valsalva maneuver.

See Appendix E for answers to review questions.

References

1. American Council on Exercise. (2000). *Group Fitness Instructor Manual.* San Diego, CA. American Council on Exercise.

2. Gray, H. (1901). *Gray's Anatomy.* New York. Crown Publishers.

3. Riposo, D. (1990). *Fitness Concepts: A Resource Manual for Aquatic Fitness Instructors.* 2nd Edition. Pt. Washington, WI. Aquatic Exercise Association.

4. Scanlon, V. and T. Sanders. (2003). *Essentials of Anatomy and Physiology.* 4th Edition. Philadelphia, PA. F.A. Davis Company.

5. Tortora, G. and S. Grabowski. (2002). *Principles of Anatomy and Physiology.* 10th Edition. Indianapolis, IN. Wiley Publishing, Inc.

6. Van Roden, J. and L. Gladwin. (2002). *Fitness: Theory & Practice.* 4th Edition. Sherman Oaks, CA. Aerobic & Fitness Association of America.

Select Images provided by;
Hillman, S. (2004). *Complete 3D Human Anatomy.* London, UK. Primal Pictures, Ltd.
Website: www.primalpictures.com

Kumm, R. (2005). *LifeART Super Anatomy 1.* Baltimore, MD. Lippincott, Williams & Wilkins.
Website: www.lifeart.com

Kumm, R. (2005). *LifeART Super Anatomy 2.* Baltimore, MD. Lippincott, Williams & Wilkins.
Website: www.lifeart.com

Kumm, R. (2005). *LifeART Super Anatomy 3.* Baltimore, MD. Lippincott, Williams & Wilkins.
Website: www.lifeart.com

Kumm, R. (2005). *LifeART Super Anatomy 5.* Baltimore, MD. Lippincott, Williams & Wilkins.
Website: www.lifeart.com

Chapter 2: Exercise Physiology

INTRODUCTION

This chapter presents a basic explanation of the physiological principles governing the body's response to exercise, how the body produces energy for exercise, how muscles contract, and the physiological responses of the body to aerobic exercise.

Unit Objectives

After completing Chapter 2, you should be able to:
1. Define and apply the physiological principles of exercise.
2. Explain the importance of muscle balance by strengthening and stretching both members of a muscle pair.
3. Describe how water promotes muscle balance.
4. Understand basic energy metabolism.
5. Describe how the metabolic energy systems work together to supply the body's energy needs.
6. Understand the sliding filament theory and the basic concept of muscle contraction.
7. Know the characteristics of fast twitch and slow twitch muscle fibers.
8. Describe isometric, isotonic, and isokinetic muscle actions.
9. Describe steady state and high intensity aerobic exercise responses.

Key Questions:
1. How do you improve your fitness level?
2. What is a muscle pair?
3. How do the metabolic systems in the body produce ATP?
4. How does a muscle contract?
5. What is the difference between fast twitch and slow twitch muscle fibers?
6. How is an isometric muscle action different from an isotonic muscle action?
7. What is steady state exercise?

Physiological Principles

There are basic physiological "principles" which need to be applied and respected in exercise programs. Understanding these concepts helps the fitness professional appreciate basic underlying physiological concepts which govern how the body changes and responds to exercise. At times, these principles are ignored or manipulated when promoting "fad" or "no-effort" exercise programs. Therefore, most of these programs do not yield effective or lasting results. These exercise principles will help you, the fitness professional, sort through exercise misconceptions and help you guide your students to appropriate and effective programs that give lasting results. Understanding these basic principles will also help you counsel clients who are "stuck" or who have reached a plateau in their fitness program.

Overload

Definition: A greater-than-normal stress or demand placed upon a physiological system or organ typically resulting in an increase in strength or function.

This principle explains the method by which you become more fit. If you simply curl the forearm repeatedly, with no additional resistance, you will see little or no change in the biceps muscle. If you curl the forearm repeatedly with an additional weight or a "greater than normal" stress or demand, you will see strength gains in the biceps and other muscles responsible for that movement. If you want to increase function or fitness, you must overload that muscle or system. The most common method for overloading the musculoskeletal system is through resistance training. The use of weights, resistance bands, or using the resistance of the water will place additional demand on the muscle groups being targeted and will result in increased function or strength. The cardiorespiratory system must be overloaded in order to achieve increases in cardiorespiratory fitness or function. The overload principle must also be employed to promote gains in flexibility.

Progressive Overload

Definition: A gradual, systematic increase in the stress or demand placed upon a physiological system or organ to avoid the risk of chronic fatigue or injury.

Improper overload in a fitness program can pose a physiological threat to the body. Doing too much, too fast may lead to injury or chronic fatigue. It is more comfortable to progress through graduated levels of additional overload with less risk of injury. For example, an unfit participant needs to participate in several programs with minimal or no equipment before adding resistance equipment. The unfit participant may also need to take brief rest beaks or bounce in place when first participating in the cardiorespiratory segment of class. Properly using progressive overload increases client compliance. Progressive overload can be achieved by incrementally increasing intensity, duration, or frequency of exercise. It is also important to allow adequate rest and recovery. Encourage your students to know the difference between pushing their bodies at a reasonable rate, and abusing their bodies by pushing too hard.

Adaptation

Definition: The ability of a system or organ to adjust to additional stress or overload over time by increasing in strength or function.

The human body becomes more fit by adapting to the additional demands or overload placed upon it. If the body repeatedly performs the same type of exercise at the same workload, that particular exercise will become easier to perform as the body adapts to the overload by increasing in strength and function. If you want to continue to increase function, you must continue to incrementally overload as the body adapts to each new challenge. Some people become discouraged by how easy their exercise session feels after they have been attending for several months or years. They no longer experience that "challenged" feeling and think they are not getting a good workout. Adaptation is one of the "prizes" of a regular exercise program. Participants should understand adaptation, realizing that becoming fit makes exercise feel easier. Participants should be cautioned not to exceed safe limits to feel challenged again. Advising them to switch to another type of exercise to be challenged (variability) is usually a healthier option.

Specificity

Definition: You only train that part of the system or body which is overloaded. Physiological adaptation is specific to the system or part of the body which is overloaded.

If you lift weights to train the biceps muscles, you will see little or no benefit for the triceps muscles, deltoid muscles, or leg muscles. In order to see improvements, that muscle, muscle group, or metabolic system has to be specifically trained.

Because of specificity, you must perform several exercises to train all of the major muscle groups in your body. Cardiorespiratory exercise also yields different results with different modes. Biking will work the muscles involved in biking, but will not effectively train the muscles and cardiovascular system for jogging. Step exercise works the musculoskeletal and cardiorespiratory system differently than water aerobics. A well-conditioned jogger may feel challenged when attempting to bike, just as a well-conditioned biker may feel challenged in a water fitness class. Exercise is specific in the way it trains the musculoskeletal system as well as the metabolic systems. Being in shape will help you better perform any kind of exercise, however, your body will perform exercises for which you have "specifically" trained with less effort and greater ease.

Variability/Cross Training

Definition: The varying of intensity, duration, or mode (cross training) of exercise sessions to obtain better muscle balance and overall fitness.

Increasing demand on a variety of muscle groups or physiological systems creates more widespread adaptation within the body. Variability is necessary because of the law of specificity. Athletes must train specifically to improve skills and performance for a particular sport. Conversely, the average adult seeking overall health and fitness should practice a variety of exercise modes, intensities, and durations to challenge the body and develop a more widespread base of overall fitness. Many people get stuck in their exercise program. Varying the workout will usually provide the challenge they crave as well as help them continue to reach their weight loss or fitness goals. It is important to remember that the body adapts specifically to any given overload. For overall health and fitness, variability is a must.

Reversibility

Definition: The body will gradually revert to pre-training status when you discontinue exercise.

Fitness cannot be stored. When you do not exercise, physiological function or strength will decrease to pre-training levels over time. Reversibility is everyone's least favorite exercise principle. You have to use it or lose it.

One encouraging point is that our bodies do store "muscle or fitness memory." Research indicates that people who have maintained fitness levels over a prolonged period of time will lose their physiological benefits at a slower rate. A person who was previously fit will find it much easier to get back in shape, as opposed to someone who has never exercised, due to many factors associated with muscle memory. Encourage your students not to use a two-week layoff as an excuse to abandon exercise completely. Getting started again may be difficult for the first few exercise sessions, but fitness will return quickly.

There is a "threshold of training," or a given overload, that must be exceeded in order to see improvements in fitness. Exceeding the safe limits of that threshold, or trying to progress too aggressively, will increase risk of injury and chronic fatigue. Often exercisers stick with one particular mode of exercise. This is particularly true of exercisers who take group exercise programs. These people often plateau or burn out. They should be encouraged to cross train to offset the body's constant desire to adapt to any specific overload. Cross training promotes muscle balance and more generalized fitness. Trying another instructor's workout, or trying a different kind of group exercise class (deep water exercise as opposed to shallow water exercise), may be enough to stimulate and challenge your body in a different way.

Muscle Balance

The muscles in the human musculoskeletal system are primarily arranged in pairs throughout the body. These muscle pairs tend to be arranged around the same joint on opposite sides. These muscles work as agonists and antagonists to affect movement at that joint. Common muscle pairs affecting gross movements would include:
- biceps and triceps–front and back of the elbow joint and shoulder joint.
- anterior deltoid and posterior deltoid–front and back of the shoulder joint.
- pectoralis and trapezius / latissimus dorsi–front and back of the torso.
- rectus abdominis and erector spinae–front and back of the torso.
- iliopsoas and gluteus maximus–front and back of the hip joint.
- hip abductors and adductors–inside and outside of the hip joint.

- quadriceps and hamstrings–front and back of the hip joint and knee joint.
- tibialis anterior and gastrocnemius / soleus–front and back of the ankle joint.

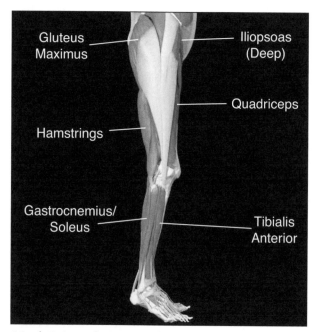

Muscle Pairs in the Lower Body.

It is important that the muscle pairs surrounding any given joint be reasonably equal in both strength and flexibility. Muscle imbalance in strength, flexibility, or both can affect the integrity at that joint and increase risk of injury. Many acute and chronic injuries can be traced to poor joint integrity as a result of muscle imbalance in either strength or flexibility. Muscle balance should be considered for the front and back, left and right sides, and upper and lower parts of the body.

The human body craves symmetry and balance. At times a weight lifter may ignore the concept of muscle balance and train only the pectoralis muscles or chest area. Often the muscles in the chest will only hypertrophy or grow in size to a certain point. After this point is reached, it is very difficult to stimulate the chest muscles to grow any larger. When only one muscle of a muscle pair is overloaded and the other ignored, the body usually triggers a physiological response to keep itself from becoming too unbalanced. It will inhibit growth in the overworked muscle. To stimulate growth most effectively, both muscles of a muscle pair should be stimulated or overloaded. Research indicates that stimulating both muscles of

the muscle pair – in the same workout – may actually enhance strength gains even more.

This principle applies not only to weight lifting, but carries over to all forms of exercise. If you train using only one type of exercise or only one certain type of program, you could be promoting muscle imbalance. Because of the law of specificity, biking places a lot of emphasis on the quadriceps muscles. Other types of exercise which actively overload the hamstrings muscles should be combined with a bike training program to maintain equality in strength in the thigh muscles and maintain integrity in the knee joint. It is very important to remember that both muscles in a muscle pair should be stretched during each workout as well to maintain equality in flexibility.

The water is a great environment in which to promote and build muscle balance. The resistance of water surrounds the exerciser and affects every movement in every direction. In addition, the effects of gravity are reduced. On land under the effects of gravity, a standing arm curl would work only the bicep muscles. The bicep would be concentrically contracted (shortened) on the way up against gravity, and eccentrically contracted (lengthened) on the way down to control the return movement. The triceps would primarily remain unloaded. In the water, both the biceps and triceps would be working to perform a standing arm curl. The biceps would be concentrically contracted on the way up against the water's resistance, and the triceps would be concentrically contracted against the water's resistance on the way down. The water promotes muscle balance by providing resistance for both muscles in a muscle pair in both directions of movement. (Remember, the use of weighted, buoyed, or rubberized equipment will change the workload and affect the way muscles in a muscle pair are loaded.)

Energy Metabolism

The conversion of energy within the human body is a very fascinating process. Providing the energy working muscles need to contract is very complicated and involves a multitude of hormones, enzymes, vitamins, and minerals. As a water exercise instructor, it is important to have a <u>basic</u> understanding of how that energy is produced in muscle tissue.

Energy

There are six forms of energy—chemical energy, mechanical energy, heat energy, light energy, electrical energy, and nuclear energy. The Law of Conservation of Energy states that "energy cannot be created or destroyed, only converted from one form to another. The total energy in an isolated system is constant." (4) This energy can be converted from one form to another. Energy production in humans starts with nuclear energy produced from the sun. All energy used by the biological world is ultimately derived from the sun. Some of this energy from the sun reaches the earth in the form of light energy. This light energy is converted to chemical energy by plants through a process known as photosynthesis. Plants use this chemical energy to build food molecules such as glucose, cellulose, proteins, and lipids. Humans are not capable of this. We must eat plants and other animals to supply our chemical energy. This food is used in the human body to supply the chemical energy needed for growth and the mechanical energy needed for muscular contractions. (see figure 2-1) It is the conversion of chemical energy to mechanical energy in the body for muscle contractions that we will focus on in this chapter. These chemical changes or reactions occurring in the body are called **metabolic respiration**.

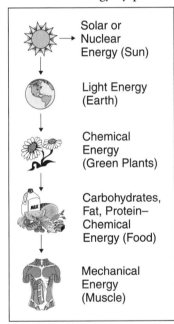

Solar or Nuclear Energy (Sun)

Light Energy (Earth)

Chemical Energy (Green Plants)

Carbohydrates, Fat, Protein– Chemical Energy (Food)

Mechanical Energy (Muscle)

Figure 2-1

Adenosine Triphosphate (ATP)

Adenosine Triphosphate, a chemical compound, is the most immediate chemical source of energy for a cell. The formation of ATP in the muscle cell involves the conversion of food stuffs. Food is consumed, digested, absorbed into the blood stream, transported to active cells (the site of energy production), and immediately used or stored. Carbohydrates are converted to glucose and stored as glycogen. Fats are converted to fatty acid and primarily stored as adipose fat tissue. Proteins are broken down into amino acids and ultimately stored as fat if not used. (see figure 2-2) This breakdown of food is not directly used to do work. Rather, it is employed to manufacture ATP, which is stored in all muscle cells.

It is the breakdown of ATP that releases energy to be used by the muscle to contract or perform mechanical work. (see figure 2-3) ATP is composed of a complex structure called adenosine, and three less complicated parts called phosphates. The phosphates are held in place by high energy bonds. When one of these phosphate bonds is broken or removed from the rest of the molecule, energy is liberated and adenosine diphosphate (ADP) and inorganic phosphate are left. The breakdown of one mole of ATP yields between 7 and 12 kilocalories of energy.

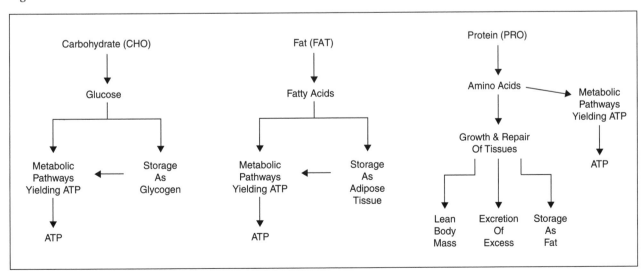

Figure 2-2

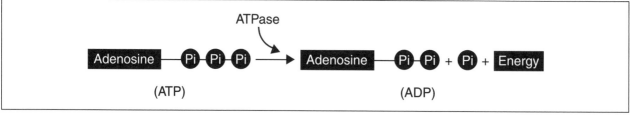

Figure 2-3

There are three systems that manufacture this energy for the muscle cells. The energy system primarily activated to supply this energy depends specifically upon the type of exercise being performed. The active muscle has available an immediate source of energy (the **ATP-PCr system**), a short-term source of energy (the anaerobic or **glycolytic system**), and a long term source of energy (the aerobic or **oxidative system**). Below is a simplified look at each system to help you gain a basic understanding of how energy is produced during exercise.

ATP-PCr System

The ATP-PCr system supplies the working muscle with an immediate source of energy. Activities with a high-energy demand over a short period of time depend primarily on ATP generated from enzyme reactions in this system. A rapidly available source of ATP is supplied to the muscles for contractions. This involves a relatively short series of chemical reactions, does not require oxygen, and both the ADP and PCr (phosphocreatine) are stored and readily available in the muscle. This is the least complicated way to generate ATP. Phosphocreatine has a high-energy phosphate bond like the one found in ATP, and both are referred to as phosphagens. PCr is broken down in the presence of the enzyme creatine phosphokinase, and the energy released from that high-energy bond is used to form ATP from ADP. (see figure 2-4)

PCr ➝ Cr + Pi + Energy

Pi + Energy + ADP ➝ ATP

Figure 2-4

This "biochemically-coupled" enzymatic reaction will continue until the stores of phosphocreatine are depleted in the muscle. The ATP-PCr system is the primary source of energy for muscle contractions

during the first few seconds of exercise. The total amount of ATP energy available from this system is very limited and would be exhausted after about 8-10 seconds of maximal exercise.

Glycolytic System

The glycolytic system, or anaerobic glycolysis, does not require oxygen, forms the by-product lactic acid which causes muscle fatigue, uses carbohydrates only, and yields 2 molecules of ATP from glucose and 3 molecules of ATP from glycogen. This metabolic system is the primary source of ATP for intermediate energy, or activities lasting more than a few seconds up to approximately two minutes. The glycolytic system, like the ATP-PCr system, does not require oxygen and involves the incomplete breakdown of carbohydrates into lactic acid.

The body breaks carbohydrates down into a simple sugar called **glucose**, which is either immediately used or stored in the liver and muscles as **glycogen**. The terms sugar, carbohydrate, glucose, and glycogen are often used interchangeably when broadly referring to energy metabolism. Anaerobic glycolysis refers to the breakdown of glycogen in the absence of oxygen. This process is chemically more complicated than the ATP-PCr system and requires a longer series of chemical reactions. The glycolytic system may be about one-half as fast as the phosphagen system, but yields slightly higher amounts of ATP (two molecules for glucose/three molecules for glycogen, as compared to one in the phosphagen system). Due to the buildup of lactic acid, a by-product in this system, the yield may actually be lower than three. When lactic acid builds in the muscle and blood, it leads to muscle fatigue and ultimately to muscle failure. Once again, the production of ATP by anaerobic glycolysis is accomplished through a "coupled" or two-part reaction. Glycogen is broken down into lactic acid and energy. This energy is used to synthesize 3 ATP from 3 ADP and 3 phosphate (Pi) molecules. (see figure 2-5)

$$\text{Glycogen} \longrightarrow \text{Lactic Acid} + \text{Energy}$$
$$\text{Energy} + 3\text{ADP} + 3\text{Pi} \longrightarrow 3\text{ATP}$$

Figure 2-5

Oxidative System

The oxidative system yields a substantially greater number of ATP, utilizes oxygen to generate ATP, and is activated to produce energy for long duration exercise. Aerobic metabolism is a slower and more complicated process. The ATP reaped from the breakdown of glucose and/or fatty acids in the presence of oxygen takes hundreds of complex chemical reactions involving hundreds of enzymes. This breakdown occurs in a specialized subcellular compartment in the muscle cell called the **mitochondrion**. The mitochondria are considered to be the "powerhouses" of the cell and are capable of producing mass quantities of ATP to fuel muscular contractions.

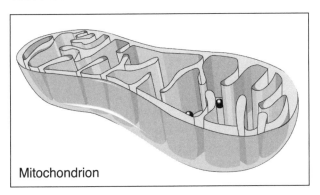

Mitochondrion

The aerobic system actually consists of three parts. The first part, aerobic glycolysis, is the breakdown of glycogen in the presence of oxygen. The difference between anaerobic glycolysis, discussed previously, and aerobic glycolysis is that oxygen prevents the accumulation of lactic acid. The precursor to lactic acid is pyruvic acid. Oxygen diverts much of the pyruvic acid into the second and third parts of aerobic metabolism (the Krebs cycle and the electron transport chain) before it is converted to lactic acid. If glycogen is used as the fuel source, 3 ATP are generated during the aerobic breakdown of glucose, and 36 ATP are generated in the electron transport system, for a total of 39 ATP. (see figure 2-6)

If fatty acids are used for fuel instead of glycogen, more oxygen is needed, but the yield of ATP is substantially higher. Fat is broken down into fatty acids and prepared for entrance into the Krebs cycle and consequently the electron transport system. This coupled reaction yields 130 ATP. (see figure 2-7)

Glycogen and fatty acids are the preferred fuel sources used in the oxidative system. Occasionally protein is used as a metabolic fuel source. Protein is typically used to provide less than five percent of energy needs. The use of protein as a fuel source usually occurs when the body has been physiologically stressed through fasting, other dietary measures, or has extremely low levels of fat and glycogen stores. When protein is used as a fuel source, it is converted to glucose through a process called gluconeogenesis. A by-product of this process is nitrogen, which is converted to urea and excreted by the kidneys. After

$$\underset{\text{(Oxygen)}}{\text{Glycogen} + 6O_2} \longrightarrow \underset{\substack{\text{(Carbon}\\ \text{Dioxide)}}}{6CO_2} + \underset{\text{(Water)}}{6H_2O} + \text{Energy}$$
$$\text{Energy} + 39\text{ADP} + 39\text{Pi} \longrightarrow 39\text{ATP}$$

Figure 2-6

$$\underset{\text{(Oxygen)}}{\text{Fatty Acid} + 23O_2} \longrightarrow \underset{\substack{\text{(Carbon}\\ \text{Dioxide)}}}{16CO_2} + \underset{\text{(Water)}}{16H_2O} + \text{Energy}$$
$$\text{Energy} + 130\text{ADP} + 130\text{Pi} \longrightarrow 130\text{ATP}$$

Figure 2-7

the amino acids are converted to glucose, they follow the same path into the Krebs cycle and electron transport system as glucose. If the body has to convert a lot of amino acids into glucose, the consequent removal of nitrogen/urea can be hard on the kidneys. Glucose is the fuel used by the brain and other vital organs. The kidneys, liver, and muscle stores can be compromised from a high protein or low carbohydrate diet.

In summary, the oxygen or aerobic metabolic system requires large amounts of oxygen to convert glycogen to 39 ATP and fatty acids to 130 ATP. The fatty acid or glycogen are broken down and prepared for the Krebs cycle and electron transport system; and carbon dioxide, water, heat, and energy are the result. The carbon dioxide is exhaled, the water and heat are eliminated through evaporation and radiation, and the energy is used in the second part of the coupled reaction to synthesize ATP.

How These Systems Work Together to Supply the Body's Energy Needs

As stated previously, specific energy systems are activated in response to specific types of exercise or activity. In times of low energy demands or physical inactivity, substrates stored as lipids or glycogens are used to supply the body's energy needs. During rest, most of your energy needs are supplied by the oxidative system, receiving oxygen through the normal breathing process. Higher demands stimulate the

cardiorespiratory system to deliver more oxygen to the mitochondria in the muscle cell to be used in aerobic energy production. It is important to realize that one system does not shut off as another is activated. All systems are being used at all times. (see figure 2-8) Which systems are being used and to what degree, is controlled and regulated by hormones. Hormones released during exercise and rest are responsible for alterations in the rate of energy production and partially for the selection of the fuel sources used.

Skeletal Muscle Tissue

Now that you know where the energy needed for muscle contractions comes from, it would be helpful to know how the ATP is actually converted to mechanical energy. To understand this, you first must know a little bit about muscle tissue and how it contracts. This too is a very complicated process, which only requires a simple understanding by the fitness instructor.

Sliding Filament Theory

Muscles are made up of bundles of fibers which are made up of bundles of **myofibrils**. (see figure 2-9) These myofibrils are made up of protein filaments. The protein filaments consist of a thick filament called myosin and a thin filament called actin. Each grouping or functional unit of actin and myosin is called a sarcomere. There are protein crossbridges between these two filaments. In the presence of certain vitamins,

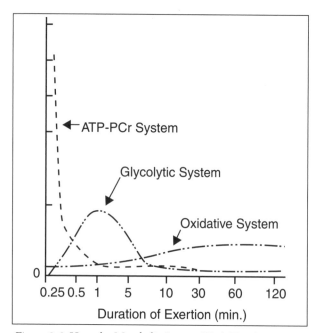

Figure 2-8 How the Metabolic Systems Work Together

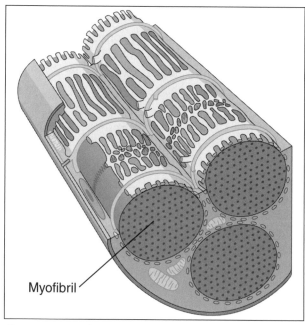

Figure 2-9 Muscle Tissue

minerals, enzymes, and of course ATP, the thin actin fibers slide over these crossbridges and shorten or contract the muscle fiber. The bands of actin and myosin do not change in length to cause the muscle to contract, but rather collectively slide over each other via the protein crossbridges. (see figure 2-10a-d)

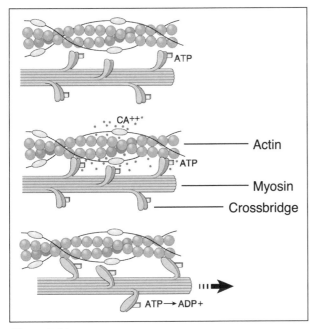

Figure 2-10a

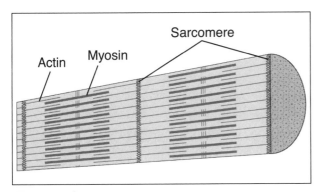

Figure 2-10b

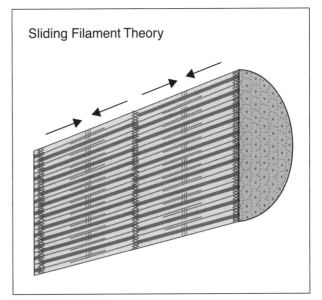

Figure 2-10c

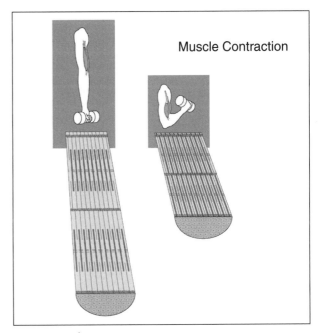

Figure 2-10d

Muscle fibers are innervated by specialized nerve cells called **motor neurons**, which originate from the spinal column and brain. This nerve connection from the brain to the muscle gives conscious control of movement or "voluntary" muscle contractions. Each motor neuron can transmit signals to a number of myofibrils. A **motor unit** consists of one motor neuron and all of the myofibrils it stimulates. If a "fine" muscle movement is required, as in the eyes or hands, a motor neuron may only be connected with five or so myofibrils. In movements requiring "gross" muscle control, one motor neuron may be associated with as many as 500 myofibrils. These motor units follow the "**all-or-none principle**" which states that all of the muscle fibers in a motor unit contract, or none contract. Although the fibers within a motor unit do not act independently, each motor unit does act independently, so this allows partial contraction of a muscle through stimulation of only part of the motor units within that muscle. The amount of tension created within a muscle depends on the number of motor units (motor neuron and its fibers) stimulated to shorten or contract.

Types of Skeletal Muscle Fibers

The duration of contraction of various muscles depends upon their function in the body. Eye movements must be rapid, so the duration of contraction of eye muscles is less than 1/100th of a second. The gastrocnemius muscle in the lower leg does not depend on rapid movement to function properly. So the duration of contraction for this muscle is about 1/30th of a second. Faster contracting muscles are made up primarily of "white muscle" or **fast-twitch** muscle fibers. Slower contracting muscles are made up primarily of "red muscles" or **slow-twitch** muscle fibers. Slow-twitch muscle fibers are slow to fatigue and are designed for submaximal prolonged exercise. They are reddish in color because they contain more mitochondria, myoglobin, and stored fat for more aerobic energy production (like dark meat in chicken). Fast-twitch muscles on the other hand, are specialized for high intensity contractions and therefore fatigue more readily. They depend more on anaerobic energy production, contain fewer mitochondria and myoglobin, and are more whitish in appearance.

It is uncertain how much of the predominant muscle fiber type is genetically predetermined in humans. There are several variations of fast-twitch muscle fibers (FT_a, FT_b, FT_c) and it is also possible that fibers may be able to take on the characteristics of another type in response to aerobic or anaerobic training. (8) It is found that long-distance runners have more slow-twitch endurance fibers and sprinters have more fast-twitch anaerobic fibers. All skeletal muscles possess both types of fibers, but predominant muscle fiber type in any given skeletal muscle is dependent upon several factors including the function of the muscle, genetics, and how the muscle has been trained.

Types of Skeletal Muscle Contractions/Actions

Skeletal muscle can generate three types of muscle actions. These three types are called **isotonic**, **isometric**, and **isokinetic** muscle actions.

Isotonic contractions are actions where the muscle shortens and lengthens, and movement occurs at the joint. Isotonic contractions cause or control joint movement. The force generated by this contraction changes with the length of the muscle and the angle of the joint. Isotonic actions consist of two parts - the shortening, or **concentric** phase, and the lengthening, or **eccentric** phase. An action is concentric when the muscle is creating tension while shortening or contracting (for example, raising a weight resisted by gravity in a forearm curl). Lowering the weight assisted by gravity, or retaining tension in a muscle as it lengthens, would be considered an eccentric muscle action. It is considered a muscle action instead of a contraction because the muscle is lengthening instead of shortening as the term contraction implies. (4) Often, the term muscle action and muscle contraction are still used interchangeably. In typical weight-lifting programs, a concentric contraction is usually followed by an eccentric contraction/muscle action. The eccentric part is often called "negative work".

Concentric and eccentric muscle actions are of particular interest in the aquatic environment. Primarily concentric contractions are utilized in aquatic exercise because the drag property of the water provides more resistance than gravity or buoyancy. As stated earlier, both parts of a muscle pair are worked concentrically in the water as opposed to one muscle being worked concentrically and eccentrically on land in gravity. It is a common misconception that eccentric contractions are significantly better at building strength in a muscle. Research indicates that eccentric training results in no greater gains in isometric, eccentric, and concentric strength than normal resistance training with dumbbells. (3) The water may not be the optimal environment for building <u>maximal</u> muscular strength (your highest strength potential) or muscle <u>hypertrophy</u> (muscle bulk), however research clearly indicates that strength gains can certainly be achieved through aquatic training. It is uncertain whether the absence of eccentric muscle actions in drag resistance exercises in the water affects the magnitude of strength gains. Eccentric actions can and should be introduced for variety through the use of buoyant, weighted, and rubberized equipment. One thing is known for certain - eccentric muscle actions cause higher levels of muscle soreness.

Isometric muscle actions occur when tension is developed in the muscle without movement at the joint or a change in the muscle length. In an isometric action, the tension remains constant because the length of the muscle does not change. An example of an isometric action would be holding a push-up in the "down" position, or trying to move an immovable object like pressing against a doorframe. Because there is no movement involved, this muscle action is often referred to as a "static" contraction.

Isokinetic muscle actions are, in a sense, a combination of isometric and isotonic contractions. Because of this, some consider isokinetic muscle actions to be a "technique" as opposed to another type of muscle contraction. (5) An isokinetic muscle action is a dynamic muscle action kept at a constant velocity that is independent of the amount of muscular force generated by the involved muscles. Therefore, with isokinetic actions, the speed of shortening and lengthening is constant. Isokinetic actions are not preformed in aqua exercise because this requires very specialized, expensive equipment. Isokinetic equipment is primarily used in physical therapy and/or athletic training facilities.

Aerobic Exercise Responses

Prolonged aerobic exercise, like a water aerobic class, elicits certain physiological responses within the body. When commencing exercise, there is an immediate demand placed upon the body for more oxygen. Unfortunately, the body cannot immediately supply increased amounts of oxygen to the working muscle. It takes time to transport the oxygen from the air, through the respiratory system, through the vascular system to the mitochondria in the muscle cell. This time of inadequate oxygen supply is referred to as **oxygen deficit**, and ATP is primarily synthesized by the anaerobic system with accumulation of lactic acid in the muscle tissue. Eventually, the body is able to supply the oxygen needed for exercise, and oxygen supply meets oxygen demand. This is referred to as **steady state** exercise. At the cessation of exercise, oxygen supply exceeds oxygen demand. Your heart rate and respiratory rate do not just drop immediately to resting rates, but do so gradually over a period of time. This time of excess oxygen supply is referred to as **oxygen debt or excess postexercise oxygen consumption (EPOC)**. During this time, extra oxygen is needed to convert waste products, like lactic acid, to be removed from muscle tissue. (see figure 2-11)

In anaerobic or high intensity exercise, the body never reaches steady state because oxygen supply never meets oxygen demand. (see figure 2-12) In this type of exercise, phosphagens are depleted, the respiratory system becomes distressed, lactic acid builds up, and muscles fatigue.

It is important to ensure your students do not work at too high an intensity level or at anaerobic levels while trying to train aerobically. Understand intensity alteration methods and guide each participant to work up to and maintain aerobic steady state. Most exercise class participants train aerobically to improve health and burn calories, unless training specifically for a particular event.

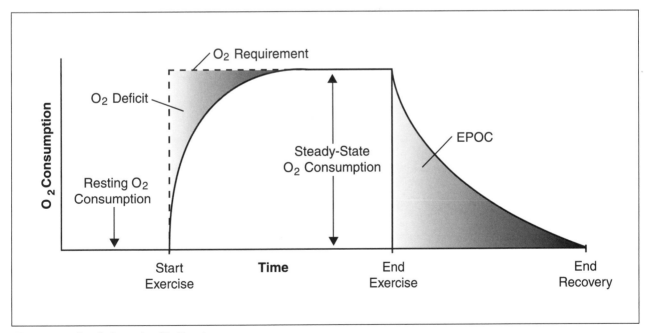

Figure 2-11 Steady State Aerobic Exercise

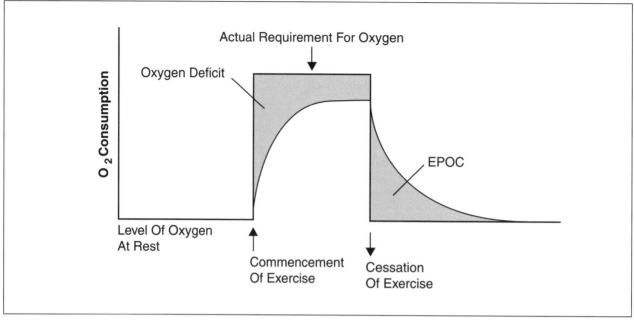

Figure 2-12 Anaerobic Exercise

The EPOC portion of an exercise program is usually referred to as recovery. During recovery, ATP, PCr, and glycogen stores are replenished. Fat is replenished indirectly through the replenishment of glycogen. Lactic acid accumulated during exercise is also removed during recovery. Replenishing energy stores and removing lactic acid requires ATP. The oxygen consumed during the recovery phase (EPOC) supplies the immediate ATP energy needed during recovery. Restoration of ATP and PCr takes only a few minutes, where as the restoration of muscle and liver glycogen can take a day or more. Light exercise and stretching during the recovery phase (active recovery) facilitates the removal of lactic acid.

The physiological status of the body during recovery supports the need for properly cooling down and stretching after an exercise session. It also supports the importance of rest in an exercise program to avoid chronic fatigue and muscle soreness. It also explains why calorie consumption, or metabolism, remains elevated for a period of time after exercise. High levels of post-exercise carbohydrates are not needed to replenish glycogen stores. Often, in the absence of readily available carbohydrates, fat stores are utilized to replenish glycogen stores.

Summary

1. There are 6 physiological principles that govern the body's response to exercise. These principles are overload, progressive overload, adaptation, specificity, variability, and reversibility.

2. The human musculoskeletal system craves symmetry in respect to flexibility and strength. Muscle balance should be a primary consideration in any exercise program to safely achieve optimum fitness levels.

3. There are 3 energy systems the body uses to synthesize ATP for muscle contractions. For immediate energy (up to 8-10 seconds), the ATP-PCr system is primarily used. For intermediate energy (10 seconds to two minutes), the glycolytic system or anaerobic glycolysis is primarily used. For long-term energy, the oxidative system supplies most of the ATP needed.

4. The chemical energy from ATP is utilized to perform the mechanical work of muscle contractions. Muscles contract via the sliding filament theory.

5. There are two basic types of muscle fibers found in human skeletal muscle: fast-twitch or white muscle fibers used for intense or explosive exercises, and slow-twitch or red muscles fibers used for moderate intensity, longer duration exercise.

6. There are 3 basic types of muscle actions: isotonic actions consisting of concentric and eccentric muscle actions, isometric actions where tension is developed without movement, and isokinetic actions that require specialized equipment.

7. Responses to aerobic exercise include oxygen deficit, steady state, and EPOC. In anaerobic exercise, the body never achieves steady state. Recovery from exercise is the time when energy stores are replenished and lactic acid and other waste products are removed.

Review Questions

1. _____ states that you only train that part of the system or body which is overloaded.
2. Name three muscle pairs in the body.
3. Which metabolic system yields the highest amount of ATP for the working muscle?
4. Protein is broken down into _____.
5. Define the "all or none" principle.
6. Which type of muscle tissue is best suited for endurance activities?
7. Concentric and eccentric muscle actions are part of an _____ muscle contraction.
8. When <u>initiating</u> exercise, the time of inadequate oxygen supply is called _____.

See Appendix E for answers to review questions.

References

1. American Council on Exercise. (2000). *Group Fitness Instructor Manual.* San Diego, CA. American Council on Exercise.

2. American Council on Exercise. (2003). *Personal Trainer Manual.* 3rd Edition. San Diego, CA. American Council on Exercise.

3. Fleck, S. and W. Kraemer. (2003). *Designing Resistance Training Programs.* 3rd. Edition. Champaign, IL. Human Kinetics Publishers.

4. Ostdiek, V. and D. Bord. (1994). *Inquiry Into Physics.* 3rd Edition. St. Paul, MN. West Publishing Company.

5. Thompson, C. and R. Floyd. (2000). *Manual of Structural Kinesiology.* 14th Edition. New York, NY. McGraw-Hill Publishers.

6. Tortora, G. and S. Grabowski. (2002). *Principles of Anatomy and Physiology.* 10th Edition. Indianapolis, IN. Wiley Publishing, Inc.

7. Van Roden, J. and L. Gladwin. (2002). *Fitness: Theory & Practice.* 4th Edition. Sherman Oaks, CA. Aerobic & Fitness Association of America.

8. Wilmore, J. and D. Costill. (2001). *Physiology of Sport and Exercise.* 3rd Edition. Champaign, IL. Human Kinetics Publishers.

Select Images provided by:

Hillman, S. (2004). *Complete 3D Human Anatomy.* London, UK. Primal Pictures, Ltd. Website: www.primalpictures.com

Kumm, R. (2005). *LifeART Super Anatomy 1.* Baltimore, MD. Lippincott, Williams & Wilkins. Website: www.lifeart.com

Kumm, R. (2005). *LifeART Super Anatomy 2.* Baltimore, MD. Lippincott, Williams & Wilkins. Website: www.lifeart.com

Kumm, R. (2005). *LifeART Super Anatomy 3.* Baltimore, MD. Lippincott, Williams & Wilkins. Website: www.lifeart.com

Chapter 3: Applied Anatomy

INTRODUCTION

This chapter will provide information needed to analyze basic movements as well as help you answer the question "WHY" when you choose exercises for the water. Instructors should have the knowledge to justify exercise choices. Exercise design is a very important factor in a successful exercise program. It is important to have the knowledge to provide an effective workout addressing cardiovascular endurance, muscular balance, neutral alignment, and good body mechanics.

Unit Objectives

After completing Chapter, 3 you should be able to:
1. Define and describe anatomical position and the anatomical movement terms.
2. Understand the three planes around which the human body moves.
3. Describe a third class lever and its application in the human body.
4. Know the types of joints in the human body.
5. Understand the functions of tendons and ligaments.
6. Describe and define abnormal curvature in the spine.
7. Understand proper postural alignment.
8. Explain center of gravity and center of buoyancy.

Key Questions:
1. What position does the human body assume in anatomical position?
2. What is the difference between flexion/ extension and abduction/ adduction?
3. What types of movement occur in the sagittal plane?
4. Can you describe how a joint serves as the fulcrum in a third class lever in the body?
5. What type of joint moves in all three planes of motion?
6. What is the difference between scoliosis and kyphosis?
7. How does center of gravity differ from center of buoyancy?

"The human body and its movements are beautiful and astounding – orderly, synchronized, adaptable, quick, and precise. The body is like an incredible machine. It actually improves with use if its movement is compatible with its design and the physical laws of motion (2)."

If your water exercise class was carefully scrutinized and evaluated, would you be able to explain why you chose a particular combination of exercises, how you decided to work certain joints and muscles, and/or what are the benefits of exercising the body in the way that you designed the workout? If you want to teach movement that is compatible with the body's design, you need to have some understanding of the way the body is designed; its movement capabilities and limitations, as well as the daily functions the human body should be able to accomplish without undue stress, impairment, or going beyond an individual's capability.

This chapter will cover **kinesiology**, the study of human motion, and **biomechanics**, the area of kinesiology that deals more specifically with the analysis of movement. Subjects like kinesiology and biomechanics can be quite daunting for the exercise practitioner. Do not be deterred, because basic movement analysis becomes an invaluable tool in the delivery of safe and effective fitness programs.

Skill in movement analysis requires practice. You need to develop keen observation skills in order to analyze all the movement and stabilizing activity that occurs during an exercise. Looking at each exercise one joint at a time will pay dividends as you become aware of exactly what each exercise is doing. This will allow you to create, sequence, and modify movements for your participants.

Anatomical Position

The first tool for movement analysis is a picture of the body in **anatomical position**. All literature about the structure and function of the human body is referenced to the anatomical position. The body is erect (or lying supine as if erect) with the arms by the sides, palms facing forward, legs together, and feet directed forward (see figure 3-1). In the anatomical position, the joints and body segments are in neutral position (not flexed, hyperextended, or rotated) except for the forearms, which are supinated (palms facing forward). This is the position of reference (neutral position or 0º) for definitions and descriptions of movements.

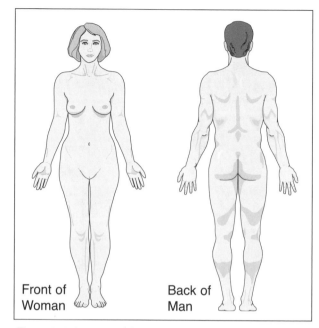

Front of Woman

Back of Man

Figure 3-1 Anatomical Position

Movement Terms

Anatomic definitions/movement terms are used to identify joint actions and describe movement of body parts. For anatomic <u>reference</u> terms, refer to Chapter 1. This chapter will define anatomic <u>movement</u> terms. These terms are usually described as pairs of opposites: **flexion/extension**, **abduction/adduction**, **medial** (internal) **rotation/lateral** (external) **rotation**, **elevation/depression**, **protraction/retraction**, **pronation/supination**, and **inversion/eversion**. These movements can occur at more than one joint in the body or may be unique to only one location. Three other terms we often meet in exercise that pertain to movement of body parts are **hyperextension**, **circumduction**, and **tilt**. Use Table 3-1 and the text and figures below to review these basic movements until you feel comfortable that you can recognize them and apply them to movement at all major joints in the body.

Flexion and **extension** can be visually described in reference to anatomical position. Flexion is moving out of anatomical position, where extension is viewed as returning to anatomical position. Flexion is generally considered to be movement in the anterior direction for the head, neck, trunk, upper extremities, and hip. However, flexion of the knee, ankle, and toes is movement in the posterior direction, simply because the lower extremities are designed differently from the upper body. Technically, flexion and extension are defined in mathematical terms. Flexion is decreasing

Table 3-1

Fundamental Movements From Anatomical Position

Action	Description
Flexion	Decreasing the angle between two bones, e.g. bending the arm at the elbow joint moving out of anatomical position. Note: Plantar flexion occurs at the ankle.
Extension	Increasing the angle between two bones, e.g. straightening the arm at the elbow returning to anatomical position. Note: Dorsi flexion occurs at the ankle.
Hyperextension	Continuing extension past neutral position, e.g. moving the head at the neck to look up.
Abduction	Movement away from the body's midline, e.g. raising your leg to the side.
Adduction	Movement toward the body's midline, e.g. returning your leg from a side leg raise.
Medial (Internal) Rotation	Rotary movement around the long axis of a bone toward the midline of the body, e.g. rotating your arm inward from the shoulder.
Lateral (External) Rotation	Rotary movement around the long axis of a bone away from the midline of the body, e.g. rotating the arm outward from the shoulder.
Circumduction	Circular movement of a limb that describes a cone. It is a combination of flexion, extension, abduction and adduction, e.g. arm or leg circles.
Elevation	Moving a body part toward the head, e.g. shrugging the shoulders upward.
Depression	Moving a body part toward the feet, e.g. pressing your shoulders downward.
Protraction	Forward movement of the shoulder girdle away from the spine. (Abduction of the scapula/shoulder blade).
Retraction	Backward movement of the shoulder girdle toward the spine. (Adduction of the scapula/shoulder blade).
Pronation	Rotating the forearm medially, or turning the palm down or backward.
Supination	Rotating the forearm laterally, or turning the palm up or forward.
Inversion	Turning the sole of the foot inward or medially.
Eversion	Turning the sole of the foot outward or laterally.
Tilt	Movements common to the head, scapulae, and pelvis, e.g. moving the top of the pelvis forward (anterior pelvic tilt), backward (posterior pelvic tilt), or to the right or left (lateral pelvic tilt).

the angle at a joint, where extension is increasing the angle at a joint. A straight arm is in anatomical or neutral position. When the arm bends at the elbow, flexion is occurring and the angle between the forearm and the upper arm is decreasing from 180º, to 90º, to 45º and less. Straightening the arm (increasing the angle from 45º, to 90º, to 180º) is extension. (see figure 3-2) Mathematical movement reference is further addressed later in this chapter.

Hyperextension is defined as going beyond neutral extension. It is important to know where hyperextension is acceptable, for example slow controlled hyperextension of the back can be a legitimate back strengthening or stretching exercise. Hyperextension can also be undesirable from the standpoint of joint integrity, for example hyperextension of the knees or elbows. Permanent lumbar hyperextension with anterior pelvic tilt

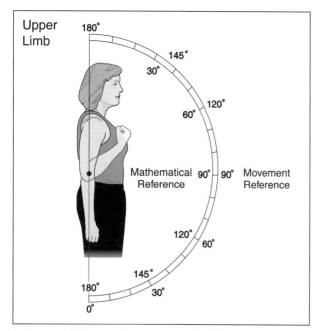

Figure 3-2 Flexion and extension at the elbow

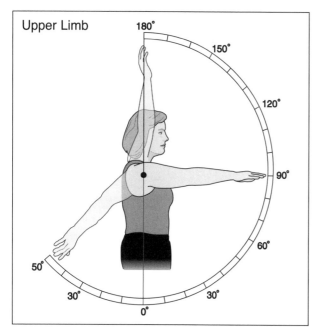

Figure 3-3
Flexion, extension, and hyperextension at the shoulder

(lordosis) is not desirable from a postural standpoint. The most acceptable joints for hyperextension are the hip, shoulder, and wrists. Hyperextension of the hip engages the gluteus maximus and the upper portion of the hamstring muscles. This movement engages these under worked muscle groups and should be included in an exercise program. Shoulder hyperextension engages several muscles in the posterior shoulder and back and should be included in exercise programs as

well. (see figure 3-3) Be aware that body alignment is crucial for safe and effective use of hyperextension exercises. For example, it is not recommended to perform hip hyperextension in combination with spine hyperextension. The pelvis should be stable in neutral position while hip hyperextension (a back kick) is performed. Movement should occur only at the hip joint and not at the lumbar spine.

Abduction and **adduction** refer to movement away from (abduction) and toward (adduction) the longitudinal axis or midline (center) of the body. These movements occur in several areas in the body, but in exercise design we tend to focus on abduction and adduction in the hips and shoulders. Jumping jacks, side steps, and a side leg lift would all be examples of abduction and adduction movements in the frontal plane, or movement to the side. (see figure 3-4)

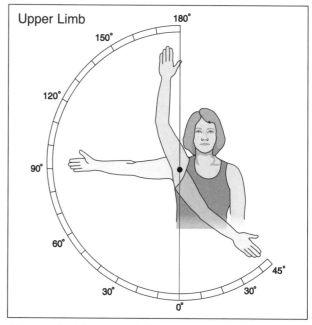

Figure 3-4 Abduction and adduction at the shoulder

Abduction and adduction movements also occur in the transverse plane or parallel to the ground. Transverse (sometimes called horizontal) abduction and adduction occur in exercise primarily at the hip and shoulder as well. Holding the arms out to the side at shoulder height and bringing the arms together in front of the body would be transverse adduction. Returning the arms from the front of the body to the sides at shoulder height would be transverse abduction.

Rotation refers to movement around the longitudinal axis of the limb or trunk for all areas of

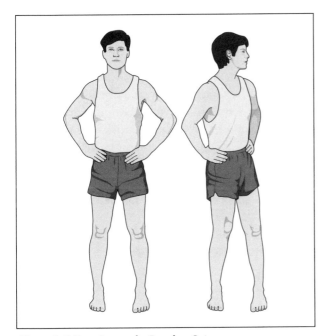

Figure 3-5 Rotation at the Lumbar Spine

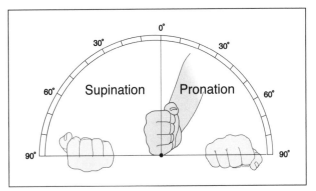

Figure 3-6 Pronation and Supination

the body except the scapula and clavicle. In exercise we use the word "turn" to indicate rotation. Rotation towards the midline is called medial (internal) rotation; movement away from midline is lateral (external) rotation. Turning the arm at the shoulder toward the center of the body is an example of medial rotation. Turning the arm at the shoulder away from the center of the body is an example of lateral rotation.

It is important to include both inward and outward rotation movements at the hips when stretching, as inward rotation is often neglected. It is recommended that outward shoulder rotation be routinely performed to stretch anterior shoulder muscles and strengthen posterior shoulder muscles to offset round shoulders. Rotation exercises against resistance for the spine will help develop internal and external oblique muscles in the abdomen. Rotation stretch exercises are often performed during the cool down to release tension in the neck.

Pronation and **supination** are terms specific to movement of the forearm. Pronation of the forearm is medial rotation (palm down or back) and supination of the forearm is lateral rotation (palm up or forward). It is beneficial to include pronation and supination exercises in the water to condition the forearm muscles including the wrist flexors and, more importantly, the wrist extensors. (see figure 3-6)

Elevation, **depression**, **protraction**, and **retraction** primarily refer to movement occurring in the shoulder girdle or scapulae. Elevation is

movement in a superior direction (towards the head). Depression is movement in an inferior direction (towards the feet). Protraction is movement of the shoulder blades forward away from the spine (abduction of scapulae), and retraction is movement of the shoulder blades back toward the spine (adduction of scapulae). Daily activities such as sitting, standing, or carrying bags on our shoulders tend to cause extensive shoulder elevation (shrugging in relation to depression) and protraction (hump back). Vertical water exercise provides an excellent medium to work on depression and retraction movements and thus offset this postural imbalance.

Inversion and **eversion** are terms specific to the ankle joint and movement of the foot. Inversion is the lifting of the medial (inner) border of the foot, or turning the sole/bottom of the foot inward. Eversion is the lifting of the lateral (outer) border of the foot, or turning the sole/bottom of the foot outward. The "lifting" is actually a form of rotation.

Circumduction is movement at a joint in a circular direction and is actually a combination of flexion, extension, hyperextension, abduction, adduction, and rotation. The proximal or near end of the bone remains relatively stable, while the distal or far end of the bone draws a circle. Common examples of circumduction would be arm circles (circumduction at the shoulder) and leg circles (circumduction at the hip). Circumduction should be performed both in a clockwise and counterclockwise direction.

Tilt is a term used to describe certain movements of the head, scapula and pelvis. The head and pelvis have anterior and posterior tilts. Anterior tilt of the head means flexion (flattening) of the cervical spine, and posterior tilt results in extension. With the pelvis, the opposite occurs. The lumbar spine flexes (flattens) with posterior pelvic tilt and goes into extension with anterior pelvic tilt. The direction of the pelvic tilt is determined from movement of the top part of the pelvis. Anterior tilt is when the top part of the pelvis moves forward. Posterior tilt is when the top part moves backward. Lateral tilt of the pelvis results in the top part of the pelvis moving to the right or left. Movements of the scapula are complex and will be dealt with later in this chapter under the Shoulder Girdle.

Table 3-2

Joint	Movement	Normal Range of Motion
Shoulder	Flexion	150 - 180°
	Extension/hyperextension	50 - 60°
	Abduction	180°
	Adduction	0° prevented by trunk
	Medial Rotation	70 - 90°
	Lateral Rotation	90°
Elbow	Flexion	140 - 150°
	Extension	0°
Radioulnar	Pronation	80°
	Supination	80°
Wrist	Flexion	60 - 80°
	Extension/hyperextension	60 - 70°
	Abduction/radial deviation	20°
	Adduction/ulnar deviation	30°
Hip	Flexion	100 - 120°
	Extension/hyperextension	30°
	Abduction	40 - 45°
	Adduction	0 - 30°
	Medial Rotation	40 - 45°
	Lateral Rotation	45 - 50°
Knee	Flexion	135 - 150°
	Extension	0 - 10°
Ankle	Plantar Flexion	40 - 50°
	Dorsi Flexion	20°

Adapted from Heyward 2002,
Advanced Fitness Assessment and Exercise Prescription

Mathematical Definitions of Movement Terms

Another important factor in movement analysis is to consider the diversity in degrees of range of motion (mathematical definitions) at each joint of the human body. In movement science, what is considered to be the degrees of normal range of motion for a few major joints is presented in Table 3-2. (also see figure 3-2) Familiarity with these "norms" is another valuable component for the instructor when designing exercises and routines or when dealing with orthopedic referrals and rehabilitations. Remember, it is important to keep in mind that movement may vary from one individual to another due to their own personal range of motion, joint structure, injury, or stress. You cannot assume that everyone will perform these ranges, but it is a good guideline, especially if participants are working to improve or regain functional capacity.

Planes and Axes

There are three planes in which the body can move. Their reference is derived from dimensions in space – forward/backward, up/down, side to side. The planes are at right angles to each other. The **sagittal plane** is vertical and extends from front to back, dividing the body into right and left parts. The **frontal plane** is vertical and extends from side to side. We can think of this plane like a "door" because it is

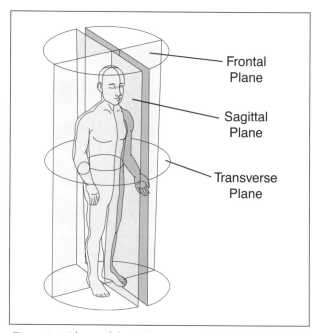

Figure 3-7 Planes of the Body

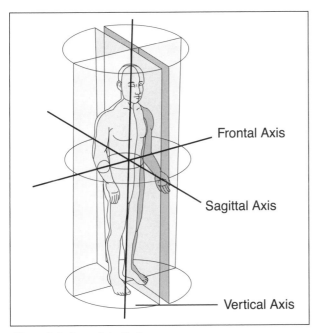

Frontal Axis

Sagittal Axis

Vertical Axis

Figure 3-8 Axes of the Body

easy to visualize if you stand in a doorway. It divides the body into an anterior and a posterior portion. The **transverse plane** is horizontal and divides the body into upper and lower portions at about waist height. (see table 3-3 and figure 3-7) Think of this plane like a "table" because transverse movements would be similar to moving on a table that was all around the body.

Movement is also referenced with imaginary lines through the body. These lines are called axes, and movement takes place around an axis. There are three basic types of axes. They are positioned at right angles to each other and occur at the intersection of two planes.

If we imagine a line from the top of our head running vertically to the feet through the center of the body, this is known as the **vertical** or **longitudinal axis**. This axis occurs at the intersection of the frontal and sagittal planes. Another line from the front of the body to the back (anterior to posterior) is called the **sagittal axis**. The sagittal axis occurs at the intersection of the sagittal and transverse planes. The third axis extends horizontally from one side of the body to the other side (medial to lateral) at about waist height and is the **frontal axis**. This axis is the cross section of the frontal and transverse planes. (see table 3-3 and figure 3-8)

The movements of abduction and adduction take place around the sagittal axis in the frontal plane; for example, opening and closing the legs to the sides (jacks). Flexion and extension take place around the frontal axis in the sagittal plane. An example would be bending forward at the waist. The movements of medial and lateral rotation and transverse abduction and adduction take place around the longitudinal axis in the transverse plane. The exceptions to these general definitions of axes and planes relate to the scapula, clavicle, and thumb.

The importance of axes and planes to the water exercise instructor is to help the instructor provide a totally balanced movement experience. For example, if the workout never includes lateral movements (frontal plane), and/or forgets extension exercises behind the body (sagittal plane), it is not balanced.

The body does not move in a pure linear design. While the whole body may be moving forward, numerous body parts can be moving in other directions and planes! Every movement is a complex

Table 3-3

Planes and Axes of the Body

Plane	Description of Plane	Axis of Rotation	Description of Axis	Common Movement *in* Plane and <u>around</u> Axis
Frontal	Divides body front and back parts	Sagittal	Runs front to back	Abduction, Adduction, and Lateral Flexion
Sagittal	Divides body into right and left parts	Frontal	Runs side to side	Flexion, extension, and hyperextension
Transverse	Divides body into upper and lower parts	Longitudinal (vertical)	Runs head to toe	Medial and lateral rotation, transverse abduction and adduction

interaction of the spatial dimensions. Water encourages multidimensional moves due to its fluid nature. It is interesting to note that more moves in the transverse plane can be achieved in the water than on land, especially in the lower torso. Support of buoyancy allows greater scope for horizontal movement. Whatever moves are created for the water, the essential reference points for exercise structure and balance are anatomical position, the planes and axes.

Levers

The body moves through the use of a system of **levers**. Bones act as lever arms, and joints function as fulcrums of these levers. Anatomical levers of the body cannot be changed, but movement can be made more efficient if you possess a basic understanding of the lever system.

Levers consist of rigid bars that turn about an axis. In the body, the bones represent the rigid bars (lever arms) and the joints are the axes (fulcrum). The axis or **fulcrum** (F) can be visualized as a pivot point. Acting on the lever are two different types of forces: **resistance** (R) and **effort** (E). Resistance (R) can be regarded as a force to overcome, while effort (E) is exerted to overcome the resistance (R). The contractions of muscles provide the force to move the levers, while resistance force primarily comes from gravity on land. On land, the resistance force may be increased with the use of training aids such as weights. In the water environment, resistance comes from fluid drag. In water, resistance may be increased by utilizing the physical laws discussed in Chapter 6 and/or by adding equipment as outlined in Chapter 7.

There are three basic types of levers: the first-class lever, the second-class lever, and the third class lever. A lever has three points which determine the type of lever and for what kind of motion it is best suited. These points are:
1. The fulcrum F (the point of rotation).
2. The point of force application or effort E (usually muscle insertion).
3. The point of resistance application R (sometimes the center of gravity of the lever arm and sometimes the location of an external resistance such as a weight)

In figures 3-9a and 3-10 the three points on the lever produce a first-class lever with the <u>fulcrum</u> (F)

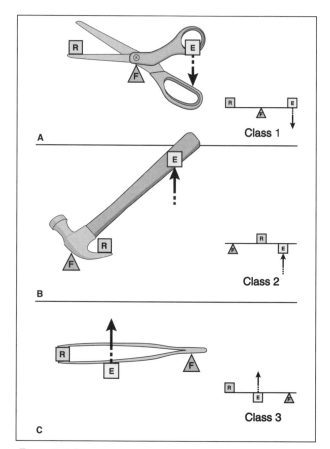

Figure 3-9 Levers

<u>between</u> the effort (E) and the resistance (R). The atlanto occipital joint (located at the base of the skull) acts as the fulcrum (F). The effort (E) is represented by the muscle contraction occurring in the upper back and neck to tilt the head backward into hyperextension. The resistance (R) is provided by the weight of the face and jaw area of the head. A common example of a first-class lever would be a see-saw/teeter-totter or scissors. There are not many first-class levers found in the human body.

In figures 3-9b and 3-10 the three points produce a second-class lever with the <u>resistance</u> (R) <u>between</u> the fulcrum (F) and the force (effort/E). In this example the body is raised to the ball of the foot. The weight of the body is the resistance (R), while the fulcrum(F) is the ball of the foot. The effort (E) occurs when the calf muscle pulls the heel upward during a contraction. A common example of a second-class lever would be a wheelbarrow or a hammer pulling out a nail. There are not many second-class levers found in the body either.

In figures 3-9c and 3-10 you can see the three points that produce a third-class lever with the <u>effort</u> (E) <u>between</u> the fulcrum (F) and the resistance (R).

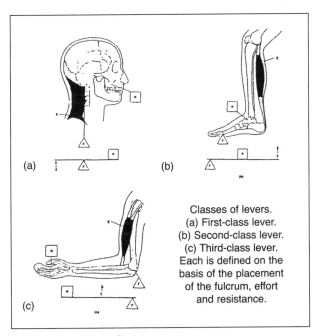

Classes of levers.
(a) First-class lever.
(b) Second-class lever.
(c) Third-class lever.
Each is defined on the
basis of the placement
of the fulcrum, effort
and resistance.

Figure 3-10 Classes of Levers

Here the weight of the forearm (or the weight held in the hand) is the resistance (R) and the contraction of the biceps muscle is the effort (E) with the elbow joint acting as the fulcrum (F). A common example of a

third-class lever would be a tweezer or the action of using a hammer driving a nail through wood. Most of the joints in the body related to exercise serve as third-class levers.

It is also important to understand the concept of mechanical advantage. Our anatomical leverage system can be used to gain a mechanical advantage that may improve simple or complex movements. The distance of the muscle insertion from the joint is important because a longer force arm requires less force to move the lever. The term force arm (FA) is the distance which exists between the joint and the muscle insertion, while the term resistance arm (RA) is the distance between the joint and the point of resistance application (R). (see figure 3-11) The mechanical advantage of a lever is the ratio of the length of the force arm to that of the resistance arm. Even the slightest variation in the location of force and resistance will affect this ratio and change the effective force of the muscle. For example, suppose there are two muscles of the same strength crossing and acting on a joint. Also, assume that one is attached farther from the joint and one is closer, creating a difference in the length of the force arm. The muscle attached farther will produce the more

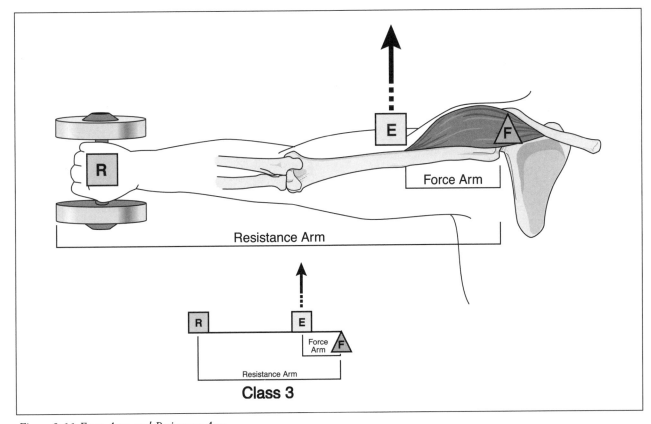

Figure 3-11 Force Arm and Resistance Arm

powerful movement because it is a longer force arm. Thus, strength of movement depends on the placement of muscle attachments. A change of simply one quarter inch in the insertion can make a considerable difference in the force applied to move a lever. (see figure 3-12)

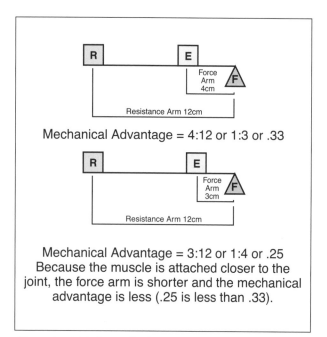

Mechanical Advantage = 4:12 or 1:3 or .33

Mechanical Advantage = 3:12 or 1:4 or .25
Because the muscle is attached closer to the joint, the force arm is shorter and the mechanical advantage is less (.25 is less than .33).

Figure 3-12 Mechanical Advantage

Participants in class come in many different shapes, and sizes. It is impossible to know that one participant has a different length force arm than another participant. So the general rule for the exercise instructor is to cater to the individual needs of the participant and continually try to make sound decisions on what amount of force and resistance will be the most beneficial to the class as a whole.

Types of Joints

Looking at the structure of joints and the interaction between the skeletal system and the muscular system will help to foster a deeper understanding of the body's capabilities. A basic knowledge of joint structure is another tool that will help the instructor make safe, effective exercise choices.

Joints are the mechanisms by which bones are held together. An anatomical joint or articulation is formed when two bony articular surfaces lined by hyaline cartilage meet, and movement is allowed to occur at the junction. The degree or range of movement possible is determined by the shape of the articular surfaces and the type of joint. Sometimes the bones are so close that there is no appreciable movement as in an immovable joint. In others the connection is quite loose, allowing tremendous freedom of movement. Joints may provide total stability, stability in one direction with freedom in the other direction, or freedom in all directions. There are three basic categories of joints based on the movement allowed at the articulation.

A. Immovable joints – bones are held together by fibrous connective tissue that forms an interosseous ligament or membrane. These joints generally hold two parts of the body together, e.g., the sagittal suture of the skull. (see figure 3-13)

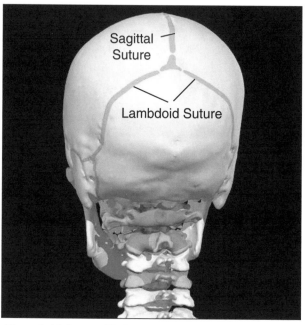

Figure 3-13 Immovable Joints

B. Slightly moveable – bones are held together by strong fibrocartilaginous membranes. The sacroiliac joint (holds the back of the pelvis to the sacrum) and symphysis pubis (holds the front lower part of the pelvis together) are slightly moveable joints. (see figure 3-14)

C. Freely moveable (synovial joints) – bones are held together by synovial membranes. The joint cavity is filled with synovial fluid which allows movement to occur with minimal

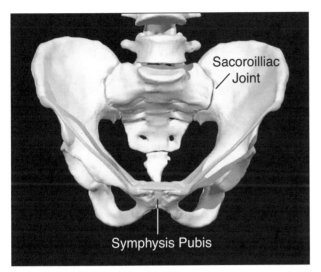

Figure 3-14 Slightly Movable Joints

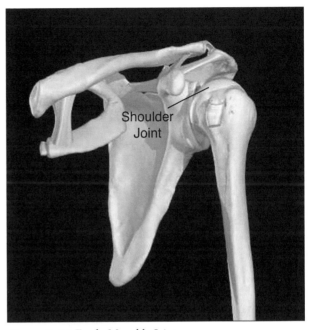

Figure 3-15 Freely Movable Joint

friction. Located between bones, ligaments, tendons, and muscles are bursae (sacs filled with synovial fluid) which also act as friction reducers for adjacent moving surfaces. Most joints in the body related to exercise are freely moveable synovial joints. (see figure 3-15)

Following are descriptions of **synovial joints** of primary interest to the exercise professional. See Tables 3-4 and 3-5 for summaries of joints, movements and movement planes.

Table 3-4

Classification of Synovial Joints

Articulation	Movement	Example
Ball and Socket or Spheroidal	All joint movements	Hip and Shoulder
Hinge or Ginglymus	Flexion and Extension	Elbow
Modified Hinge	Flexion, Extension, and slight Rotation	Knee and Ankle
Ellipsoidal or Condyloid	All except Rotation and Opposition	Radiocarpal (wrist)
Pivot or Trochoid	Supination, Pronation and Rotation	Atlantoaxial (base of skull) and Radioulnar (forearm)
Saddle	All except Rotation	Thumb- first joint
Plane or Gliding	Gliding	Intertarsal (ankle) and Intercarpal (wrist)
Combined Hinge and Plane	Flexion, Extension and Gliding	Temporomandibular (jaw)

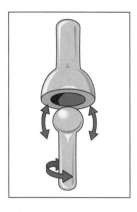

Spheroidal or Ball and Socket

Examples: Hip joint and Shoulder joint

A ball-shaped surface articulates with a cup-shaped surface. Movement, including flexion/extension, abduction/adduction, rotation, and circumduction, is possible around innumerable axes. The hip joint is the articulation of the acetabulum of the pelvis with the head of the femur. (see figure 3-16) The shoulder joint (glenohumeral joint) is the articulation of the head of the humerus with the glenoid cavity of the scapula.

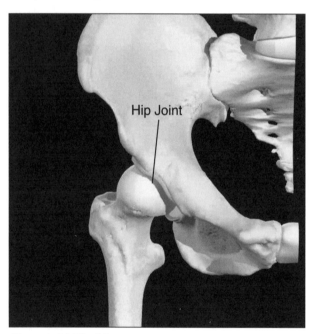

Figure 3-16 Hip Joint

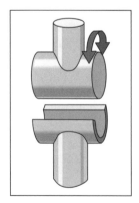

Hinge or Ginglymus

Examples: Elbow joint, Knee joint, and Ankle joint

A hinge joint involves two articular surfaces that restrict movement largely to one axis. Hinge joints usually have strong collateral ligaments. Flexion and extension are the primary movements. The elbow joint is the articulation of the humerus with the ulna and radius. (see figure 3-17) Hyperextension is limited by the olecranon process of the ulna. The knee joint is formed by the articulations of the condyles of the femur with the condyles of the tibia and by the patella articulating with the patellar surface of the femur. (see figure 3-18) Hyperextension of the knee is abnormal. Some lateral and medial rotation is possible when the knee is flexed. The extended knee is essentially locked and rotation is not possible. The ankle is the articulation of the tibia and fibula with the talus. (see figure 3-19)

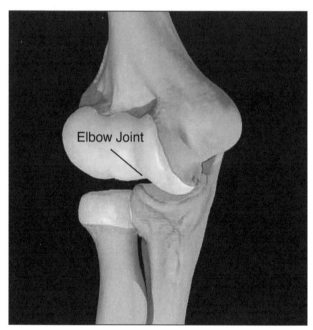

Figure 3-17 Elbow Joint

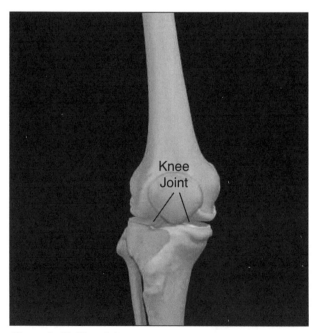

Figure 3-18 Knee Joint

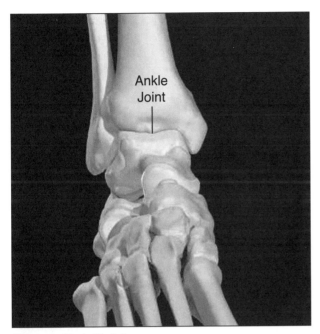

Figure 3-19 Ankle Joint

frontal axis. Abduction and adduction occur around the sagittal axis. Circumduction (wrist circle) is possible by combining the radioulnar joint and the midcarpal joint, but the movement is not as free as a true ball-and-socket joint. (see figure 3-20)

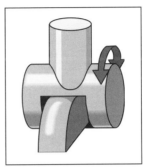

Saddle

Example: First Carpometacarpal joint (thumb)

Each joint surface has a convexity at right angles to a concave surface. All movements except rotation are possible at this joint. The thumb joint is formed by the articulation of the trapezium with the first metacarpal. (see figure 3-21)

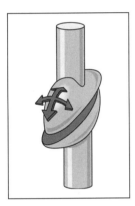

Ellipsoidal or Condyloid

Example: Radiocarpal (wrist) joint

This joint is formed by an oval convex surface placed near an elliptical concave surface. This articulation provides movement around two axes. Wrist extension and flexion occur around the

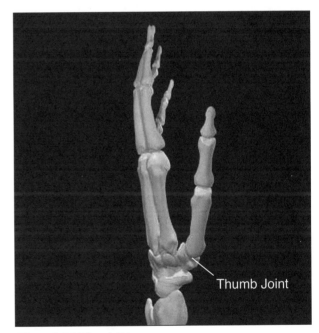

Figure 3-21 Thumb Joint

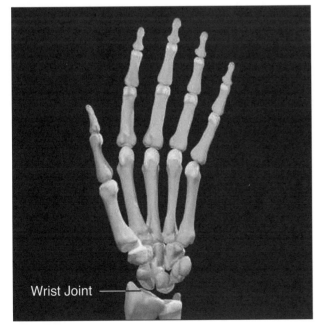

Figure 3-20 Wrist Joint

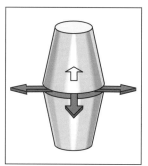

Plane or Gliding

Example: Intertarsal joints (in the foot) or intercarpal joints (in the wrist)

These joints are formed by the proximity of two relatively flat surfaces. This allows gliding movements to occur. The intertarsal joint is the articulation of the talus and the calcaneus. (see figure 3-22)

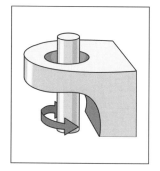

Pivot or Trochoid

Example: Superior Radioulnar joint

This joint is formed by a central bony pivot surrounded by an osteo-ligamentous ring. Rotation is the only movement possible. Pronation and supination of the forearm occurs at the radioulnar joint. (see figure 3-23)

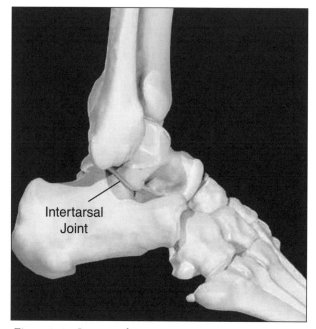

Figure 3-22 Intertarsal Joint

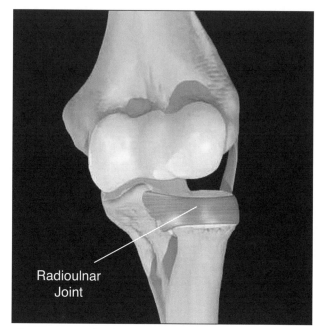

Figure 3-23 Radioulnar Joint

Table 3-5

Joints, Possible Movements, and Planes

(Tortora and Grabowski)

Joint	Movement	Plane
Vertebral Column (intervertebral joints-cartilaginous and gliding) (cervical & lumbar spine)	Flexion, Extension, and Hyperextension	Sagittal
	Lateral Flexion	Frontal
	Rotation	Transverse
	Circumduction	Multiplanar
Hip (ball and socket)	Flexion, Extension, and Hyperextension	Sagittal
	Abduction and Adduction	Frontal
	Rotation	Transverse
	Circumduction	Multiplanar
	Transverse Abduction and Adduction	Transverse
Knee (hinge)	Flexion and Extension	Sagittal
Ankle (hinge)	Dorsi and Plantar Flexion	Sagittal

Shoulder (ball and socket)	Flexion, Extension, and Hyperextension	Sagittal
	Abduction and Adduction	Frontal
	Rotation	Transverse
	Circumduction	Multiplanar
	Transverse Abduction and Adduction	Transverse
Elbow (hinge)	Flexion and Extension	Sagittal
Radioulnar (pivot)	Pronation and Supination	Transverse
Wrist (condyloid)	Flexion, Extension, Hyperextension	Sagittal
	Abduction and Adduction	Frontal
	Circumduction	Multiplanar

See Appendix C to study pure movement analysis, movement analysis on land with gravity, and submerged movement analysis

Interaction Between the Skeletal and Muscular Systems

It is important to look at the interaction between the skeletal system and the muscular system in order to understand movement. Bones can do nothing without muscles. Plus joint motion alone does not accurately indicate all of the muscles involved in a movement.

Muscle comprises the largest portion of the body's total mass. Movement results when muscular tension created by our muscles pulls on a system of levers across a joint, thereby moving the muscle's insertion closer to its origin. Even the simplest of human movements is a complex, coordinated effort of activation (contraction) of certain muscles (agonists), deactivation (relaxation) of others (antagonists), or a co-contraction of both agonists and antagonists.

The amount of movement within a specific joint is limited by several factors. Apart from bony limitations, there may be ligament limitations. For example, the iliofemoral ligament (connecting pelvis to thigh bone) limits trunk extension when the femur is fixed. For example, it is hard to hyperextend at the hip when both feet are on the ground. There are also muscle limitations. The connective tissue components of skeletal muscle have limited elastic properties. If a movement is forced beyond its natural limitation, our body immediately responds with pain or a reflex mechanism to stop the movement.

Of particular note for exercise instructors are the areas of the body where muscles span more than one joint. Biarticular muscles span two joints where multiarticular muscles act on three or more joints. Involvement at one joint can cause limited motion in another joint; for example, try making a tight fist with the finger flexors while your wrist is actively flexed. Similar to this is passive insufficiency. The length of a muscle prevents full range of motion at the joint or joints that a muscle crosses. An example would be passive insufficiency of the hamstring muscles. It is easier to pull your knee to your chest when your knee is bent than when your leg is straight. In other words, you have greater range of motion at the hip when the knee is flexed than when the knee is extended.

Some muscles act as guiding muscles (assistors) to rule out undesired motion or help the prime mover. These muscles are called synergists. A good example is the synergistic action of the hamstring group. The individual muscles in this group are rarely referred to because they are nearly always working as a team. Some muscles contract to stabilize (or fixate) a joint or bone so that another body part can exert force against a fixed point. This happens a great deal around the shoulders. Shoulder muscles will stabilize so that specific movements can be done with our hands. It is important to include activity for the stabilizing muscles. The water is a great place to work on the trunk stabilizers, particularly in deep water where control of the body is totally focused on the dynamic stabilization of the trunk muscles. This is one of the reasons such big improvements are often seen in postural alignment following a consistent water exercise program.

Table 3-6 presents an overview of the muscles most involved in primary movements of the body parts. Some of these muscles are not included in

Chapter 1 and are included for advanced study if you choose. A comprehensive look at each of these muscles is beyond the scope of this manual, but we will focus on key movement considerations for major areas of the body. See the figures following the chart for muscle locations.

Table 3-6

Major Movements and Muscles Involved

Body Part	Joint Motion	Muscles primarily Involved
Scapula	Fixation	Trapezius, serratus anterior, rhomboids, levator scapulae.
	Adduction	Trapezius (middle fibers), rhomboids.
	Abduction	Serratus anterior.
Upper Arm (shoulder joint)	Flexion	Anterior deltoid, pectoralis major, biceps brachii.
	Extension	Latissimus dorsi, triceps.
	Adduction	Latissimus dorsi, teres major, pectoralis major.
	Abduction	Middle deltoid, supraspinatus.
	Transverse Add.	Pectoralis major, anterior deltoid.
	Transverse Abd.	Posterior deltoid, infraspinatus, teres minor.
	Medial Rotation	Latissimus dorsi, teres major.
	Lateral Rotation	Infraspinatus, teres minor.
Forearm (elbow and radioulnar joint)	Flexion	Biceps brachii, brachioradialis, brachialis.
	Extension	Triceps brachii.
	Supination	Supinator, biceps brachii.
	Pronation	Pronator teres, pronator quadratus.
Trunk (lumbar spine)	Flexion	Rectus abdominis, internal and external obliques.
	Extension	Erector spinae.
	Rotation	Internal and external obliques.
	Lateral Flexion	Quadratus lumborum.
Upper Leg (hip joint)	Flexion	Iliopsoas, rectus femoris in quadriceps.
	Extension	Gluteus maximus, all 3 hamstrings.
	Adduction	Adductor longus, magnus, and brevis, and gracilis.
	Abduction	Gluteus medius and minimus.
Lower Leg (knee joint)	Flexion	Hamstrings.
	Extension	Quadriceps.
Foot (ankle joint)	Dorsi Flexion	Anterior Tibialis, extensor digitorum longus.
	Plantar Flexion	Gastrocnemius, soleus, posterior tibialis.
	Inversion	Posterior tibialis, anterior tibialis.
	Eversion	Peroneus group, extensor digitorum longus.

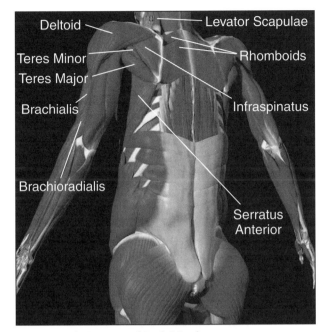

Figure 3-24a Location of Back Muscles

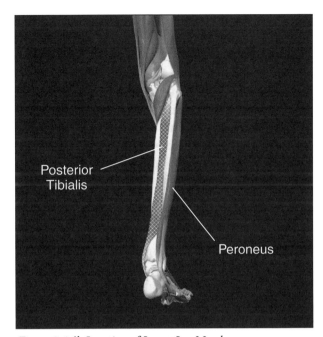

Figure 3-24b Location of Lower Leg Muscles

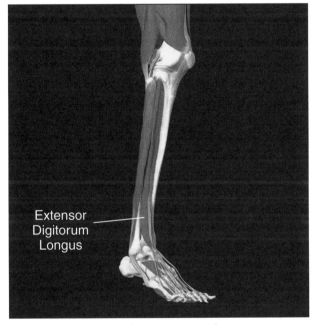

Figure 3-24c Location of Lower Leg Muscles

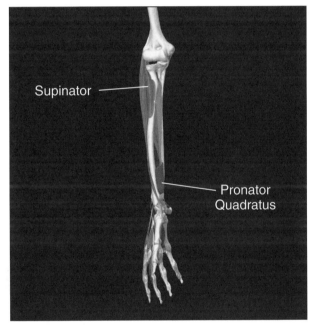

Figure 3-24d Location of Forearm Muscles

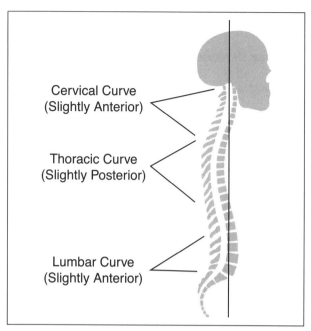

Figure 3-27 Normal Curves of the Spine

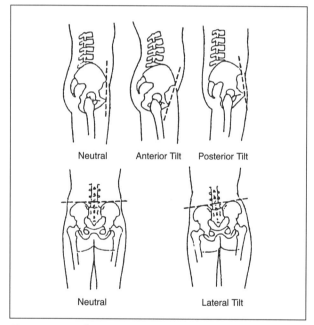

Figure 3-28 Pelvic Positions

Maintaining or retraining the normal curves of the spine can be a primary focus in exercise programs. A large percentage of the population has back problems, and many of these problems are caused or made worse by imbalances in muscular strength, flexibility, or body mechanics. Because we are vertically oriented creatures, these imbalances become exaggerated by the pull of gravity. For example, weak abdominals allow the anterior pelvic

tilt to move further forward, causing lumbar hyperextension. Prolonged sitting causes tight hip flexors, and again the anterior tilt is pushed beyond the norm, forcing the lumbar spine into hyperextension. This increased lordotic curve is a contributing factor to low back pain. Similarly, an exaggerated posterior pelvic tilt eliminates the normal curve of the lumbar spine and can also cause low back pain. Abdominal exercises are recommended for correction of extreme anterior tilt to improve posture. Strength in the erector spinae muscles will help control unnatural posterior pelvic tilt. The general exercise guidelines are to stretch tight muscles and strengthen weak muscles.

We may also see abnormal curvatures of the spine. The three most common ones are **scoliosis**, **kyphosis**, and **lordosis**. (see figures 3-29a and b) Scoliosis refers to a lateral bending of the spine. The shoulders and pelvis will appear uneven, and the rib cage may be twisted. Kyphosis (humped back) refers to an exaggerated curve in the thoracic region. The head is often too far forward (forward head) with rounded shoulders and sunken chest. Lordosis (bent backward) is an increased, concave curve in the lumbar region of the spine. Lordosis is often accompanied by an increased anterior pelvic tilt. The abdomen and the buttocks will protrude and the arms hang further back. These conditions may be considered permanent, in which case exercise will not correct them.

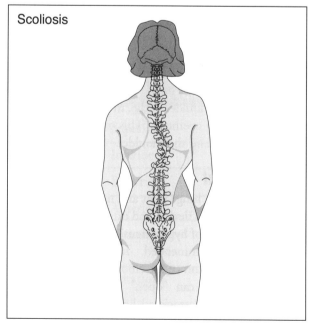

Figure 3-29a Postural Deviations

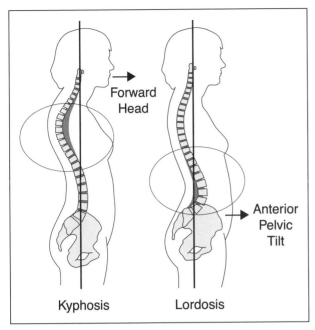

Figure 3-29b Postural Deviations

Our aim is to establish (and continually reestablish) the normal curves of the spine. We call this neutral posture, or neutral spinal alignment. It is the recommended position for minimal stress on the spine and the safest position for injury prevention when the limbs are engaged in activities. In neutral posture the pelvis is upright, not tilted in any direction. The spine is in neutral – not flexed or extended. There is a natural, slight inward curve of the low back (see

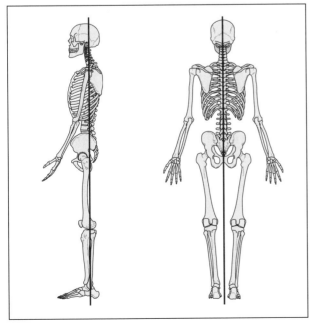

Figure 3-30 Neutral Posture

figure 3-30). When doing resistance training, including water exercise, the body should always be set in neutral posture before overloading specific muscle groups. If a participant cannot achieve neutral posture, he/she may require referral to a physician. Neutral alignment occurs easily if there is muscular balance. Unfortunately, many of our daily habits put inappropriate stress on our muscles and cause imbalances. Examples would include tucking the telephone in your neck or sitting at the computer for hours. Even in exercise programs imbalances are seen, especially if the participant only utilizes hip flexor exercises such as knee lifts and front kicks only, ignoring the back of the body. Achieving muscular balance can be helped by regular exercise that includes cross training. The instructor should plan to provide ways to balance muscle strength and flexibility from right to left sides, from front to back, from upper body to lower body, as well as balancing strength ratios in opposing muscle pairs within the exercise program.

The density of water necessitates the careful positioning of the spine in the "ready position" for the challenges of resistance training. This is particularly relevant with the popularity of flotation and other resistance equipment for water exercise. This equipment provides an additional challenge to balance and coordination, and if the participant cannot control neutral posture while exercising with equipment, the equipment should be removed.

The Hip Joint

The hip joint is a ball-and-socket joint like the shoulder, but has greater stability mainly because of its weight bearing role. The hip socket is deeper, and the head of the femur is a more complete sphere than the head of the humerus. The hip joint also has several strong ligaments. Just as the shoulder joint interacts with the shoulder girdle, the hip joint interacts with the pelvic girdle. Movements of the hip joint can either refer to the flexion of the thigh as moving the leg towards the pelvis (for example, a front kick) or the pelvis moving towards the thigh (for example, bending forward from the hips). Movement at the hip joint includes flexion, extension and hyperextension, abduction and adduction, lateral and medial rotation, and circumduction. The important point for instructors to remember is that some of the muscles crossing the hip joint also have attachments on the spine (such as the iliopsoas), so hip movements can affect changes in the lumbar spine.

The Knee Joint

The knee is a modified hinge joint, designed to primarily perform flexion and extension, with a small degree of rotation possible when the knee is bent. It is possible for the knee to achieve a few degrees of hyperextension. However, hyperextension is considered an unnatural movement of the knee, and instructors should certainly not use exercises that encourage knee hyperextension. The main muscles acting on the knee are the quadriceps and hamstrings. The patella bone, or kneecap, acts as a pulley to increase the effective strength of the quadriceps by increasing leverage or mechanical advantage. Water exercise can provide the important muscle balance needed between the quadriceps and the hamstrings.

Posture and Alignment

The importance of neutral spinal alignment has been discussed in relation to the spine and injury prevention. Neutral spinal alignment is also part of the body's control mechanism for **balance**. The ability to maintain the body's balance during many exercises is important for proper exercise execution as well as injury prevention. From a mechanical perspective, maintaining balance involves controlling the position of the body's **center of gravity**. In a symmetrical, equally dense object, the center of gravity would be located in the object's geometric center. In the human body, the position of the body parts determines where the center of gravity will be at any one time. Each time the body moves, there is a redistribution of body mass and the center of gravity shifts. Movement of large body parts (legs) will have a greater effect on center of gravity than moving smaller body parts (arms).

To maintain balance, a vertical line that passes through the body's center of gravity to the ground must fall within the base of support. The base of support includes the area of the body in contact with the ground, which is in most cases the feet, plus the area between these points. Keeping the base wide and the body low to the ground helps ensure that the line of gravity stays within the base of support. When you lean in any direction, the center of gravity shifts with you. If you lean too far, the center of gravity may move outside the base of support and cause the exercise participant to lose balance and possibly fall over.

As you enter the water, center of gravity still applies, especially in shallow water. You still have a base (the feet) in contact with the pool bottom. As you reach in different directions, your center of gravity may move outside the base of support, causing you to be off-balance, ending up horizontal and floating. As an instructor you may actually design moves to place the body horizontal or to take advantage of buoyancy to extend range of motion. However, the theory of balanced alignment is still the key consideration in exercise design, and off-balance moves invariably lead to problems such as loss of coordination and compromised alignment. Plus, a lot of shallow water exercisers are not swimmers and do not want their feet to leave the bottom of the pool.

The deeper the water, the more **center of buoyancy** takes over from center of gravity. Center of buoyancy can be defined as the center of the volume of the body displacing the water. Center of buoyancy is usually located in the chest region near the lungs. It does vary according to body composition of the participant. In the vertical position, the center of buoyancy and center of gravity will be in a vertical line, but the distance between them will depend on fat deposits in the body, size of chest cavity, and amount of muscle. A person with a lot of fat floats easily and a muscular person sinks. Fat and air have greater water-displacement volume than bone, organs, and muscle.

Exercise design for water should encourage control of the center of buoyancy and gravity because it is strongly linked to neutral posture. Keep the shoulders over the hips with the pelvis upright. Reestablish neutral position frequently, and consider visiting neutral alignment between changes of movement pattern and changes of direction. Allowing time for water turbulence to settle by offering a centering activity between traveling moves would help your students remain in alignment.

The introduction of buoyancy equipment for the ankle and foot has added a whole new challenge to alignment in deep water exercise. The fact that this equipment wants to float to the surface further challenges the trunk stabilizing muscles. The abdominals and erector spinae have to be active all the time (dynamic stabilization) to keep the shoulder/hip alignment with the legs deep below the body. This adds considerable postural training benefits to deep water exercise. See more about Deep Water Exercise in Chapter 16.

Summary

1. A basic understanding of movement analysis is necessary for safe and effective programming. A clear understanding of what each exercise accomplishes and why certain movements are included in a program will maximize a program's benefits.

2. Anatomical movement terms are referenced to anatomical or neutral position. Pertinent movement terms would include flexion/extension/hyperextension, abduction/adduction, medial/lateral rotation, circumduction, tilt, supination/pronation, inversion/eversion, elevation/depression, and retraction/protraction.

3. The human body moves around three axes and three planes which are situated at right angles. It is important to include movement around all three axes in all three planes to achieve muscle balance.

4. The skeletal and muscular systems work together as a system of levers to move the human body. Most movements related to exercise result from third-class levers involving associated bones, joints, and muscles.

5. There are several types of joints in the human body. Movement at any joint is determined by the type of joint, bones surrounding the joint, how muscles cross the joint, and associated soft tissue. It is important to know the muscles associated with each joint, the type of joint, and possible safe movement options at each joint.

6. Posture and alignment are critical in the prevention of chronic musculoskeletal disorders as well as acute injury. Proper posture and alignment should be taught and promoted in any aquatic exercise program.

Review Questions

1. _____ is moving away from the midline of the body.
2. Flexion and extension are performed primarily in the _____ plane.
3. In a third class lever, the _____ is between the _____ and _____.
4. What type of joint is the elbow?
5. Name the three normal curves in the spine.
6. In deep water, you primarily manipulate your center of _____.

See Appendix E for answers to review questions.

Components of Physical Fitness

Physical Fitness is broadly defined as the ability of the body's physical parts to function, and is measured by the level at which these physical parts are capable of functioning. A person possessing a high fitness level would have a body capable of functioning physically at optimal levels. A person possessing a poor fitness level would have physical weaknesses or limitations that would affect the body's ability to function at optimal levels. Measurement of functional capacity and fitness level are discussed in Chapter 10.

Physical Fitness is achieved through regular exercise. When developing or participating in an exercise program, it is essential to consider all of the components necessary for optimal physical fitness.

The five major components of Physical Fitness are:
- Cardiorespiratory Endurance
- Muscular Strength
- Muscular Endurance
- Flexibility
- Body Composition

It is important for a fitness instructor to understand all of the components that affect a person's fitness level as well as have the ability to design a program that will promote or enhance all five components.

Cardiorespiratory Endurance

Cardiorespiratory Endurance is defined as the capacity of the cardiovascular and respiratory systems to deliver oxygen to the working muscles for sustained periods of energy production. Cardiorespiratory fitness describes the body's physical capacity to perform large muscle movement over a prolonged period of time. Large muscles are found in the legs, trunk, and arms and are responsible for gross motor movement. Cardiorespiratory fitness is often termed "aerobic fitness."

Research clearly indicates that the aquatic environment is suitable for increasing and maintaining cardiorespiratory fitness, as long as you adhere to the American College of Sports Medicine (ACSM) guidelines for aerobic exercise.

Muscular Strength

Muscular Strength is defined as the maximum force that can be exerted by a muscle or muscle group against a resistance. The muscle is expected to exert this maximum force one time or in one effort.

Resistance of some kind is needed to train for muscular strength. Free weights and weight machines are commonly used on land to train for muscular strength. When training for strength gains, a routine is employed that utilizes heavy weight lifted for fewer repetitions. Although no optimal number of sets and repetitions has been found to elicit maximal strength gains, the accepted range indicated by research appears to be somewhere between 2 and 5 sets of 2 to 10 repetitions at an all out effort. (7) Many people are unable to train for muscular strength because they cannot meet the demands it places on the musculoskeletal system due to orthopedic or structural problems. Some people do not like to strength train for fear of building too much muscle girth or because they find it physically uncomfortable.

Equipment is utilized for strength training in the water to maximize or increase resistance just as on land. On land the resistance is usually determined by the amount of "weight" being lifted. In the water, resistance is determined by the amount of resistance, buoyancy, drag, or weight the equipment provides, as well as the velocity or speed at which the movement is performed. (see Chapter 7)

Muscular Endurance

Muscular Endurance is defined as the capacity of a muscle to exert force repeatedly or to hold a fixed or static contraction over time. It is assessed by either measuring the length of time the muscle can hold a contraction, or the number of contractions performed in a given length of time.

Once again, there is no optimal number of sets and repetitions for building muscular endurance. As with strength gains, programs should be individualized and varied to achieve the best results. When focusing on endurance gains, multiple repetitions are usually prescribed in sets of 20 repetitions or more. (12) These sets differ in intensity from the "all-out" effort in strength lifting. By the end of the set, the muscle should feel fatigue, but not necessarily be exhausted. Using the resistance of the water is an excellent way to promote and maintain muscular endurance. Resistance can be progressively increased by applying more force against the water's resistance, increasing surface area, and adding equipment.

Note: Although it is possible to specifically train for muscular strength or endurance, these two components of fitness are not independent of each other. It is impossible to train for strength and not have endurance gains as well, just as it is impossible to primarily train for endurance and not experience strength gains.

Flexibility

Flexibility is defined as the ability of limbs to move at the joints through a normal range of motion. Having reasonable joint flexibility is important in the reduction of risk of injury as well as for general body mobility. Loss of flexibility can lead to impaired movement and the inability to perform activities of daily living (ADL). Loss of flexibility occurs as a natural part of the aging process or as the result of trauma, injury, or surgery. In order to maintain flexibility, the joints must be taken through their normal range of motion on a regular basis.

Exercise is a series of muscle contractions which will leave a muscle shortened unless it is intentionally stretched after an exercise session. The post-stretch phase of an exercise program is the best time to stretch to maintain and improve flexibility because the muscles are warm and pliable and pumped with oxygenated blood. Stretching after exercise is critical for every type of exercise program, including aquatic fitness programs.

It is also imperative to stretch correctly when warming up and cooling down. **Ballistic stretching** (bouncing, tugging, or overstretching the muscle) can cause the muscle to tighten instead of relax. Ballistic stretching activates the **muscle spindle**, a specialized receptor in the muscle known as a proprioceptor, which monitors muscle length change and the speed of length change. If you tug or pull on the muscle, it may activate the muscle stretch reflex arc. This stretch reflex is a neurological loop which actually tightens/contracts the muscle or increases muscle tension. It is an involuntary response designed to help protect muscle tissue from tearing when being overstretched. Ballistic stretching can actually oppose the desired effect of stretching by tightening rather than lengthening the muscle. (see figure 4-1)

Static stretching involves stretching to the point of pain, backing off slightly, and holding the elongated position. Holding a static stretch for 15-60 seconds is most beneficial during the post stretch. Proper static stretching does not activate the stretch reflex, and therefore muscles relax and lengthen. Static stretching is the preferred method for enhancing flexibility for the general population.

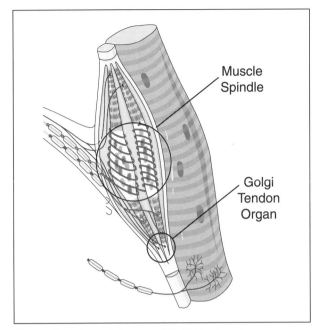

Figure 4-1 Muscle Spindle and Golgi Tendon Organ

Rhythmical stretching is moving body parts through full range of motion in a slow controlled manner. Instead of stopping and holding a static stretch, you may pause briefly in an extended or stretched position before continuing through full range of motion. For example, a slow front kick with a pause in front will help to lengthen the gluteal and hamstring muscles. Participants need to respect their normal range of motion and not overstretch to avoid activating the stretch reflex arc. If water temperatures are cool, instructors may choose rhythmic stretching over static stretching in the pre-stretch segment of the workout. This way adequate heat can be generated to keep participants comfortable and maintain warmth in muscle tissue during the warm up stage of the workout.

Another proprioceptor, the **Golgi tendon organ** is found in the tendons of your muscles. The Golgi tendon organ is a receptor that monitors tension in the muscle. If the Golgi tendon organ senses that too much tension is being created in the muscle, and the tension generated may damage related soft tissue, the muscle responds by relaxing. This involuntary response produces the desired effect of releasing tension or relaxing the muscle to avoid excessive or dangerous tension. The Golgi tendon organ safeguards you from lifting excessive loads that you may not be conditioned to safely execute. (6) (see figure 4-1)

Body Composition

Body Composition is defined as the body's relative percentage of fat as compared to lean tissue (bones, muscles, and organs). Body composition is discussed in Chapters 10 and 13. As a primary component of fitness, it is important to realize its role in overall physical health. It is desirable to build and maintain a reasonable level of lean muscle tissue. Adequate levels of muscle tissue increase stamina and strength as well as boost metabolism. Having too high a relative percentage of fat increases your risk of heart disease, cancer, as well as other metabolic diseases. Carrying a lot of subcutaneous fat can actually impair physical performance as well as inhibit quality of life (see Chapter 12).

The water is a wonderful environment in which to develop a favorable body composition as well as overall physical fitness. Aerobic exercise in the aquatic environment not only promotes fat loss, but promotes the development and maintenance of lean tissue. Working against the three-dimensional resistance of the water builds muscle density.

Muscle **hypertrophy** is the term used to describe an increase in the size, girth, or function of muscle tissue. Muscle **atrophy** is the term used to describe the loss or wasting of muscle tissue or function through lack of use or disease.

Skill-Related Components of Fitness

In addition to the five major components of physical fitness, there are several "skill-related" components of fitness as well. The skill-related components of physical fitness are: (10)

• **Balance**: the maintenance of equilibrium while stationary (static balance) or moving (dynamic balance).
• **Coordination**: the integration of many separate motor skills or movements into one efficient movement pattern.
• **Speed**: the rate at which a movement or activity can be performed.
• **Power**: a function of strength and speed. The ability to transfer energy into force at a quick rate.
• **Agility**: the ability to rapidly and fluently change body positioning during movement.
• **Reaction time**: the amount of time elapsed between stimulation and acting upon the stimulus.

The average exerciser is not overly concerned with developing these "skill-related" components. Athletes

primarily train for these components in order to enhance performance in their sport. The skill-related components do usually improve with regular exercise even though you may not be specifically training for them. Many of these components are utilized during an aquatic fitness class, during transitions, in pace changes, in one-footed moves, etc., and are developed and improved through practice and repetition. Skill or "functional training" is becoming more popular as a method of training to improve quality of life and improve activities of daily living (ADL).

Guidelines for Exercise

"Lifestyle" diseases have become prevalent in many developed countries due to the population becoming more sedentary, physically inactive, diet changes, and exposure to more environmental hazards. Several long-term or epidemiological research studies starting in the 1940's and continuing through the present have been and are being conducted in the United States to attempt to find which lifestyles increase or decrease your risk of various diseases. One of the most famous epidemiological studies is the Framingham Study. In this study, several generations of families in the town of Framingham, Massachusetts, have been studied to develop "risk factors" for disease-cardiovascular disease in particular.

A sedentary lifestyle, or physical inactivity, was determined to elevate risk for cardiovascular disease and cancer as well as contribute to elevating risk for many other diseases. (Other risk factors are discussed in Chapter 10.) Once determined, research studies were then conducted collecting metabolic and other data to determine how to exercise, or what kind of exercise would significantly lower risk. The guidelines developed by the American College of Sports Medicine (ACSM) printed initially in 1975, and revised several times since, have emerged as the primary guidelines utilized by the exercise profession. These guidelines are very similar to what is published by the American Medical Association and the American Heart Association.

ACSM "makes the following recommendations for the quantity and quality of training for developing and maintaining cardiorespiratory fitness, body composition, and muscular strength and endurance in the healthy adult." (2)

to train for strength and not have endurance gains as well, just as it is impossible to primarily train for endurance and not experience strength gains.

Flexibility

Flexibility is defined as the ability of limbs to move at the joints through a normal range of motion. Having reasonable joint flexibility is important in the reduction of risk of injury as well as for general body mobility. Loss of flexibility can lead to impaired movement and the inability to perform activities of daily living (ADL). Loss of flexibility occurs as a natural part of the aging process or as the result of trauma, injury, or surgery. In order to maintain flexibility, the joints must be taken through their normal range of motion on a regular basis.

Exercise is a series of muscle contractions which will leave a muscle shortened unless it is intentionally stretched after an exercise session. The post-stretch phase of an exercise program is the best time to stretch to maintain and improve flexibility because the muscles are warm and pliable and pumped with oxygenated blood. Stretching after exercise is critical for every type of exercise program, including aquatic fitness programs.

It is also imperative to stretch correctly when warming up and cooling down. **Ballistic stretching** (bouncing, tugging, or overstretching the muscle) can cause the muscle to tighten instead of relax. Ballistic stretching activates the **muscle spindle**, a specialized receptor in the muscle known as a proprioceptor, which monitors muscle length change and the speed of length change. If you tug or pull on the muscle, it may activate the muscle stretch reflex arc. This stretch reflex is a neurological loop which actually tightens/contracts the muscle or increases muscle tension. It is an involuntary response designed to help protect muscle tissue from tearing when being overstretched. Ballistic stretching can actually oppose the desired effect of stretching by tightening rather than lengthening the muscle. (see figure 4-1)

Static stretching involves stretching to the point of pain, backing off slightly, and holding the elongated position. Holding a static stretch for 15-60 seconds is most beneficial during the post stretch. Proper static stretching does not activate the stretch reflex, and therefore muscles relax and lengthen. Static stretching is the preferred method for enhancing flexibility for the general population.

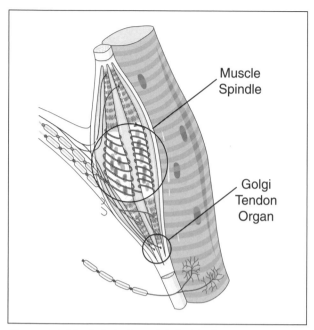

Figure 4-1 Muscle Spindle and Golgi Tendon Organ

Rhythmical stretching is moving body parts through full range of motion in a slow controlled manner. Instead of stopping and holding a static stretch, you may pause briefly in an extended or stretched position before continuing through full range of motion. For example, a slow front kick with a pause in front will help to lengthen the gluteal and hamstring muscles. Participants need to respect their normal range of motion and not overstretch to avoid activating the stretch reflex arc. If water temperatures are cool, instructors may choose rhythmic stretching over static stretching in the pre-stretch segment of the workout. This way adequate heat can be generated to keep participants comfortable and maintain warmth in muscle tissue during the warm up stage of the workout.

Another proprioceptor, the **Golgi tendon organ** is found in the tendons of your muscles. The Golgi tendon organ is a receptor that monitors tension in the muscle. If the Golgi tendon organ senses that too much tension is being created in the muscle, and the tension generated may damage related soft tissue, the muscle responds by relaxing. This involuntary response produces the desired effect of releasing tension or relaxing the muscle to avoid excessive or dangerous tension. The Golgi tendon organ safeguards you from lifting excessive loads that you may not be conditioned to safely execute. (6) (see figure 4-1)

Body Composition

Body Composition is defined as the body's relative percentage of fat as compared to lean tissue (bones, muscles, and organs). Body composition is discussed in Chapters 10 and 13. As a primary component of fitness, it is important to realize its role in overall physical health. It is desirable to build and maintain a reasonable level of lean muscle tissue. Adequate levels of muscle tissue increase stamina and strength as well as boost metabolism. Having too high a relative percentage of fat increases your risk of heart disease, cancer, as well as other metabolic diseases. Carrying a lot of subcutaneous fat can actually impair physical performance as well as inhibit quality of life (see Chapter 12).

The water is a wonderful environment in which to develop a favorable body composition as well as overall physical fitness. Aerobic exercise in the aquatic environment not only promotes fat loss, but promotes the development and maintenance of lean tissue. Working against the three-dimensional resistance of the water builds muscle density.

Muscle **hypertrophy** is the term used to describe an increase in the size, girth, or function of muscle tissue. Muscle **atrophy** is the term used to describe the loss or wasting of muscle tissue or function through lack of use or disease.

Skill-Related Components of Fitness

In addition to the five major components of physical fitness, there are several "skill-related" components of fitness as well. The skill-related components of physical fitness are: (10)

- **Balance**: the maintenance of equilibrium while stationary (static balance) or moving (dynamic balance).
- **Coordination**: the integration of many separate motor skills or movements into one efficient movement pattern.
- **Speed**: the rate at which a movement or activity can be performed.
- **Power**: a function of strength and speed. The ability to transfer energy into force at a quick rate.
- **Agility**: the ability to rapidly and fluently change body positioning during movement.
- **Reaction time**: the amount of time elapsed between stimulation and acting upon the stimulus.

The average exerciser is not overly concerned with developing these "skill-related" components. Athletes primarily train for these components in order to enhance performance in their sport. The skill-related components do usually improve with regular exercise even though you may not be specifically training for them. Many of these components are utilized during an aquatic fitness class, during transitions, in pace changes, in one-footed moves, etc., and are developed and improved through practice and repetition. Skill or "functional training" is becoming more popular as a method of training to improve quality of life and improve activities of daily living (ADL).

Guidelines for Exercise

"Lifestyle" diseases have become prevalent in many developed countries due to the population becoming more sedentary, physically inactive, diet changes, and exposure to more environmental hazards. Several long-term or epidemiological research studies starting in the 1940's and continuing through the present have been and are being conducted in the United States to attempt to find which lifestyles increase or decrease your risk of various diseases. One of the most famous epidemiological studies is the Framingham Study. In this study, several generations of families in the town of Framingham, Massachusetts, have been studied to develop "risk factors" for disease-cardiovascular disease in particular.

A sedentary lifestyle, or physical inactivity, was determined to elevate risk for cardiovascular disease and cancer as well as contribute to elevating risk for many other diseases. (Other risk factors are discussed in Chapter 10.) Once determined, research studies were then conducted collecting metabolic and other data to determine how to exercise, or what kind of exercise would significantly lower risk. The guidelines developed by the American College of Sports Medicine (ACSM) printed initially in 1975, and revised several times since, have emerged as the primary guidelines utilized by the exercise profession. These guidelines are very similar to what is published by the American Medical Association and the American Heart Association.

ACSM "makes the following recommendations for the quantity and quality of training for developing and maintaining cardiorespiratory fitness, body composition, and muscular strength and endurance in the healthy adult." (2)

Mode of Training:

Mode describes the <u>type of exercise</u> being performed. Activities which utilize large muscle groups, can be maintained continuously, and are rhythmical and aerobic in nature are recommended. Aerobic activities would include walking-hiking, running-jogging, cycling-biking, cross-country skiing, dancing, rope skipping, rowing, stair climbing, swimming, deep water exercise, shallow water exercise, skating, and some endurance sport activities.

Frequency of Training:

Frequency is <u>how often</u> you should exercise or train. Although cardiorespiratory fitness improvements may be seen in deconditioned individuals with exercise 2 times/week, optimal training frequency appears to be 3-5 times/week. Training less than two days per week does not generally show a meaningful change in functional capacity. Moderate to somewhat vigorous exercise, 3-5 times/week is generally prescribed for healthy adults. The value in training more than five times per week is small in regard to improvements in maximal oxygen consumption. It is generally believed that the increased risk of chronic fatigue and injury is not worth the small gains achieved in functional capacity with excessive daily training.

Intensity of Training:

Intensity is <u>how hard</u> you should exercise. Intensity is measured in several ways. It is important for a fitness instructor to understand the various ways in which intensity can be measured even though only one or two ways may be actually utilized in class.

In research and medical settings cardiorespiratory fitness is often measured as a percent of maximal oxygen uptake. An intensity level of between (40/50)-85% of oxygen uptake reserve (VO_2R) is considered sufficient to elicit a cardiorespiratory response. For the average adult, 50-85% is generally prescribed. Intensity levels as low as 40% can be prescribed for very deconditioned individuals. VO_2max is determined with specialized equipment that measures the amount of oxygen the subject exhales. The difference between the amount of oxygen breathed in and exhaled is the amount of oxygen being utilized by the body. To find the maximum amount of oxygen a subject can utilize, the subject runs on a treadmill until he or she reaches exhaustion. At this point of exhaustion, the maximum amount of oxygen the body

is capable of utilizing is determined. Intensity measurement by utilizing a percentage of VO_2max is not practical for use in an exercise class but is important to fitness instructors for understanding research and medical studies.

More common ways to measure exercise intensity utilize a percentage of a person's **maximal heart rate** (HRmax) or **heart rate reserve** (HRR). A person's maximal heart rate is determined the same way a VO_2max is determined. A person runs on a treadmill with a heart monitor until exhaustion, at which point a maximal exercise heart rate is determined. Since measuring maximal heart rate in this manner is not practical, we utilize an <u>estimated</u> maximal heart rate instead. The equation "220 minus age" is accepted in the exercise profession as a reasonably accurate estimate of maximal heart rate. An intensity range of (64/70)-94% of estimated HRmax (220 minus age) is recommended for aerobic training.

A more accurate way to measure intensity utilizing heart rate would be to use the heart rate reserve method also known as Karvonen's formula. Karvonen's formula personalizes heart rate measurement by factoring in the individual's resting heart rate. A true **resting heart rate** (HRrest) is found by taking your heart rate for 60 seconds, three mornings before rising, and averaging the three. Heart rate reserve is calculated by taking 220 minus age, minus resting heart rate, multiplying by the desired percentage, and then adding back the resting heart rate. Karvonen's formula for a person 40 years of age with a resting heart rate of 65 is calculated in the example.

"For most individuals, intensities within the range of 60-80% HRR or 77-90% HRmax are sufficient to achieve improvements in cardio-respiratory fitness, when combined with appropriate frequency and duration of training." (2) Deconditioned individuals may see cardiorespiratory improvements working at lower training thresholds. "The HRR method is recommended for prescribing exercise intensity rather than the HRmax method because the HRR method more accurately depicts the intensity relative to oxygen consumption." (2) Working at too high a heart rate may be an indication that the person is training anaerobically as opposed to aerobically. As discussed in Chapter 2, anaerobic metabolism results in the by-product lactic acid which leads to muscle fatigue.

A fitness instructor should be aware there are several factors which can affect training heart rate.

Example of Karvonen's Formula

	220		220
	-AGE		-40
	———		———
	HRmax		180
	-HRrest		-65
	———		———
	HRR		115
HRR	115	HRR	115
X .60*	X .60*	X .80*	X .80*
———	———	———	———
( )	69	( )	92
+HRrest	+65	+HRrest	+65
———	———	———	———
Minimum	134	Maximum	157
training threshold		training threshold	

*For most individuals 60-80% HRR is recommended. Very deconditioned individuals may need to begin around 40% and conditioned individuals may work near 90% intensity. (2)

These factors include stress, caffeine, medication, general health, and environmental factors. In the aquatic environment, heart rate can be additionally affected by the water's temperature, compression, reduced gravity, partial pressure, the dive reflex, and reduction of body mass. (see table 4-1) It is recommended that a 6-second heart rate count be utilized in the water. Informal data collected indicated that a 10-second heart rate may not be as accurate due to how fast the water can cool the body. Research clearly shows a reduced heart rate in the water as compared to the same intensity of exercise on land. **According to initial research, if an aquatic exercise heart rate is to be used to measure intensity, a 13% or 17 BPM recommended deduction should be taken from the minimum and maximum training thresholds. It is important to remember that these recommendations are general, and the aquatic effect on heart rate is actually very individual. Additional research has indicated that the aquatic suppression of heart rate is dependant on the factors listed in Table 4-1, as well as fitness level and age. Some research has indicated an 11 BPM deduction, and some research has suggested that the aquatic suppression of heart rate is even greater in deep water.** Because of the multiple factors involved, determination of target heart rate in the water can be difficult. At this time, it may be prudent to use a

deduction of 11-17 beats per minute for shallow water exercise. For deep water exercise, a 17 beat per minute deduction is recommended. You may want to consider using a percentage deduction (approximately 13%) as opposed to a straight beat per minute deduction as in most cases this will raise the lower target number and lower the upper target number better reflecting a proper heart rate deduction and target range for most clients. Using perceived exertion combined with exercise heart rate may help you better individualize and adjust a target range for a client in the water.

Many fitness professionals, both land and water instructors, are utilizing **rating of perceived exertion** to measure exercise intensity. Intensity level in this method is subjectively determined by the participant. Students are advised to increase their respiration rate, break a sweat (depending on water temperature), and to feel like they are working "somewhat hard" to "hard" (between 12 and 16) according to Borg's scale of perceived exertion. (see table 4-2) Even though perceived exertion is considered to be a subjective measure of intensity, many studies have shown a correlation between perceived exertion and working heart rate range. For most people, perceived exertion is a viable way to measure intensity without involving the additional factors which could affect working heart rate measurements. In personal training, both perceived exertion and heart rate are often combined to monitor intensity.

Another subjective intensity measurement is the "**talk test**." It is believed that a person is working above maximum threshold, at too high of an intensity for exercise if he/she cannot talk while exercising. This method proves useful for some exercise settings and with certain class populations.

Duration of Training:

Duration is <u>how long</u> you exercise. A duration of 20-60 minutes of continuous or intermittent (10-minute bouts accumulated through the day) training is recommended. Duration is "inversely" related to intensity. (↑ Intensity = ↓ Duration where as ↓ Intensity = ↑ Duration.) Higher intensity exercise carries a higher risk of musculoskeletal injury and a lower compliance rate. It is recommended that higher intensity exercise be performed for shorter duration to reduce the risk of injury and fatigue for the average adult. Improvement is similar for higher intensity-shorter duration compared to lower intensity-longer duration when the energy expenditure of the activities is equal. Longer duration, low to moderate intensity

Table 4-1

Theories why aquatic heart rates may be lower than heart rates achieved during comparable land exercise:

Temperature	Water cools the body with less effort than air. This reduced effort means less work for the heart, resulting in a lower heart rate.
Gravity	Water reduces the effect of gravity on the body. Blood flows from below the heart back up to the heart with less effort, resulting in a lowered heart rate.
Compression	The water is thought to act like a compressor on all body systems, including the vascular system, causing a smaller venous load to the heart than equivalent land exercise. The heart has to work less to return blood from the limbs.
Partial Pressure	A gas enters a liquid more readily under pressure. The gas would be oxygen and the liquid blood. It is believed more efficient gas transfer may occur due to water pressure and reduce the workload of the heart.
Dive Reflex	This is a primitive reflex associated with a nerve found in the nasal area. When the face is submerged in water, this reflex lowers heart rate and blood pressure. The reflex is stronger in some individuals than others. Some research suggests the face does not even need to be in the water for the dive reflex to occur. Some experience its affects when standing in chest deep water.
Reduced Body Mass	Research indicates that a reduction in body mass (you weigh less in the water) may at least be partially responsible for lower aquatic heart rates.

Table 4-2

Borg Scale for Rating of Perceived Exertion

6-20 Category Scale		1-10 Category-Ratio Scale (used for older adults and special populations)	
6	No Exertion at all	0	Nothing at all
7	Extremely Light	0.3	
8		0.5	Extremely Weak, Just Noticeable
9	Very Light	0.7	
10		1	Very Weak
11	Light	1.5	
12		2	Weak
13	Somewhat Hard	2.5	
14		3	Moderate
15	Hard (heavy)	4	
16		5	Strong
17	Very Hard	6	
18		7	Very Strong
19	Extremely Hard	8	
20	Maximal Exertion	9	
Recommended intensity to improve cardiorespiratory fitness is considered to be between 12 and 16 on the 6-20 scale and 4 and 5 on the 1-10 category-ratio scale.		10	Extremely strong
		11	
		•	Absolute Maximum

exercise is recommended for the non-athletic adult due to the lower injury rates and higher compliance rates associated with this kind of exercise.

Muscular Fitness:

The ACSM makes the following recommendations for resistance training. (2)

• Choose a mode that is comfortable throughout the full pain free range of motion.
• Perform a minimum of 8-10 separate exercises to develop that total body strength and endurance in a time-efficient manner. Total exercise training programs over one hour are associated with higher drop out rates.
• The traditional recommendation is 8-12 repetitions. Choose a range between 3 and 20 repetitions that can be performed at a moderate repetition duration (using approximately 3 seconds for concentric and for eccentric).
• Exercise each muscle group 2-3 nonconsecutive days/week.
• Vary your exercise program and allow enough time between exercises to use proper form and technique for each set.
• Maintain proper control during resistance training and breathe normally avoiding breath-holding.
• People with high cardiovascular risk and chronic disease should terminate each exercise as the concentric portion becomes difficult (RPE 15 to 16).

Flexibility:

Following are ACSM recommendations for achieving and maintaining flexibility. (2)

• Warm up to elevate muscle temperature.
• Do a static stretching routine including all major muscle groups focusing on those with reduced range of motion.
• Stretch to the end of range of motion inducing tightness, not discomfort. Hold the stretches for 15-30 seconds, performing 2-4 repetitions.
• Stretch 2-3 days/week, ideally 5-7 days/week.

In summary, a well-rounded exercise program including cardiorespiratory, resistance, and flexibility training is recommended for healthy individuals. It is important to design a program to include the proper amount of physical activity to achieve maximal benefit with minimal risk and investment of time. Another consideration in program design is progression. Progression is gradually increasing intensity, duration,

and frequency over time to reduce the risk of injury and improve exercise compliance. It is recommended that the unconditioned exerciser start with lower intensity exercise and gradually add time as endurance increases. Starting out with too much too fast can result in injury or poor compliance. The beginner exerciser should be advised to start slow and progress comfortably. Proper warm up and cool down is important. Excessive soreness and/or fatigue are sure signs of overexertion. Exercise should be exertive but leave you feeling refreshed, not fatigued. Muscle soreness can be a result of omitting stretching, stretching improperly, or of muscle injury.

Types of Aerobic Conditioning

There are several types of aerobic conditioning commonly used in group or individual exercise settings. The most common form of aerobic training is continuous training. Interval and circuit training are also becoming more popular as training alternatives. All three types of training can be used to add variety to your exercise program.

Continuous Training: Continuous training resembles a bell curve. After warming up, a relatively constant level of training is maintained in the target training zone for a prescribed length of time. Most group exercise programs typically use the continuous training format. (see figure 4-2)

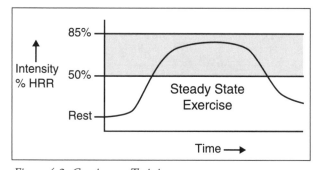

Figure 4-2 Continuous Training

Interval Training: Interval training consist of "harder" bouts of exercise interspersed with "easier" bouts or "work" and "recovery" cycles. The goal of most interval programs is to maintain easy and hard intervals within the recommended training zone. (see figure 4-3) For the most part, interval programs done within the training threshold can be very intense and cardiovascular in nature. Some interval programs include exercise bouts below the minimum training threshold to train low-level or beginner exercisers. Some beginner exercisers cannot tolerate continuous training within the training threshold but can comfortably do short bouts above and below the minimum threshold. Interval training adds variety to your workouts.

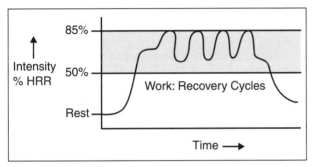

Figure 4-3 Interval Training

Circuit Training: Circuit training is usually done in a station format. Stations may be all aerobic in nature, all for muscular strength and endurance, or a mixture of the two. Usually equipment is utilized. Some circuits are designed to elicit a cardiorespiratory response, and some are designed to alternate aerobic work with muscular endurance training. Circuits can be designed in numerous ways and can add variety and cross training to any exercise program.

Many inventive instructors intersperse different methods of training into their programs to add variety and keep their students stimulated. Interval and circuit training have a very different "feel" as compared to continuous training, and can provide a very challenging workout. Utilizing interval training for 10 minutes during the cardio portion of class or utilizing circuit training during the toning portion of class can be fun for your students as well as broaden your abilities as an instructor. Additional information on how to incorporate these methods for training into a class format is available in Chapter 9.

Benefits of Regular Exercise

Increasing functional capacity or physical fitness results in several physiological and psychological benefits. Many of these benefits have been confirmed through research. Some benefits, such as the psychological benefits, are harder to isolate and confirm. Beyond improved physical appearance, safe and effective physical training can improve your health and enhance the quality of your life.

Health Benefits of Regular Exercise

The reason most often cited by people who want to start a regular exercise program is a desire to "improve physical appearance." Many want to lose weight, gain weight, or increase muscle mass or tone. Regular fitness training does improve physical appearance and is instrumental in achieving and maintaining weight loss. (see Chapter 13) When the majority of beginning exercisers get past their initial reasons for starting an exercise program, they continue to exercise because of how it makes them "feel." This good feeling is the result of physical and chemical changes that occur in the body. Because of these physical and chemical changes, exercise reduces your risk for cardiovascular disease, cancer, and many other diseases.

Regular aerobic exercise increases the functional capacity of the respiratory and cardiovascular systems. The respiratory system becomes more efficient by increasing the volume of air inhaled and exhaled with each breath (tidal volume). Intercostal (breathing) muscles become more fit, and the ability of the lungs to hold air increases. The heart muscle becomes stronger with use, and the heart's ability to eject more blood with each beat (stroke volume) increases. Because the heart can eject a greater volume of blood with each beat, the heart beats less to supply blood to the body. A fit person has a lower resting heart rate. Regular exercise also strengthens the walls of the blood vessels and promotes the development of capillary beds and a better blood supply to the body. The body's ability to extract oxygen from blood increases as well, elevating cardiorespiratory endurance levels.

Exercise is beneficial for the musculoskeletal system. Regular exercise strengthens the skeletal system and increases bone density. Muscles and tendons tugging on the bones at their attachments strengthen bone and connective tissue and help reduce risk of osteoporosis. Repetitive use of the muscles in aerobic training combined with resistance training actually increases the girth and density of muscle tissue. This increased function of skeletal muscle is apparent in muscular strength and endurance gains. If proper flexibility training is included, the skeletal muscles not only become stronger but more flexible as well. Strong, flexible muscles protect joints from injury and enable the body to move and function with ease.

The efficiency of the endocrine system, nervous system, and lymph system also improves with regular exercise. The endocrine system becomes more efficient at regulating hormones, and the lymphatic system becomes more efficient at protecting the body from disease. Motor pathways are developed and enhanced, allowing the nervous system to better regulate the quality of movement and other nervous functions. Metabolic functions improve favorably altering blood lipid levels and metabolism, making it easier to lose fat and improve body composition.

Many organs, such as the liver, intestines, and kidneys, benefit as well. Regular exercise enhances blood flow, fluid transfer, and oxygenation in the body. The body's functional capacity drops 5-10% per decade between the ages of 20-70. Muscle tissue and flexibility are also lost in the aging process. Regular exercise promotes the maintenance of functional capacity, muscle tissue, and flexibility at any age. The health benefits of exercise are truly staggering. Our bodies evolved as active machines, made to move and be physically active. Physical inactivity and lack of use can have detrimental health effects. Regular physical activity protects the body from injury and disease.

Psychological Benefits of Regular Exercise

Although psychological benefits are difficult to isolate and confirm, health professionals are under a general impression that exercise training may improve psychological function. Exercise is regularly prescribed to reduce depression and anxiety. Regular exercisers report reduced stress and tension, improved sleep habits, increased energy, increased productivity, improved self-image and self-esteem, and an increased sense of self-control. Corporate fitness programs show that regular exercisers are more productive, have lower absenteeism, fewer accidents, lower health care costs, and fewer hospital days and days of rehabilitation.

Overall, regular exercisers experience increased feelings of general well being and enhanced quality of life. People who are fit can more readily handle the physical, emotional, social, and psychological rigors of their jobs, personal life, and home life.

Physical Activity vs. Physical Fitness

Not everyone is interested or motivated to begin a regular exercise program to improve physical fitness. Some participants may not be interested in or able to comply to an intense physical fitness program. Some participants want to at least begin with moderate activity instead. It is becoming increasingly apparent that moderate physical activity can produce favorable health benefits. As fitness professionals, we are encouraged and challenged to provide moderate

activity based programming for participants who may want to improve their metabolic profile (resting heart rate, blood pressure, blood lipids, blood sugar, and body weight) as opposed to improving physical fitness components (cardiovascular and muscular fitness). By offering opportunities for increasing moderate physical activity, health benefits are achieved, and it is hoped that many of these participants will eventually move on to regular exercise programs.

An estimated 250,000 deaths per year in the United States can be attributed to lack of regular physical activity. The relationship between regular exercise, physical fitness, and enhanced health is well substantiated. In addition, research studies accumulated over the past several decades clearly show the beneficial relationship between health and regular, moderate intensity physical activity as well. Only a small percentage of adult Americans (~22%) are believed to be active at the recommended level to provide health benefits. It is believed that ~24% of adult Americans are sedentary and engage in little or no physical activity. The remaining ~54% would benefit from increased regular physical activity in addition to the ~24% who are inactive. Overall, participation in regular physical activity has remained relatively low. Perhaps this low participation rate can be at least partially attributed to the overemphasis placed on regular intense exercise. It is important to recognize that lower intensity, regular activity yields substantial health benefits. The American College of Sports Medicine and the U.S. Centers for Disease Control and Prevention, in cooperation with the President's Council on Physical Fitness and Sports, reviewed the accumulated scientific evidence and formulated the following conclusions and recommendations:

1. Scientific research clearly demonstrates that regular, moderate-intensity physical activity provides substantial health benefits.

2. Physical activity appears to provide some protection against several chronic diseases such as coronary heart disease, adult onset diabetes, hypertension, certain cancers, osteoporosis, and depression.

3. "Significant health benefits can be obtained by including a moderate amount of physical activity (e.g., 30 minutes of brisk walking or raking leaves, 15 minutes of running, or 45 minutes of playing volleyball) on most, if not all, days of the week. Through a modest increase in daily activity, most Americans can improve their health and quality of life." (2)

4. "Because most Americans fail to meet this recommended level of moderate-intensity physical activity, almost all should strive to increase their participation in moderate or vigorous physical activity."

5. "Additional health benefits can be gained through greater amounts of physical activity. People who can maintain a regular regimen of activity that is of longer duration or of more vigorous intensity are likely to derive greater benefit." (2)

6. The dose-response relationship between physical exercise and health should be emphasized. (2) Encourage at least moderate amounts of daily physical activity.

If a person wishes to increase functional capacity or physical fitness, he or she should participate in a vigorous exercise program following the guidelines set forth by the ACSM for intensity, duration, frequency, and mode. The health benefits of regular exercise have been well substantiated. Unfortunately, the majority of the American adult population is not motivated to pursue a regular exercise program despite the substantiated health benefits. Fitness professionals should bear this in mind and plan programs that encourage moderate intensity activities and opportunities to their clients and members, as well as vigorous exercise programs. People are encouraged to walk to work, take the steps instead of the elevator, turn off the TV, garden, walk, dance, rake leaves, and gradually increase accumulated active time spent over the course of each day.

As a fitness class instructor, personal trainer, water therapist, or any other type of aquatic fitness professional, it is imperative that you recognize and promote not only vigorous exercise, but moderate level physical activity as well. As more fitness professionals realize the benefits of moderate activity and develop programs accordingly, the participation level in physical activity should rise. Not all people are motivated to exercise or will adhere to vigorous programs, at least not initially. So as professionals we need to provide alternatives. Moderate intensity programs are a viable alternative for a potentially untapped market of clients, with health benefits confirmed. We are in a better position to involve and help more people than ever before.

Summary

1. Regular exercise programs need to include all five major components of physical fitness. It is essential to build cardiorespiratory endurance, muscular strength and endurance, flexibility, and a favorable body composition. Developing all five components promotes overall fitness and good health.

2. Guidelines for mode, intensity, duration, frequency, resistance training, flexibility, and progression should be addressed in any physical fitness program in order to obtain optimal benefits and functional capacity. These guidelines ensure an effective exercise program for increasing physical fitness and reducing risk of chronic disease.

3. Aerobic conditioning could include continuous, interval, and circuit training.

4. Benefits of regular exercise fall into two basic categories. Health benefits of regular exercise have been substantially documented with scientific data. Psychological benefits are more difficult to isolate and confirm but are generally acknowledged by the medical community.

5. A fitness professional should understand the difference between physical fitness/ exercise programs and moderate intensity physical activity and the health benefits of each. Programs should be developed to include regular exercisers as well as those who want moderate activity.

Review Questions

1. _____ is defined as the maximum force that can be exerted by a muscle or muscle group against a resistance.

2. Which proprioceptor is found in the tendons of your muscles and measures muscle tension?

3. Name the 6 skill-related components of fitness.

4. What is the difference between maximal heart rate and heart rate reserve?

5. How does compression lower your heart rate in the water?

6. What are the recommended guidelines for duration of training?

7. Describe circuit training.

8. List 5 benefits of regular exercise.

See Appendix E for answers to review questions.

References

1. American College of Sports Medicine. (1990). *The Recommended Quantity and Quality of Exercise for Developing and Maintaining Cardiorespiratory and Muscular Fitness in Healthy Adults*. MSSE, 22:2, pp. 265-275. American College of Sports Medicine.

2. American College of Sports Medicine. (2006). *Guidelines for Exercise Testing and Prescription*. 7th Edition. Baltimore, MD. Lippincott, Williams & Wilkins.

3. American Council on Exercise. (2000). *Group Fitness Instructor Manual*. San Diego, CA. American Council on Exercise.

4. American Council on Exercise. (2003). *Personal Trainer Manual*. 3rd Edition. San Diego, CA. American Council on Exercise.

5. Anderson, R. (1993). Is Exercise/Increased Activity Necessary for Weight Loss and Weight Management? *Medicine, Exercise, Nutrition and Health. Volume 2.*

6. Beachle, T. and R. Earle. (2004). *NSCA's Essentials of Personal Training*. Champaign, IL. Human Kinetics Publishers.

7. Fleck, S. and W. Kraemer. (2003). *Designing Resistance Training Programs*. 3rd. Edition. Champaign, IL. Human Kinetics Publishers.

8. Howley, T and D. Franks. (2003). *Health Fitness Instructor's Handbook*. 4th Edition. Champaign, IL. Human Kinetics Publishers.

9. Riposo, D. (1990). *Fitness Concepts: A Resource Manual for Aquatic Fitness Instructors*. 2nd Edition. Pt. Washington, WI. Aquatic Exercise Association.

10. Sova, R. (2000). *AQUATICS: The Complete Reference Guide for Aquatic Fitness Professionals*. 2nd Edition. Pt. Washington, WI. DSL, Ltd.

11. U.S. Centers for Disease Control and Prevention and ACSM. (1993). *Summary Statement: Workshop on Physical Activity and Public Health. Sports Medicine Bulletin, Volume 28, No.4.* President's Council on Physical Fitness.

12. Van Roden, J. and L. Gladwin. (2002). *Fitness: Theory & Practice*. 4th Edition. Sherman Oaks, CA. Aerobic & Fitness Association of America.

13. Wilmore, J. and D. Costill. (2001). *Physiology of Sport and Exercise*. 3rd Edition. Champaign, IL. Human Kinetics Publishers.

Select Images provided by:
Kumm, R. (2005). *LifeART Super Anatomy 3.* Baltimore, MD. Lippincott, Williams & Wilkins. Website: www.lifeart.com

Chapter 5: The Aquatic Environment

INTRODUCTION

Exercise professionals face many challenges in their attempts to provide programming for participants. The aquatic fitness profession is faced with the additional challenges of working in the aquatic environment. Water temperature, water resistance, pool structural considerations, pool chemicals, acoustical factors, and the risk of electrical shock become additional concerns. The aquatic fitness instructor must learn how to manage the aquatic environment as well as his/her class.

Unit Objectives

After completing Chapter 5, you should be able to:
1. Compare the body's ability to dissipate heat in land and aquatic exercise.
2. Know the importance of generating body heat during the thermal warm up and stretches.
3. Explain precautions that should be taken by students and instructors in relation to air and water temperatures and humidity. Know water temperature appropriate for various class formats and populations.
4. List problems and possible solutions associated with slippery, rough, or sloped pool bottoms; water depth; pool edges, gutters, or sides; water quality; acoustical factors; and the use of electrical appliances.
5. Discuss the benefits of wearing shoes when leading or participating in aquatic exercise.

Key Questions:
1. What are the primary ways the body dissipates heat in aquatic exercise?
2. How do you keep participants from chilling when entering the pool and during stretching?
3. What are ideal water temperature ranges for various aquatic exercise program formats?
4. How can you overcome environmental difficulties in a pool setting to improve the quality of your aquatic fitness instruction and insure the safety of your participants?

Heat Dissipation in the Aquatic Environment

Water cools the body faster than air. Because participants are surrounded by water, most don't experience the negative effects of heat when exercising vigorously in the pool. Heat, a by-product of metabolism, is eliminated from the body through **radiation** (heat lost through vasodilation of the surface vessels), **evaporation** (sweat evaporating from the skin cooling the body), and in the water, primarily through **conduction** (the transfer of heat to a substance or object in contact with the body) and **convection** (the transfer of heat by the movement of a liquid or gas between areas of different temperatures). On land as well as in the water, a great deal of heat is dissipated and radiated from the head. Restricting heat dissipation (for example, through the use of bathing caps or shower caps) can lead to heat related illness (see Chapter 11). The body can still dissipate heat in the water through peripheral vasodilation and/or sweating. In most aquatic fitness programs, water temperature is well below normal body temperature. Because the cooler water surrounds the body, heat dissipation through conduction and convection is facilitated.

Chilling can be a problem for some participants due to the facilitated cooling effects of the water. There are several products (i.e. neoprene vests) on the market for participants to wear to help conserve core temperature and body heat. Humans are warm-blooded and have a stable body temperature of about 98.6 degrees Fahrenheit (37 degrees Celsius). When the body is placed in water below this temperature, the water will draw heat from the body. Participants can be comfortable in the water if they generate additional body heat, for example, through exercise. In therapy settings or other programs where the participant does not generate sufficient body heat through movement, additional measures must be taken to keep participants warm if the pool temperature cannot be increased.

Aquatic environments and pool temperatures can vary from facility to facility as well as from day to day. Aquatic instructors need to watch participants for overheating or chilling and adjust the programming and exercise intensity accordingly.

Water Temperature

Water varying from 83-86 degrees Fahrenheit (28-30 degrees Celsius) is the most comfortable temperature for typical water fitness programs. This temperature range is considered tepid and allows the body to react and respond normally to the onset of exercise and the accompanying increase in body temperature. Cooling benefits are still felt as body heat rises due to vigorous activity. Yet there is little risk of overheating.

In cool water, under 78 degrees Fahrenheit (26 degrees Celsius), physiological responses in the body will be altered. With a cooler water temperature, metabolic rate and heart rate will slow down, circulatory functions become slower, and the majority of body fluids will remain in the trunk area to keep the essential organs warm and functioning. If circulation is reduced to the extremities, muscles will remain cold and inflexible, increasing risk of injury. Ischemia (lack of oxygen) will occur in the muscles of the extremities due to reduced blood flow. This will cause muscle cramping, most notably in the calf area.

It should be noted that swimming and other forms of non-impacting exercise could be performed in slightly lower temperatures. The effect of impacting, as in shallow water exercise, seems to cause higher susceptibility for cramping and chilling. Even though water temperatures at 76 and 77 degrees Fahrenheit (22 –25 degrees Celsius) may be borderline acceptable for swimming, these temperatures may be too cool for vertical impacting exercise programs, and may lead to injury.

On the other hand, trying to achieve the benefits of physical fitness in water temperatures near or above 90 degrees Fahrenheit (32 degrees Celsius) can be detrimental as well. This range is too warm for vigorous exercise programs that generate a lot of body heat. Increased internal heat, increased metabolic and heart rate, and increased circulation and fluid distribution result from vigorous aerobic exercise. If the water is too warm, the possibility of overheating may occur. Heat dissipation is hindered and the body is not as efficiently cooled. This temperature range is better suited for therapeutic-type activities, such as water massage or range-of-motion and strength/rehabilitation exercises for musculoskeletal injuries. This water temperature also works well for water Tai Chi, Ai Chi, Pilates, Yoga, arthritis, and stretching programs. Table 5-1 indicates recommended temperatures for various programs.

Working in water temperatures from 83 to 86 degrees Fahrenheit (28-30 degrees Celsius) allows the body to react naturally to achieve the benefits of physical fitness without the worry of conserving heat or overheating. Physiological changes due to water temperature are minimal in this range, and the body can stabilize internal temperatures to a comfortable level.

Participants should be encouraged to begin large muscle movements as soon as they enter the pool to adjust from the change in air temperature to water temperature. They should also be encouraged to maintain some type of movement to generate heat for the majority of time they are in the water. Even slight pauses will begin the cooling process. If a traditional aerobic class is being taught, participants should be encouraged to maintain some type of movement during the stretch portion of the class to keep core temperature from dropping. For example, during static stretching of the lower extremities, keep the upper extremities moving to generate heat, or vice versa. The amount of movement needed to maintain core temperature is dependent upon the water temperature.

Vigorous aquatic exercise programs that produce significant body heat are best suited for tepid water temperatures. As discussed above, 83-86 degrees Fahrenheit (28-30 degrees Celsius) is an appropriate temperature range for this type of activity. Programs that require slow, controlled movement, such as strength, toning, or stretching programs, will require slightly higher water temperatures. You should avoid teaching vigorous exercise programs in pools with temperature extremes above 90 degrees Fahrenheit (28-30 degrees Celsius) and lower extremes below 80 degrees Fahrenheit (27 degrees Celsius).

Many facilities now have the luxury of having a warm water/therapy pool and a fitness pool. This makes programming simple in regards to water temperature. These facilities can offer a wide range of programming in the appropriate water temperature. Often, pool managers with only one pool will choose a mid-range temperature that can be used for many types of programs. For example, a pool temperature of 84 degrees Fahrenheit (29.1 C) will be acceptable for vigorous programs such as swimming and shallow or deep water aerobics. This temperature may still be acceptable for therapy and arthritis programs if the participants wear vests to conserve body heat. A mid-range temperature will increase programming options that will, in turn, increase facility usage and income.

Encourage participants to listen to their own bodies. If they are too warm, slow down; if they are too cold, increase activity and/or intensity levels. Every body is different and will respond differently to aquatic exercise. Encourage your participants to find the comfort level best for them no matter what the pool temperature.

Table 5-1

Recommended Water Temperature / Aquatic Exercise Association Standards and Guidelines for Aquatic Fitness Programming

• Swim Team & Lap Swim	78 – 82 F / 25.5 – 27.5 C
• Resistance Training	83 – 86 F / 28 – 30 C (minimum range)
• Therapy & Rehab	91 – 95 F / 33 – 35 C
• Multiple Sclerosis	80 – 84 F / 26.5 – 29 C
• Pregnancy	78 – 84 F / 25.5 – 29 C (avoid pools 85 or higher)
• Arthritis	83 – 88 F / 28 – 31 C (minimum, Arthritis Foundation)
	86 – 90 F / 28 – 32 C (low level class, ATRI)
• Fibromyalgia	86 – 96 F / 30 – 35.5 C
• Older Adults, mod-high	83 – 86 F / 28 – 30 C
• Older Adults, low	86 – 88 F / 30 – 31 C
• Children, fitness	83 – 86 F / 28 – 30 C
• Children, swim lessons	82+ F / 27.5+ C (varies with age, class length)
• Obese	80 – 86 F / 26.5 – 30 C

Humidity and Air Temperature

Air temperature and humidity are additional environmental concerns. In indoor pools, it is recommended that the air temperature be 3-4 degrees higher than the water temperature; humidity levels are commonly above 50 percent.

The combined high humidity and air temperatures usually have little effect on the participants in the water unless the combination is extreme. High air temperatures can contribute to participant overheating, and cool air temperatures can contribute to participant chilling. The air temperature and humidity directly affect the instructor teaching from deck. Air temperatures commonly in the upper 80s, combined with humidity of 50-60 percent, can create extreme conditions for an instructor. When on deck, the instructor should take precaution to avoid overheating and dehydration. Drink plenty of water and cool the body by submerging or splashing. Use verbal, hand, and leg cues to avoid overexertion. Demonstrating leg movements by utilizing a chair or stool on deck to avoid impact can help protect the instructor from musculoskeletal injuries and overheating.

If you teach in an outdoor pool, you will have the challenge of facing unpredictable temperatures. Remember that high temperatures and lots of sun can contribute to overheating in participants and especially the instructor on deck. Humidity combined with air temperature can make conditions more extreme. Cool air temperatures, especially combined with wind, can contribute to instructor and participant chilling, even if the water is warm. When the air temperature is cool, the instructor may want to advise that participants keep their head dry. In addition, the instructor may want to avoid going from the pool to the deck to instruct, to prevent chilling from being wet in the cool air on deck. An instructor must remain flexible and versatile to provide programming that works with fluctuating environmental conditions.

Water Resistance

The viscosity and resistance of the water presents a unique challenge to instructors in aquatic exercise programming. A full understanding of the properties of water is very important to safe and effective program planning. An entire chapter will be dedicated to this subject. For additional information on water resistance, please refer to Chapter 6.

Pool Considerations

Pools come in many shapes, sizes, and depths. The depth of the water, as well as pool slope, pool gutters, and the surface of the pool bottom, can create additional programming considerations in aquatic exercise.

Pool Depth and Slope

Some pools, such as lap pools, vary little in depth. Other pools may begin at 3 feet (1m) and end at 10 feet (3.05m) or more. Lap pools limit programming to shallow water exercise with a maximum depth usually being around 4.5 feet (1.4m). In this depth shallow water aerobics, water walking and / or jogging, aquatic step, strength, toning, and stretching programs can be offered. A section of the pool with a depth of 3.5 feet to 4.5 feet (1 to 1.4 meters) is considered ideal, and will usually accommodate most shallow water exercisers comfortably at the recommended mid-rib cage to armpit depth.

A pool with a slight slope is ideal for accommodating participants of varying heights. Almost all pools have some degree of slope, and it is good practice to have participants face different directions while exercising. This will help offset musculoskeletal and alignment imbalances that may occur due to working on a sloped surface. If pool slope is severe, shallow water programs may not be viable. A steep slope can cause slipping, uneven footing, equipment instability and poor body alignment.

Pools with a substantial amount of water at 6.5 feet (1.08m) and deeper can provide ideal conditions for deep water exercise programs. Deep water programs include deep water aerobics, jogging, toning, and stretching. Programs that utilize deep water are independent of pool slope.

Water depth affects a participant's impact level, control of motion, and body alignment. In a shallow water program, exercising in water that is too shallow (waist level or below) will increase impact and reduce the participant's ability to utilize his or her arms effectively in the water. Exercising in water that is too deep (above armpit depth) will compromise control of motion and body alignment. In a deep water program, exercising in water that is too shallow will affect body alignment and restrict movements due to the participant striking the pool bottom. Pool depth and programming are further addressed in later chapters.

As a safety measure, be sure to inform participants of pool depth, even when clearly marked on the pool or deck, as they enter the pool area. This will prevent a non-swimmer from getting into deep water and will alleviate the need for an unwanted rescue.

Pool Bottom

Pools are constructed of many types of materials including concrete, ceramic tile, metal, vinyl, and plastic. The type of material used to construct the pool and how it is finished (painted, coated, etc.) determines the surface of the pool bottom. The pool bottom surface is of little concern to deep water exercisers or swimmers. It can, however, affect the quality of a shallow water workout. If the pool bottom is rough, it can cause participants to lose a layer of skin from the soles of their feet. If the pool bottom is slippery, it becomes very difficult to push against the pool bottom to change direction or elevate a movement.

Wearing shoes can be very beneficial to aquatic fitness participants. Shoes provide extra shock absorbency, assure good footing, protect skin on the feet, and provide added weight or resistance. Wearing shoes improves the quality of the workout by allowing for better footing and better control when moving and changing directions. This control allows the participant to utilize the properties of the water more effectively. Shoes also provide safety for students when entering and exiting the pool and while walking on deck and/or in the surrounding environment that could be slippery.

Even with the reduced gravity environment of the water, participants still experience some degree of impact during shallow water programs. Shoes help with impact stress produced from bounding-type movements by providing some degree of cushioning and support. Shoes are beneficial for participants who have orthopedic problems or those who need to wear orthotic devices even while exercising in the pool.

Constant friction and impact can be harmful to the soles of the feet producing injuries, especially for the diabetic participant or individuals with delicate skin or skin disorders. Wearing shoes can help protect the bottom of the feet and avoid contact with the

rough surfaces found most often in concrete pools. Wearing shoes will also help to avoid slipping or stepping on a foreign object in the pool (earring, etc.) that could cause injury.

All shallow water exercise participants should be encouraged to wear some type of aquatic shoe to minimize the risk of injury in and out of the pool and to increase their ability to work effectively in the water. There are a variety of shoes available on the market in a variety of price ranges. Most sporting shoe stores now carry aquatic fitness shoes. Help your participants choose shoes best suited for their use.

AEA recommends all aquatic fitness instructors wear shoes and use a mat while teaching on deck. Wearing the appropriate shoes for deck teaching is vital to instructor safety. If you teach completely on deck, wear appropriate athletic shoes to provide cushioning and support. If you teach on deck and in the water or enter the water to cool off, you need to wear an appropriate water fitness shoe to minimize impact and provide the support needed for both environments.

Deck Surfaces

Most pool deck surfaces are made of materials that are non-resilient in nature. Deck surfaces can be slippery when dry or wet and an instructor needs to take precautions for the safety of students and self. Again, wearing appropriate shoes, using a mat when teaching, and verbally instructing and cautioning students of hazards can help avoid slips and falls for the instructor and participants.

Pool Gutters and Ladders

Pool gutters can affect how students enter and exit the pool, hold on to the side of the pool, as well as provide options for various toning and stretching exercises. Be aware of the design and do not force exercises or positions that may put participants at risk when working along the pool side. Be aware that some pools slope where the bottom meets the side and you may not be able to comfortably stand by the side to do toning exercises. On the other hand, that slope may be great for doing a post workout calf stretch.

Many pools now have ramps, walk-in access, chair lifts, or shallow areas where participants can exit or enter the water in accordance with the Americans with Disabilities Act. Some pools still require the use of ladders to enter and exit the pool, and this may restrict the type of participants you can accommodate in class.

Some participants may require assistance, or may not be able to get out of a pool by climbing a ladder. Make sure the ladder is well attached, not cracked or broken, and does not pose a hazard to your participants. Some instructors use ladders to attach equipment or to use as a station for toning exercises in a circuit station. Be sure the area around the ladder is free of potential hazard and that pool entry/exit is not restricted.

Water Quality

Public and private pools offering group fitness programs should have their pools maintained by a licensed pool operator/manager with the appropriate credentials as designated by state, national, or international codes. These individuals are trained and licensed to keep the public safe in an aquatic environment. For more information on appropriate guidelines for the maintenance of pools and details on becoming a Certified Pool and Spa Operator®, please check with the National Swimming Pool Foundation (NSPF), www.nspf.org.

Swimming pools vary in sizes, shapes and locations, but they all work in the same basic way. To provide a safe environment for individuals, pools require a combination of water filtration and chemical treatment to continually clean a large volume of water. There are seven essential components needed for a typical swimming pool. These components include:
- A large basin to hold the water and bathers.
- A motorized pump to move the water from one component of the pool to another.
- A water filter to clean the water and remove debris.
- A chemical feeder to add chemicals that disinfect the water so it does not carry disease pathogens.
- Drains in the basin and skimmers to feed into the pump system.
- Returns back into the basin for the water that has been pumped through the filtration and disinfectant systems.
- A system of plumbing pipes to connect all of these elements. (see figure 5-1)

Pool disinfectant systems are required for public health and are essential for four reasons:
- They eliminate dangerous pathogens, such as bacteria, which thrive in water. This reduces the potential for the spread of disease from bather to bather.
- To balance the chemistry of the water to avoid damage to the various parts of the pool.

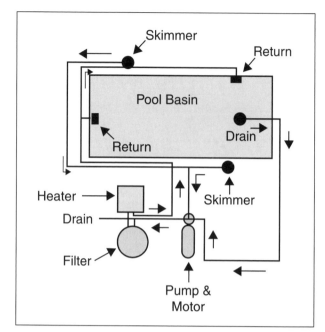

Figure 5-1 Pool Components

- To balance the chemistry of the water to avoid irritation to bather's skin and eyes.
- To balance the chemistry of the water to keep it clear so it does not become cloudy.

The most popular disinfecting agent used in pool systems is **chlorine**. Chlorine is an unstable chemical compound and care must be taken during storage and use in the pool area. An alternative sanitizer is **bromide**, which works essentially the same way as chlorine with slightly different results, but is not as widely used.

Sometimes individuals complain of throat or eye irritation, suit fading, skin irritations, or their hair turning colors in the pool. There are many factors that can cause these things to happen. Incorrect chlorine levels are often suspected, but do not usually cause these complaints. Following are a list of factors that could cause these symptoms to occur:
- Improper water chemistry balance of acidity and alkalinity (pH).
- Wind and sun reflection.
- Excessive debris or turbidity present in the water due to a disrupted or unclean filtration system.
- Diatomaceous earth not adhering to the septum of the filter and therefore not filtering properly.
- Dirty hair and lint baskets/traps.
- Settled debris not vacuumed out.
- High total dissolved solid levels.
- Improper filter size for the bather load.
- Inadequate turnover of the filtering system.

- The presence of copper oxides in the water.
- The presence of chloramines in the water.
- Improper handing of pool chemicals.

The big irritator in water is often **chloramines** (combined available chlorine). Chloramines are formed when the free chlorine in the water combines with other elements such as ammonia. When these are formed, the ability of the chlorine to kill bacteria is 100 times slower than free available chlorine. The chloramines cause eye irritation and the unpleasant odor often attributed to chlorine.

You may come across an ozonation pool disinfectant system. This system allows ozone to act as the primary oxidizer and disinfectant. Ozone is fed into the pool water prior to the chlorine injection process. Ozone destroys many organic compounds and microorganisms that would typically react with chlorine, resulting in a reduction of the chlorine demand and total dissolved solids. Lower chlorine demand allows the pool operator to achieve disinfection of the water with minimal chlorine residual, and the reduction of total dissolved solids improves the water clarity. The reduction of chlorine usage will minimize the amount of chlorine off-gas that causes corrosion in swimming pool environments. Ozone will also break down chloramines.

Air Quality

Air temperature, humidity levels, and circulation are important issues for indoor pool facilities and influence both comfort and safety of employees and clients. Lifeguard Lung Disease is a condition directly affected by air quality and ventilation concerns found with indoor pool facilities, especially those with water spray features; see Chapter 11, Injury Prevention, for more information.

As an instructor, it is considered your responsibility to check the pool area carefully prior to class. Make sure to inform students of any problems or concerns that could result in injury. Student safety is of the utmost importance. Arriving at least ten minutes early for class to conduct a quick safety check is time well spent.

Pool hazards should be recorded in writing and forwarded to the facility manager or pool operator. Always document any injuries in writing as well, using an injury incidence report (see Chapter 15), and take the name of a witness. If hazards are not corrected, an additional complaint should be filed. If the facility will not correct the hazard, keep your recorded complaints in your files and work around the hazard if possible. If you and your students cannot work around the hazard safely, it may be unadvisable to teach at that facility until the problem is corrected.

Acoustical Factors

Acoustics in pool areas are generally poor and can alter the quality of instruction. Often you may compete with echo from high ceilings and concrete walls as well as noise from blower fans, filtration systems, whirlpools, swim lessons, birthday parties, and other individuals using the same pool. It can be very difficult for the instructor to communicate cues and instructions. Poor acoustics can cause student frustration (they can't hear) as well as voice injury for the instructor. (Voice injury is discussed further in Chapter 11.)

Experiment with different teaching locations around the pool before starting your class. Due to construction or layout, it may be less noisy in one area than another, or your voice may carry more clearly from some locations. Sometimes students can hear you better when you instruct from deck, and other times they can hear you better when you are in the pool. Make the necessary adjustments to reduce frustration from additional noise, but do not compromise participant or instructor safety.

Make the best of your situation by learning how to effectively use hand and arm signals and other non-verbal cueing techniques. There are great microphone systems available for use in the aquatic environment, and often these systems will enhance the quality of class and reduce risk of voice injury for the instructor. With the growing popularity of aquatic fitness, many companies have designed and manufactured sound systems and PA systems specifically for use in the aquatic environment. These systems vary in cost and are a worthy investment for facilities and instructors.

Electrical Shock

Electricity and pool water can be a deadly mix. Many instructors use boom boxes, microphones, pace clocks, and other electrical devices to teach aquatic fitness programs. Instructors should use extreme caution when using electrical appliances to minimize the risk of shock or electrocution. Keep electrical appliances away from the pool unless they are approved for poolside use. Approved appliances will be double insulated or designed to reduce the risk of shock. They will be labeled with a sticker from NSF International, Underwriters Laboratories, etc., as safe to use around water.

Make sure that prior to use, any electrical outlet, light, or other electrical fixture is properly installed and grounded according to code. Do not take any chances with faulty or damaged outlets. Do not use the appliance where it can get wet. Make sure the cord and appliance will not be submerged or splashed, and place it on a table or chair above, as opposed to on the pool deck. Dry off before touching electrical appliances, cords, or outlets. Wear rubber-soled shoes to prevent tissue burns or disruption in electrical heart signals if shocked. Refer to the National Electrical Code (NEC) published by the National Fire Protection Association for additional information and safety tips.

Many instructors use waterproof, battery-operated boom boxes in the pool area. Many facilities recognize the danger and will not allow electrical appliances in the pool area. Rechargeable batteries are used to reduce the cost of battery replacement. Other facilities have sound systems installed away from the pool area. This eliminates the risk of shock and electrocution.

In summary, use the following as a checklist for choosing a pool for aquatic fitness programs.

- Will the pool's water and air temperature be appropriate for the types of programs you wish to teach?
- Will air temperature and humidity levels allow you to safely teach and demonstrate from deck?
- Is there enough space at the appropriate depth to accommodate a reasonable sized class? What would be your class maximum for that pool at that depth? (Approximately 4 x 8 feet or 32 square feet / participant recommended for shallow water, 32-36 square feet / participant for deep water.)
- Is the pool bottom and slope appropriate for the type of class you wish to teach?
- Is there an adequate space for you to teach and demonstrate from the deck?
- Will your targeted class population be able to safely enter and exit the pool?
- Will the pool gutters and sides limit the type of programming you plan to conduct?
- Is the pool deck kept clean and free of hazards?
- Are the pool chemicals properly monitored and kept in accordance with local board of health and state standards?
- Is the pool area properly ventilated?
- Will the pool acoustics work for the type of program you plan to teach?
- Is there a safe source for electricity for a sound system, or will you need to plan to use a battery-operated system?
- Are pool conditions conducive and is there adequate storage space for any equipment you plan to use? (Additional information in Chapter 7.)
- Is there a lifeguard on duty during your class and is there appropriate life saving equipment in the pool area? (Additional information in Chapter 11.)

Chances are slim that all of these parameters will be perfectly met. All of these factors will, however, have some impact on the way you teach your aquatic program. Choose your facility and pool based on the parameters that are absolutely necessary for you to conduct a safe and effective class for the target population and type of programming you wish to teach. Determine if you can make program adjustments or modifications to allow for the unmet parameters. For example if a pool meets your physical specifications, but acoustics are poor, experiment with different sound systems and placement, microphones, or types of music until you find something that is acceptable as opposed to perfect.

Summary

1. Exercising in water is different than exercising on land. Water temperature, heat dissipation, and pool factors affect programming in the aquatic environment.

2. Be familiar with the pool and facility. Check pool slope, the surface of the pool bottom, water temperature, and acoustical factors before teaching your class. Design a safe and effective program to fit your aquatic environment.

3. The aquatic fitness instructor must also be aware of the potential hazards associated with the aquatic environment. These hazards provide risk of injury to both the instructor and participants. It is important to document and report hazards to upper management.

4. Use electrical appliances according to acceptable safety standards.

Review Questions

1. How is radiation different than convection in heat dissipation?
2. What are the possible pitfalls of doing vertical exercise in water under 80 degrees (27 C)?
3. What is an ideal water temperature range for a typical cardiorespiratory aquatic fitness class?
4. What is ideal water depth range for a pool to conduct a shallow water aquatic fitness program?
5. What is usually the primary irritator in the aquatic environment in a chlorinated pool?

See Appendix E for answers to review questions.

References

1. Aquatic Exercise Association. (2005). *Standards & Guidelines for Aquatic Fitness Programming*. Nokomis, FL. Aquatic Exercise Association.

2. Harris, T. (2005). *Introduction to How Swimming Pools Work*. www.howstuffworks.com/swimming-pool. HowStuffWorks, Inc.

3. Howley, T and D. Franks. (2003). *Health Fitness Instructor's Handbook*. 4th Edition. Champaign, IL. Human Kinetics Publishers.

4. Kinder, T. and J. See. (1992). *Aqua Aerobics, A Scientific Approach*. Peosta, IA. Eddie Bowers Publishers.

5. Lindle, J. (2001). Is Your Indoor Pool Environment Safe? Nokomis, FL. *AKWA*. 15:4, pp. 3-4. Aquatic Exercise Association.

6. Moor, F, E. Manwell, M. Noble and S. Peterson. (1964). *Manual of Hydrotherapy and Massage*. Nampa, ID. Pacific Press Publishing Association.

7. Osinski, A. (1988). Water Myths. Nokomis, FL. *The AKWA Letter*. 2:3, pp. 1-7. Aquatic Exercise Association.

8. Osinski, A. (1993). Don't Court Disaster: Use Electrical Equipment Safely. Nokomis, FL. *The AKWA Letter*. 7:3, pp 1, 14-15. Aquatic Exercise Association.

9. Sharkey, B. (1989). *Physiology of Fitness*. 3rd Edition. Champaign, IL. Human Kinetics Publishers.

10. Sova, R. (2000). *AQUATICS: The Complete Reference Guide for Aquatic Fitness Professionals*. 2nd Edition. Pt. Washington, WI. DSL, Ltd.

Chapter 6: The Physical Laws

INTRODUCTION

Chapter 6 provides information needed to gain a clear understanding of "how the water works," or more importantly, "how to work the water." Your body reacts to movement differently in the water as compared to movement on land, which is affected primarily by gravity. In the water, the level of exertion is a function of:

- *the speed of movements,*
- *the rate of change in speed (acceleration),*
- *the surface area (frontal resistance) in the direction of the motion,*
- *the individual's and fluid's inertia,*
- *and the number of times you change direction.*

You will refine your effectiveness as an fitness professional as you familiarize yourself with the physical laws and properties of a liquid environment. Increasing your knowledge of principles that govern water exercise will allow you to maximize the benefits your clients receive in your programs and keep them coming back for more.

Unit Objectives

After completing Chapter 6, you should be able to:
1. Define Newton's laws of inertia, acceleration, and action/reaction; explain how each applies to aquatic exercise and describe ways to increase and decrease intensity using the principles of these laws in aquatic movement.
2. Describe how the water's viscosity causes resistance to motion in the aquatic environment.
3. Describe and demonstrate how intensity is altered in aquatic exercise by altering frontal surface area/ frontal resistance.
4. Demonstrate hand positions that will increase and decrease intensity in aquatic exercise.
5. List the alternatives to using speed to increase intensity in aquatic exercise. Explain the advantages to using these alternative methods.
6. Explain and demonstrate how the limbs are used as levers in aquatic exercise and how the length of the lever affects the intensity of the movement.
7. Describe how buoyancy, hydrostatic pressure, surface tension, and turbulence contribute to the aquatic exercise experience.

Key Questions:
1. How is motion in the aquatic environment affected by the water's viscosity?
2. How do body, water, and limb inertia affect intensity in aquatic exercise?
3. How does changing the body's position when traveling affect intensity?
4. Which hand position is most effective for pulling water and adding to the upper torso training effect?
5. Why is simply increasing the speed of movement not the best alternative for increasing intensity in the aquatic environment?
6. How can you apply the concept of acceleration in aquatic movement?
7. What influence does the combination of arm and leg movements have on the intensity of aquatic exercise?
8. Why is a knee lift a less intense movement than a front kick?

One of the most common shortcomings found in a beginner aquatic fitness professional is the inability to put together programming that utilizes the water to its fullest extent. Unfortunately, this is sometimes the case in an experienced aquatic fitness professional as well. Instructors who simply "plop" their land-based program into the pool soon discover that it's just not the same in the water. Ineffective utilization of the aquatic environment sometimes leads to a disillusioned perspective of water exercise by both the instructor and clients.

Aquatic fitness professionals with strong swimming backgrounds can have the same experience if they try to apply water principles in a fitness class in the same manner as they would for swimming. Vertical water exercise is different than horizontal exercise or swimming. An effective aquatic fitness professional learns not only how to deal with the fluctuating aquatic environment as learned in Chapter 5, but also how to manipulate and utilize the unique properties of the water to provide an effective workout.

Chapter 6 will define and explain Newton's laws of motion, the properties of viscosity and buoyancy, and the utilization of levers, frontal resistance, and hand positions to manipulate the intensity of an aquatic workout. In addition, practical application for each principle will be applied to an aquatic fitness workout. It is important to understand that these laws and principles can be employed to increase the effectiveness of shallow water aerobics, water walking, deep water exercise, aquatic step, one-on-one aquatic training, water therapy, sports specific training, and even the utilization of equipment in the aquatic environment.

Motion

Motion occurs when there is a change in location in space. Motion is a relative rather than an absolute term. For example, if you were seated on a moving train, the person seated next to you, in relation to you, would not be moving. But to the person standing in the train station watching the train go past, both you and the person seated next to you would be moving or in motion. Your motion in a pool accounts for part of your exertion, but the motion of the water relative to your motion can also affect your workload.

Motion of the body can be a direction or linear motion, for example, forward and backward or right to left. Motion can also occur within the body, for example, flexion and extension or abduction and adduction of a limb, which is a rotational motion because it is performed around an axis of rotation. Rotational motion has a contrast to linear motion. In linear motion, the entire body moves the same distance. However, if you flex or "rotate" your knee, your foot travels the greatest distance, which results in it having the greatest velocity of the lower leg relative to the knee. (see figure 6-1) The ability of muscles to cause joint movements or rotational motion is a combination of the distance of the muscle attachment point from the joint, the magnitude of the muscle force, and the direction of action or angle of pull of the muscle. (Mechanical advantage is described in Chapter 3.) Normally, the body automatically learns which muscles to use to produce the most efficient rotational motion.

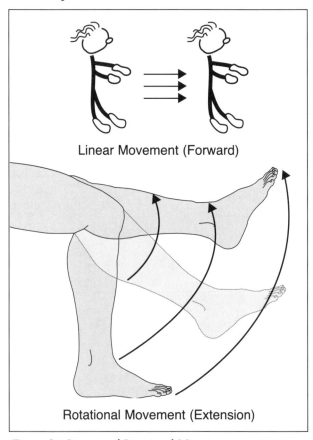

Linear Movement (Forward)

Rotational Movement (Extension)

Figure 6-1 Linear and Rotational Movement

Basic concepts of motion were developed by Aristotle and Galileo. They developed concepts and terms such as speed, velocity, and acceleration which are now terms and concepts used in every day life. Aristotle's model of falling bodies developed the concept that an object falls with a constant speed that depends on its weight and the medium through which it falls. Unfortunately, this concept was not true. A heavy object falls at the same speed as a light object in a vacuum and often in air as was documented by Galileo. Because of the friction (see viscosity) in water, an object does fall faster through air than through water. Galileo further developed Aristotle's incomplete concepts of motion to include the effects of friction and gravity.

The human organism is capable of running, jumping, hopping, dancing, walking, bending, twisting, and moving in many ways. Our body was designed to be an active, moving machine. Motion for the human machine takes the form of physical activity or exercise and is essential to normal functioning and health.

Exercise professionals study motion or movement in the human body in order to determine safe, effective, and efficient ways to move the entire body or its parts. Safe movement may save the body from an injury, or chronic disease and wear over time. Effective means that the movement is accomplishing its desired intention. That intention may be to increase cardiorespiratory endurance, flexibility, muscular strength, or the ability to maneuver a grocery cart in a crowded store. Efficient movement is the best way, quickest way, or the least "costly" way (from a movement perspective) to achieve your desired intention safely. Motion of the body or its parts in water is affected by the water's viscosity, buoyancy, and even somewhat by gravity.

Research studies on joint motion when walking in a pool have shown that individuals will have more than 30% higher joint motions (range of motion) than when walking on land. The added range of motion is very beneficial for therapy and for seniors.

Newton's Laws of Motion and Related Concepts

Sir Isaac Newton was a great 17th-century scientist who extensively studied the laws of gravity and motion. He took Galileo's ideas about motion and sought systematic rules that govern and change motion. We exert forces every day to move objects, move our body, change direction, and to stand upright and move against gravity. The forces that cause motion can be analyzed by applying Sir Isaac Newton's three laws of inertia, acceleration, and action/reaction. In addition, the concepts of drag, viscosity, frontal resistance, hand positions, and altering intensity with speed are discussed.

The Law of Inertia

Inertia: An object will remain at rest or in motion with constant velocity (speed and direction) unless acted on by a net external (unbalanced) force. (4)

This law basically states that an object remains stationary unless a force causes it to move. When a force is applied that is greater than resisting forces, such as friction, the object will begin to gain speed in the direction of the applied force. If the object is moving at a constant speed in a particular direction, it will require a force to change either the speed or direction of the object. This tendency to resist changes in the state of motion is described as an object's inertia.

The mass of the object will affect the amount of force required to change its speed or direction. Mass relates to both weight and inertia. The force of gravity on a mass generates its resistance to change in direction and speed. So an object with more mass will require more force to overcome its inertia.

A weightless object floating in outer space or neutrally buoyant in the water will still exhibit inertia even though it doesn't have weight. Because of inertia, an object will move forever in the same direction and speed in outer space until you apply a force. This is not true on land because of friction and the fact that gravity is a force that pulls the object downward. Nor is it true in the water due to the water's friction and viscosity. An example of the effect of inertia on land would be that it takes more force to push a car than it does a grocery cart because the car has more mass and friction. If the same force was applied to both, the grocery cart would have more acceleration because it has less mass and friction than the car. (see figure 6-2)

In the human body, the muscles attach to the outside of the bones. When we contract our muscles, the external force, or contracting muscle attached to the bone, moves the bone. If both muscles in a muscle pair contracted on either side of the joint at the same time, the net external rotational motion could be zero and the bone would not move. Because our muscles act as agonists and antagonists, one muscle contracts to provide the force while the other muscle relaxes and movement occurs at the joint. Our bones and muscles make up a system of levers to give us mechanical advantage, and to maximize muscular forces so we can move more efficiently. It has been shown that the efficiency is related to both the agonist's strength and the ability to relax the antagonist.

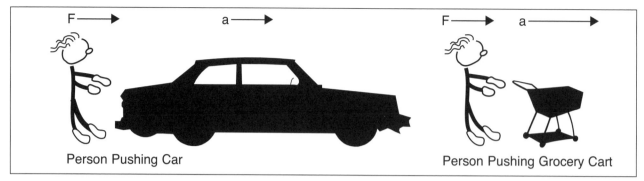

Figure 6-2 Force and Acceleration. If the same force is applied to pushing a car and a grocery cart, the grocery cart would have greater acceleration because it has less mass and friction.

In water exercise, there are basically three objects that move and are affected by the law of inertia: movement of the entire body (total body inertia), movement of the water (water inertia), and movement of the limbs (limb inertia).

Total Body Inertia

Total body inertia can contribute to exercise intensity if traveling is incorporated into the choreography. It requires more effort to overcome inertia to start, stop, or change a movement for the entire body than it does to continue with the same movement. You can visualize the example of a train. The engine has to produce a great deal of force to get the train moving. Once it is moving, the engine only has to provide enough energy to overcome air and ground resistance from the wheels on the track. It takes more force to start or stop a train than it takes to keep it moving at a constant speed. In other words, the engine doesn't have to work quite as hard once the train is moving.

Just as with the train, it takes more force to start the body moving and stop the body from moving than it does to continue the same movement. Jogging 16 counts forward and back requires force to initiate the jog forward, stop the jog, change the direction to backward, and stop the jog. (Of course limb inertia is happening as well.) This movement could be made even more intense by jogging 8 counts forward, 8 counts back, 8 counts forward, and 8 counts back. This combination would require more force or energy because you would stop and change direction twice as much. By jogging 4 counts forward, 4 counts back, 4 counts to the right, 4 counts to the left, and 8 counts in your own circle, you would be increasing intensity by overcoming inertia even more to start, stop, and change direction.

The Water's Inertia

If the class is moving in a particular direction for a time and then turns around, it will feel like it is moving upstream. Because of class motion, the water has begun to move with the class. But when the class turns, the inertia of the water makes it continue in the original direction at its previous speed. The class turns but the water keeps going.

The water's inertia can be used to increase exercise intensity. If many steps are taken forward in a straight line, the water will begin to move in that direction. When you then reverse body direction, you will be trying to stop and then reverse the water motion, just as you have with the body motion. This combined effect will increase exercise intensity. If you jog forward and then straight back, you are not only applying force to overcome body inertia, but to overcome the water's inertia as well. Incorporating traveling movements in your choreography will increase energy expenditure by increasing total body inertia <u>and</u> the water's inertia.

Limb Inertia

In the human body, muscles attached to bones provide the external force that moves the skeleton. On land, the muscular effort required to move a limb back and forth is due to inertia- you have to apply force to make the limb move, change direction, and stop. Our movement is limited by joint structure and soft tissue, so we have a limit to how far a limb can travel before it has to stop or change directions. In flexion and extension of the leg, you must first start the motion, stop the motion, start the motion in the opposite direction, stop the motion, and repeat. As you perform this movement faster (for example a jog), it requires more force and energy, as long as you maintain the same range of motion, because you are overcoming inertia more often. The effect of inertia is clearly felt when hand weights are utilized during land aerobics. An overextension injury can result if the participant cannot control the inertia of the hand weight (stop the motion) if the muscles become exhausted at the end of class.

Air is not very viscous and does not offer much resistance unless the movement speed is very fast. The primary resistance to movement felt on land is when the motion is against gravity or friction with respect to the ground. The primary resistance to the limbs in the water is from drag, which relates to a combination of viscosity of the water and the relative speed of the motion between the limb and the water. When you move your total body in a straight line, the drag forces produce an inertial effect of starting, changing direction, and stopping a volume of water. This effect is added to other effects from viscosity, but does not relate to just velocity. Because the water offers resistance, even more force or energy is required to initiate and change movement. Force is applied to start a jumping jack and abduct the legs. Force is used to stop the movement, initiate adduction, and stop adduction. Therefore, additional energy is required to move the limb or body from a state of rest to movement or exercise. Once a limb is moving in a straight line at a constant speed in the water, the major energy requirements are due to drag. Additional energy will be required when you either try to stop the limb motion or change its direction.

> *Note: Increased speed of complete motion increases the energy expenditure of a movement only if you keep exactly the same range of motion. If you decrease the range of motion when you increase music tempo, energy expenditure will be reduced.* Often participants will cheat and make a movement easier by taking it through a smaller range of motion when tempo increases.

When utilizing the law of inertia (total body, water, and limb inertia) in exercise programming, there are two important factors to consider. The first factor is your participants. They must be reasonably fit and skilled at water exercise in order to follow more complicated patterns which change movements and directions. The second factor involves acoustics in your pool setting. Participants can become very frustrated attempting to follow more complex patterns when they cannot understand the verbal cues. In poor acoustical situations, instructors are often more successful using traveling moves to overcome inertia. Traveling with fewer movement changes to increase intensity is easier to cue with body language.

It is important for an instructor to know how to utilize the law of inertia to increase and decrease intensity. A less fit student can be instructed to jog 24 counts in place, instead of traveling forward and backward, to decrease intensity. More fit students can incorporate traveling movements and combinations to create inertia through starting, stopping, changing direction, and using the water's inertia to increase intensity. Understanding the law of inertia will enable you to help your students individualize the program to meet their specific goals and abilities.

Before continuing to Newton's second and third laws of motion, it is important to understand the properties of drag, viscosity, frontal resistance, hand positions, and intensity alterations using speed. These concepts are closely related and further explain Newton's laws of motion.

Drag

Movement in water tends to slow down quickly. It turns out that **drag**, the resistance you feel to movement in the water, is a function of fluid characteristics (viscosity), frontal shape and size, and the relative velocity between a person and the water. This results in a very different loading to the muscles during exercise in the water compared to land exercise. On land, your muscle load decreases when you come up to speed. In the water however, you have a constant muscle load provided by the water through full range of motion.

Viscosity

Viscosity refers to the friction between molecules of a liquid or gas, causing the molecules to tend to adhere to each other (cohesion) and in water, to a submerged body (adhesion). Water is more viscous than air, just as molasses is more viscous than water. Viscosity increases as temperature decreases. Air, water, and molasses are more viscous when cold. A change in water viscosity is not noticeable in the small temperature fluctuations we experience in water exercise.

This friction between molecules, or the water's viscosity, is what causes resistance to motion. Since water is more viscous than air, water provides more resistance to motion than air. As Galileo discovered, friction or viscosity causes an object to fall slower through water than air. He found that a combination of the surface area of an object and its speed determines the resistance to the motion caused by the fluid viscosity (drag). During exercise additional resistance increases the intensity of the movement, and therefore requires greater muscular effort. Greater energy expenditure causes higher caloric expenditure.

When you walk forward in the water for a few feet, the viscosity (cohesion and adhesion) of the water allows you to get a "block" of water to move with you. Viscosity can also make it more difficult to walk at a specific pace next to a wall rather than some distance from the wall. When you walk closer to the wall, you experience more friction which impairs your forward movement.

There are many ways to alter the resistance of the water. **Streamlined flow** is continuous, steady movement of a fluid. (see figure 6-3) The rate of movement at any fixed point remains constant. A swimmer attempts to streamline the body by reducing frontal surface area and creating smooth, efficient stroke mechanics to minimize friction or resistance as he or she travels through the water. A streamlined swimmer can go farther faster, with less energy expenditure. Proper stroke mechanics and streamlined flow are advantageous to a competitive swimmer.

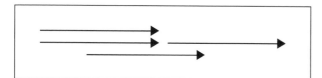

Figure 6-3 Streamlined Flow

The purpose of vertical water exercise is to increase energy expenditure. Resistance can be increased by creating additional drag and impedance with **turbulent flow**. (see figure 6-4) Turbulent flow is irregular movement of a fluid with movement varying at any fixed point. It creates rotary movements called **eddies**, is less efficient, and increases the water's resistance. (see figure 6-5) You can increase turbulent water flow around the body and its limbs by applying Newton's laws of motion through increasing frontal resistance, changing the length of the lever or limb, and by changing hand position. These principles are discussed below.

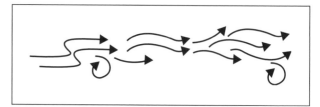

Figure 6-4 Turbulent Flow

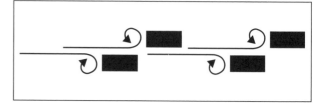

Figure 6-5 Eddies

Frontal Resistance

Frontal resistance is another factor affecting exercise intensity. Frontal resistance results from the horizontal forces of the water. In air, the primary force acting on the body is the downward vertical force of gravity. The horizontal resistance of air can be felt when trying to walk forward against a strong wind. In most exercise settings, horizontal resistance of the air is minimal and unnoticeable. In water, gravity is not the primary force acting on the body because the vertical downward pull of gravity is offset by the upward vertical force of buoyancy. However, the horizontal resistance of water is very noticeable due to water's viscosity. In a sense, walking through water can be compared to walking through a brisk windstorm.

The size of the frontal surface area of an object presented against the water's horizontal resistance affects the amount of energy required to move the object through the water. Most boats are tapered in the front so they can slice through the water, creating less turbulence and eddies. Reduced surface area allows for more streamlined movement and requires less energy to move the boat. (see figure 6-6) In water exercise, presenting a smaller frontal surface area to the intended line of travel will make movement easier. For example, the surface area of the side of the body is typically smaller than the surface area of the front of the body. Movement sideways would thus create less frontal resistance than moving forward. To further increase resistance via frontal surface area, you could walk forward with the arms out to the side, palms forward. Traveling forward with side knee lifts would be more intense than traveling forward with front

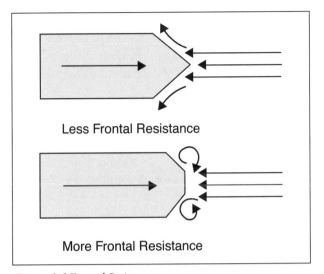

Figure 6-6 Frontal Resistance

knee lifts because the side knee lifts increase the width of the body's frontal surface area.

An object or body must be traveling in order to encounter frontal resistance. Stationary movement of the body (i.e. jogging in place) is not as affected by the water's horizontal resistance, just as a stationary boat is not. However, the size of the surface area of the limbs and hands moving against the water's resistance in stationary movements will affect intensity. Hand and limb position will be discussed below.

Hand Positions – Shape Factors

Surface area created by the positioning of the hand while moving the arm through the water will affect the amount of effort required by the associated working muscles. The hand can serve as a paddle to scoop more water or can be positioned to minimize its pull in the water. The size of the surface area of the hand as it moves through the water and its shape determine how much water the hand will pull and how much resistance will be created. A hand closed in a fist or a hand sliced sideways through the water will create minimal resistance. The hand position used for most swimming strokes (an open, slightly cupped hand with the fingers relaxed and slightly spread) is most effective at pulling the water. Many beginner aquatic exercisers will ignore or not understand hand positioning in the water and therefore not utilize the water most effectively for toning upper torso muscles. It is important to teach students to position their hands to "work the water" and increase the effectiveness of their workout. Conversely, less

demanding hand positions are useful for participants with weak upper torsos, shoulder or joint problems, arthritis, or any other musculoskeletal condition that would be aggravated by adding of resistance.

Intensity Alterations with Speed

Often the terms "speed" and "velocity" are used interchangeably. Speed is not always the same as velocity. Technically, speed measures the rate at which we move or travel, and velocity involves not only speed, but also direction. In movements that involve only one direction, speed and velocity are practically synonymous.

In water exercise, the resistance of the water increases with the speed or velocity of movement. Many instructors who are unfamiliar with the water's properties will exclusively utilize speed to increase intensity. Although increasing speed does increase intensity, it is highly questionable as to whether it is the most effective way to alter intensity. Applying the principles and laws described in this chapter would increase intensity in a more diverse, safe, and effective way.

When speed is increased, range of motion can be compromised. The most effective way to train a muscle is through a full range of motion. It is also difficult to push against the water's resistance in all directions of movement when using fast, ballistic movements. Many participants are not able to maintain movement at speeds high enough to alter or influence intensity. The instructor often confuses the effects he/she feels with the effects on the class. The only way for a student larger than the instructor (inertia, frontal resistance) or less conditioned than the instructor to "keep up with the instructor" is by reducing range of motion, unless they can apply enough force against the water's resistance to keep up. The instructor needs to offer alternatives that provide a full range of motion with individually styled modifications based on the physical laws. The options include hand position (drag shape), lever arms (bent arms and legs), adding impact (acceleration), using impeding or assisting arms (action/reaction), and traveling (total body inertia). There are other options and combinations of options as well.

Altering intensity with these options would not compromise range of motion or safety. Students could work through a full range of motion against the water's resistance in all directions and promote muscle balance. Utilizing the laws and principles of the water can help individualize intensity alterations through a variety of adjustments, and is a much better option than merely adjusting speed.

The Law of Acceleration – Changing Velocity Also Affects Effort

Acceleration: The reaction of a body as measured by its acceleration is proportional to the force applied, in the same direction as the applied force, and inversely proportional to its mass.

Newton's second law of motion is acceleration. The law of acceleration describes how fast an object will change its direction or speed when a force is applied. Acceleration is how fast you change velocity. If you change velocity over a year's time, you would need only 0.00000003 amount of the force needed for the same change over a minute's time. It expresses the exact relationship between force and acceleration. For a given body or mass, a larger force will cause a proportionally larger acceleration. All objects have mass and objects with a larger mass require a greater external force to change speed at the same rate as a smaller object. As mentioned previously, it would take a lot more force to push a car than it would to push a grocery cart because the car has more mass. The direction of the acceleration of an object is the same direction as the force acting on it. (4)

The greater a vertical force applied to the object over a fixed distance, the higher the object will go. (This is expressed by the equation Force = mass x acceleration or F = ma.) In simple terms, this indicates that the harder you push off the bottom of the pool, the higher you will be able to jump. You can increase intensity using the Law of Acceleration by applying more force to the pool bottom to jump higher at the same tempo.

A heavier object, containing more mass will not go as high as a lighter object when the same force is applied. In other words, a heavier person will not jump as high when they apply the same force. To jump as high, they will have to apply more force to move the heavier mass the same height. This change of motion, or acceleration (jumping up) is dependant upon the magnitude of the force applied and the mass of the object. (This can be expressed by the equation

acceleration = Force ÷ mass or a = F/m.) As an instructor, it is important to remember that not every student has the same mass or the same ability to apply muscular force. A muscular person may have a lot of mass, but will still be able to generate a lot of force to move the heavy mass. A deconditioned person with a lot of fat mass, may not be able to apply very much muscular force to jump very high.

Another concept in acceleration is that it will take more muscular force to move the same mass farther in the same period of time. This concept is very useful for increasing intensity without increasing the tempo of movement. For example, it will require more force/muscular effort to leap two meters to the right every beat of music than it would to leap one meter to the right every beat of music. (see figure 6-7) So another way to increase intensity using the law of acceleration is to encourage your students to travel farther, leaping farther or taking larger steps, with each beat, applying more muscular force.

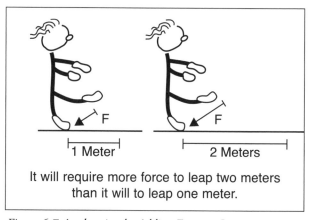

It will require more force to leap two meters than it will to leap one meter.

Figure 6-7 Acceleration by Adding Force to Cover More Distance

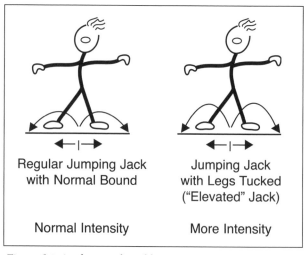

Figure 6-8 Acceleration by Adding More Force to Elevate the Movement

The concept of acceleration also applies to "elevated" moves as described in Chapter 8. These moves require more force to move the legs through a greater range of motion, or a greater distance, in the same period of time. One example would be the difference between a regular jumping jack and a jumping jack where the legs tuck up on the outward movement. (see figure 6-8) To increase intensity even more, the student could tuck the knees up on both the out and in movement.

The table below shows how a regular jumping jack can be made more intense using more force to increase acceleration.

Regular jumping jack, with normal bound on the out and in movements.	Regular intensity
Jumping jack with the legs tucked on the out movement and a normal bound on the in movement. or Jumping jack with a normal bound on the out movement and the legs tucked on the in movement.	More intense
Jumping jack with the legs tucked on the out and in movements.	Most intense

Another example of this concept could be applied when jumping forward and backward. More force needs to be applied to move the legs a greater distance with tuck jumps than with a normal bound forward and back. So tucking the legs as if jumping over a log is more intense than jumping forward and back with a normal bound <u>at the same tempo</u>. (see figure 6-9) More force is required to accelerate the legs through a greater range of motion at the same tempo.

The law of acceleration can be utilized to affect exercise intensity in two ways: 1) by pushing harder (applying more force) against the water's resistance with the arms and legs as you start a movement to come up to speed and 2) by pushing harder (applying more force) against the pool bottom to propel the body up or forward.

Applying more force against the water's resistance provides toning benefits for the muscle groups

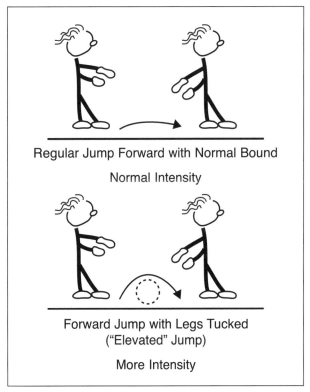

Figure 6-9 Acceleration by Adding More Force to Elevate the Movement

performing the movement. It also requires more effort and energy expenditure. Casually pushing the arms forward along the water's surface (easy) while doing cross country ski legs requires less effort than alternately pulling the arms forcefully and deep along the sides of the thighs (hard) while doing cross country ski legs. (see figure 6-10)

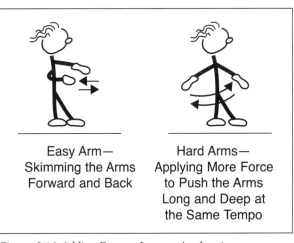

Figure 6-10 Adding Force to Increase Acceleration

Many instructors get confused, thinking that acceleration means simply increasing speed, like pressing the accelerator in your car. This is not completely true.

Think about acceleration as <u>applying more force</u> to move your limb through a greater or harder range of motion at the same tempo.

It is important to understand how to utilize the law of acceleration to both increase and decrease intensity. Movements utilizing less force against the water's resistance or the pool's bottom at the same tempo will require less effort. Examples for <u>decreasing</u> intensity would include <u>skimming</u> the arms through the water (easy), <u>reducing range of motion</u>, taking <u>smaller steps</u>, or <u>impacting less</u>. Movements which position the limbs to <u>work harder against the water's resistance</u> and movements which require you to <u>push harder off the pool bottom</u> to jump higher or take larger steps at the same tempo will <u>increase</u> intensity.

The Law of Action/Reaction

Action/Reaction: For every action there is an equal and opposite reaction.

Newton's third law makes an important statement about force. A force can be described generally as an interaction between two bodies. Newton discovered that forces occur in pairs. For example, you cannot play tug-o-war without people on the other end of the rope. There would be no force for you to pull against and there would be no tension in the rope. In order to apply force on the rope, you need to have people on the other side to provide the other force against which you pull. If you want to play one-man tug-o-war, you could anchor the other end of the rope to a pole to provide the force against which you would pull. Another example would be pushing against a wall. When you push against a wall, it pushes back with equal force. (see figure 6-11) Forces occur in pairs, and Newton named these paired forces "action" and "reaction."

In the viscous environment of the water, this law becomes very apparent. When you push your feet against the bottom of the pool, the reaction is for your body to be pushed upward. More force applied in the action will produce a more forceful reaction. (So you can see how action/reaction is associated to acceleration. Acceleration talks about the amount of force, where action/reaction talks about the paired force.) Hence, the harder you push with your feet against the pool bottom, the higher you will spring up. This is not unique to the water, and the same reaction

occurs when you push your feet against the ground in air. The unique properties of the water make action and reaction noticeable with every movement, unlike air. In the water, when you sweep your hands to the left (action), it results in the body moving to the right (reaction). When you push your arms forward (action), it results in the body being pushed backward (reaction). (see figure 6-11) This viscous environment presents an additional challenge when attempting to combine arm and leg movements.

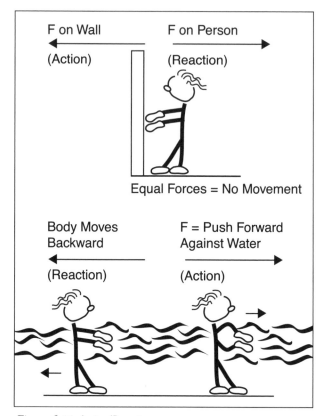

Figure 6-11 Action/Reaction

It is possible for an instructor to pair arm and leg movements that are acceptable but are not utilizing the water to its fullest extent. For example, an instructor could combine a knee lift with a lateral bent arm sweep downwards (pulling bent arms down to the waist). This movement is commonly performed in land programs. This move would work in the water but could be performed more effectively. Analyzing the movement using the law of action/reaction shows an upward lift of the body (reaction) as the leg pushes off the bottom of the pool (action) to propel the body and lift the knee. The upward lifting of the knee (action) would provide limited resistance to the upward movement produced from the jump by causing a downward reaction. Overall, the primary tendency or reaction of the body in a knee lift would be upward movement. Now incorporate the movement of the arms with the legs. When the arms sweep downward (action), the body tends to move upward (reaction). The downward sweep of the arms causing an upward movement, would be "assisting" the upward movement produced by the legs. As stated previously, this movement is perfectly acceptable.

But if the instructor wants to increase intensity, a more effective combination of the legs and arms should be considered. If the arm movement is changed, to have the arms sweep up (action) during the knee lift, the result would be a downward force (reaction) on the body. More turbulence and resistance would be created with this move because the upward reaction of the knee lift would be opposing the downward reaction of the arm sweep. When the arms and legs are used to create opposing reactions, the arms are considered to be "impeding" the leg movement. So "assisting" arm movements would create less turbulence and resistance and be less intense, where "impeding" arms would create more turbulence and resistance and be more intense.

The limbs can also be used to assist or impede movement when traveling in the water as well as in stationary movement. Front crawl arms or sweeping the arms back would assist forward movement of the body. Back crawl arms or sweeping the arms forward would assist a jog backwards. Arm movements can be combined with leg movements to assist progress in the intended direction or impede progress in the intended direction of travel. Pushing both arms forward in front of the body while jogging forward would make forward movement more intense or difficult. The reaction of the body to move backward as the arms are pushed forward opposes the reaction of the body to travel forward as the feet are pushed backward against the pool bottom to jog.

The legs can also assist or impede traveling movement. An example would be a kick while traveling forward and backward. The upward and forward action of the leg causes a downward and backward reaction of the body. A front kick emphasizing the upward movement of the leg assists traveling movement backward and impedes movement when traveling forward.

When the arms work in opposition to the legs, more turbulence and resistance are created and the move is more intense. The same is true when the arms are used to impede movement of the legs when traveling. Arms that assist the legs when traveling, or work with the legs in stationary movement create less turbulence and resistance and decrease intensity. The fitness level and abilities of your participants should be considered when utilizing the law of action/reaction. If your students are not strong enough or skilled enough to use impeding arms to increase intensity and still maintain body position and alignment, then assisting arms would be a more prudent choice. Safety and alignment are primary considerations when combining arm and leg movements. Providing options and encouraging self-monitoring will allow students of different fitness levels to exercise within the same class.

Levers

The principle of levers was discussed in Chapter 3. This system of levers (with bones serving as lever arms, joints serving as fulcrums, and the muscles providing the force) is what allows movement in the human body. As discussed in Chapter 3, the ratio between the length of the force arm and the resistance arm is what determines mechanical advantage. Even the smallest change in this ratio will increase or decrease the amount of force required by the muscle to move the limb. Although it is not possible to change the length of the force arm (where the muscle attaches to the bone), it is possible to change the length of the resistance arm or the length of the limb. The leg can be made longer by extending the knee and plantar flexing the ankle, and the arm can be made longer by extending the elbow and holding the wrist in neutral position with the hand open.

In exercise, the length of the resistance arm of the lever affects intensity or the amount of energy required by the muscle to move the limb or body part. A knee lift, or shortened resistance arm, requires less effort from the iliopsoas muscle than a straight-leg kick. In a knee lift, the water's resistance along the length of the limb from the hip joint to the knee joint must be overcome. In a kick, the amount of the water's resistance from the hip joint to the toes along the full length of the leg must be overcome. It is easy to understand why a kick would require more muscular effort than a knee lift. The same is true of movements performed with the arms. A lateral lift of the arms with the elbows bent (shorter resistance arm) would require less effort than a lateral lift of the arms with the elbows extended (longer resistance arm). (see figure 6-12)

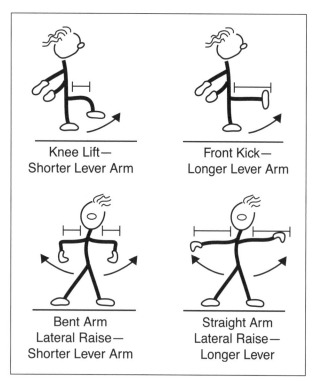

Knee Lift—
Shorter Lever Arm

Front Kick—
Longer Lever Arm

Bent Arm
Lateral Raise—
Shorter Lever Arm

Straight Arm
Lateral Raise—
Longer Lever

Figure 6-12 Lever Arms

A straight leg results in more inertia. Therefore a straight-leg strut requires more energy than a bent-knee jog because the foot is farther from the hip joint. In water, this effect is exaggerated because of the water's viscosity. It also means that a larger person with longer limbs must perform more muscular work than a shorter limbed person to move the same range of motion (90 degrees) in the same time. The longer limbed person would have more inertia effects to overcome because the foot would be further from the hip or rotation joint.

Long-lever moves can be used in water exercise to increase intensity. It is advisable to begin or warm up with shorter levers and then gradually progress to longer levers through the course of the workout to avoid excessive stress on "cold" joints. Most instructors progress to and use longer levers during the higher intensity portion of the workout. It is also important to remember that although increasing the lever arm increases intensity, there is no advantage to working with locked or hyperextended limbs. Maintaining a slight bend in the limb, or "soft joints," actually provides a slight advantage through creating more eddy swirls which increases turbulence. Maintaining soft joints also keeps strain out of the soft tissue in the joint and better insures the intended muscle will provide the effort.

Use Table 6-1 to review the properties and laws of motion in the water that affect and determine muscular effort or intensity. It is important to learn

Table 6-1

Increasing and Decreasing Intensity in Water Exercise		
Law or Principle	**To Increase Intensity:**	**To Decrease Intensity:**
Law of Inertia *Total body inertia, water inertia, and limb inertia.*	Combine movements to start, stop, and change direction, add traveling movements. Use fewer repetitions in a combination.	Repeat the same move for several repetitions, remain in place.
Law of Acceleration *Force and mass.*	Push harder against the water's resistance or harder against the pool bottom to jump higher or take larger steps.	Skim the arms through the water, reduce range of motion, take smaller steps, impact less.
Law of Action/Reaction *Opposing forces.*	Use impeding arms, legs, or combinations.	Use assisting arms, legs, or combinations.
Frontal Resistance *Frontal surface area.*	Increase the size of the frontal surface area presented in the line of travel.	Decrease the size of the frontal surface area presented in the line of travel.
Hand Positions *Slice, fist, open, and cupped.*	Cup the hand with the fingers slightly apart.	Slice the hand through the water or make a fist.
Levers *Long and short levers.*	Use long levers with extended arms and legs.	Use shorter levers with flexed arms and legs.

and understand the options available when creating your choreography. Learning these principles and the effects they have on increasing or decreasing workload for each participant in your exercise program will enhance the effectiveness of your instruction, and is the cornerstone to effective vertical aquatic exercise.

Buoyancy

Archimedes' principle describes the buoyant property of water.

Archimedes' Principle: The loss of weight of a submerged body equals the weight of the fluid displaced by the body.

When standing in water, you are subjected to two opposing forces — the downward vertical force of gravity and the upward vertical force of **buoyancy**. The magnitude of buoyancy is dependent upon the size and density of the submerged body. Since the loss of weight is equal to the weight of the water displaced, the weight and size of the submerged body would determine its buoyancy. A compact, more dense body (a small muscular person) would displace a relatively small amount of water; however, the difference between the weight of the water displaced and the weight of the body might be relatively small. If the weight of the body is more than the weight of the water displaced, the person will sink. If the weight of the body is less than the weight of the water displaced, the person will float. (see figure 6-13) Most people are buoyant to varying degrees, depending on their body size, density, lung capacity, and percentage of fat. Only a small percentage of the population are true "sinkers."

Buoyancy provides many benefits for water exercisers. Buoyancy decreases the effects of gravity and reduces weight bearing or compression of joints. Many people who cannot exercise on land bearing their full weight can exercise comfortably and vigorously in the water. Buoyancy is also dependent upon the depth of immersion, as being immersed deeper will displace more water. A body immersed to the neck bears approximately 10% of its body weight. A body immersed to the chest bears approximately 25-35%, and a body immersed to the waist bears about 50%. These percentages will vary with body composition and gender. Control of motion is impaired the deeper you

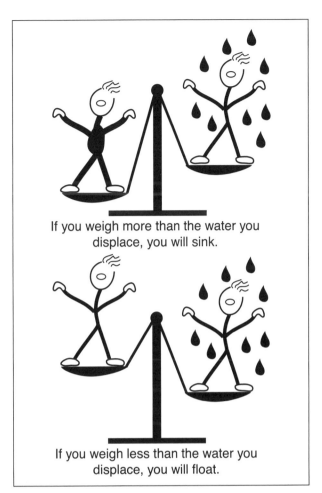

If you weigh more than the water you displace, you will sink.

If you weigh less than the water you displace, you will float.

Figure 6-13 Buoyancy

immerse. Most people can exercise comfortably at chest or armpit depth because they still experience enough body weight to effectively control their movements. Movement speed and control are substantially impaired when immersed to the neck while trying to work in contact with the pool bottom.

If the center of gravity (typically in the hip/waist area) and the center of buoyancy (typically in the chest area) are vertically aligned, the body is relatively stable in the water. If center of gravity and center of buoyancy are not vertically aligned, the body will roll or turn until this balance is achieved. When the body or limbs are moved, this vertical alignment can be altered. Repeatedly taking participants out of alignment and off balance can increase the risk of musculoskeletal injury. Care should be taken when planning transitions and traveling movements in the water to keep the body in alignment or realign the body between movements.

When suspended in the water, your body turns around your center of buoyancy. Although center of gravity is not as important a consideration when suspended, proper alignment of the body remains important. In vertical suspended exercise, proper body alignment increases the effectiveness of the workout and reduces risk of injury.

Just as gravity assists or resists movements on land, buoyancy can assist or resist movement in the water. Since the force of buoyancy is vertically upward, any buoyed movement toward the surface of the pool is buoyancy "assisted." Any movement of a buoyant object toward the pool bottom would be buoyancy "resisted." Any floating movement on the surface of the water would be buoyancy "supported." When moving the body in the water without equipment, you tend to work more against the water's resistance as opposed to its buoyancy. When equipment is added, buoyancy and gravity become more important and affect muscle use. Equipment use is discussed further in Chapter 7.

Hydrostatic Pressure

Hydrostatic pressure is defined as the pressure exerted by molecules of a fluid upon an immersed body. According to Pascal's Law, pressure is exerted equally on all surfaces of an immersed body at rest at a given depth. Pressure increases with depth and the fluid density of the water. Sea water would exert more pressure at a given depth because it is more dense than fresh water.

This hydrostatic pressure affects internal organs of the body as well as the body's surface or skin. Hydrostatic pressure can decrease swelling and pressure, especially in the lower extremities which are immersed deeper. It offsets the tendency of blood to pool in the lower extremities during exercise and aids venous return to the heart. It can also help to condition the muscles used to inhale and exhale as pressure is exerted on the chest cavity. However, people who have respiratory disorders may have difficulty breathing in the water because of hydrostatic pressure.

Although hydrostatic pressure has no direct relationship to intensity in water exercise, it does have an effect on bodily systems and organs. As mentioned above, this pressure can affect the vascular and respiratory systems. As mentioned in Chapter 4, it is believed that hydrostatic pressure may be at least partially responsible for lower working heart rates in the water. Hydrostatic pressure also exerts "even" tactile

input and assists with increasing awareness of body parts, which is of benefit in the therapeutic setting.

Surface Tension

Surface tension is described as the force exerted between the surface molecules of a fluid. This surface tension creates a "skin" on top of the water which may be difficult for special population participants to "break" through. Some participants may need assistance when getting out of the water due to the surface tension of the water.

As a limb breaks through the surface of the water into the air, the change of viscosity and breaking the tension of the surface of the water can result in ballistic movements and torque for the joints involved. It is recommended that movements be performed under the water's surface or over the water's surface, but not interchangeably between the two. The additional torque and ballistic movement will increase risk of overuse or acute injury to the joints involved, usually the shoulder. Certain swimming strokes such as the front crawl and back crawl, involving circumduction at the shoulder joint without equipment, are an exception to this recommendation.

Drag and Turbulence

For swimmers and boaters, drag and turbulence are a hindrance. But for the aquatic instructor, drag and turbulence are major beneficial tools for individualizing exercise in a group environment by allowing the instructor to increase or decrease intensity. The following discussion is an attempt to better explain the constant interaction of the physical laws and aquatic class planning.

Drag is the force you feel that opposes your movements in the water. As previously stated, this force is affected by the frontal surface area of the object, the velocity of the object, and also by the shape of the object. Most muscles produce motions around joints which are opposed in the water by moments and inertia. Moments are the product of the force and the distance of the force from the moving joints. The velocity of an object (for example, the hand) is also a function of the distance from the moving joint. This combination of effects can be illustrated in that drag caused by the hand becomes extremely important in affecting the work done by the shoulder and/or elbow muscles. The work of the shoulder muscles due to the drag on the hand is therefore affected by both the change in velocity of the hand movement (a function of the distance from the shoulder) and by the distance of the hand from the shoulder.

The drag shape of the hand is another effect to discuss. This effect is due to both frontal surface area and shape. Everyone can feel the effect of frontal surface area when using a slicing versus a flat hand. The effect of shape can be easily felt from a cupped hand versus a flat hand. A cupped shape has a higher drag coefficient than a flat shape with the same area if the cupped hand is facing the direction of motion. The drag force is increased by approximately 40 percent. Drag coefficient is further discussed in Chapter 7.

Lines of people water walking are just like bike racers. The people behind the first person in line feel much less drag and work less. Motion patterns that prevent prolonged drag "shielding" increase the work effort of the majority of the class. Lines of people walking, where the lines are close to each other but in opposite directions, also increase the average exertion. If a group of people have formed a circle and are walking one direction around the circle, then the water close to the people is accelerated to the same velocity as their movement. When the group reverses direction, the law of inertia says that the water tries to continue to move in the original direction. The people then must apply more force against the pool bottom and the water (acceleration) in order to change the water's direction from clockwise to counter clockwise. More water turbulence would be created if you have two concentric circles walk in opposite directions.

The Aquatic Exercise Association encourages aquatic fitness professionals to become familiar with the laws and physical properties of water. You are also encouraged to utilize these laws and properties to create safe and, as important, "effective" water exercise programs for clients or participants. Dynamic programming will develop your skills as an instructor as well as develop your participants' skills and fitness levels. The best way to appreciate these laws and concepts is feeling them in class. When you are working with clients, take time to think about your experience and the laws. As you are able to make these connections, the laws will be something you "own" rather than something you need to learn.

Summary

1. Viscosity is the property that is primarily responsible for providing resistance when exercising in water.

2. Newton's laws of motion (inertia, acceleration and action/reaction) can be effectively utilized to increase or decrease intensity of exercise. The water's viscous properties make these laws more prevalent in aquatic exercise program design as compared to land exercise program design.

3. Intensity can additionally be altered by changing frontal resistance when traveling, changing the length of the lever or limb, and altering hand positions.

4. The properties of buoyancy, hydrostatic pressure, and surface tension do not dramatically affect intensity but are important in understanding water exercise programming.

5. Utilizing speed or velocity to increase or decrease exercise intensity is not as effective as using Newton's laws of motion and the physical properties of the water to alter intensity.

6. Drag is the primary force we work against in the water. Understanding how to utilize drag effectively increases your skills as an instructor.

References

1. Grolier. (1990). *The New Book of Popular Science Volume 3.* Danbury, CT. Lexicon Publishers.

2. Kinder, T. and J. See. (1992). *Aqua Aerobics, A Scientific Approach.* Peosta, IA. Eddie Bowers Publishers.

3. Miller, F. (1977). *College Physics.* 4th Edition. New York, NY. Harcourt Brace Jovanovich, Inc.

4. Ostdiek, V. and D. Bord. (1994). *Inquiry Into Physics.* 3rd Edition. St. Paul, MN. West Publishing Company.

5. Shoedinger, P. (1994). *Principles of Hydrotherapy.* Aquatic Therapy Symposium. Charlotte, NC. Aquatic Therapy and Rehabilitation Institute.

6. Sova, R. (2000). *AQUATICS: The Complete Reference Guide for Aquatics Fitness Professionals.* 2nd Edition. Pt. Washington, WI. DSL, Ltd.

7. World Book. (1993). *The World Book Encyclopedia.* Chicago, IL. World Book, Inc.

Review Questions

1. By adding the element of travel in aquatic choreography, you are increasing intensity using the law of _____.
2. What is the difference between linear and rotational movement?
3. Friction between the molecules of a liquid or gas is referred to as _____.
4. Which movement is more intense based on frontal resistance: an alternating side leg lift traveling forward, or an alternating side leg lift traveling to the side?
5. True or False? Considerably increasing speed in the water reduces range of motion for most movements.
6. Would pushing the arms forward while jogging forward in the water increase or decrease intensity?
7. Will you sink or float if you weigh more than the water you displace.
8. What is the primary force that causes resistance in the aquatic environment: buoyancy, gravity, or the water's viscosity/drag?

See Appendix E for answers to review questions.

Chapter 7: Aquatic Fitness Equipment

INTRODUCTION

As the experienced instructor becomes more familiar with the aquatic environment, he/she will undoubtedly learn to appreciate the versatility available in water fitness programming. The unique physical properties of water make it a far more interesting and mentally challenging medium to work with than its counterpart, air. Adding aquatic equipment to your workout can add to that programming challenge. Aquatic exercise equipment increases your programming potential by adding deep water programming, resistance training, and variety. Open effective new training possibilities to your students with aquatic equipment by understanding how the equipment works.

Unit Objectives

After completing Chapter 7, you should be able to:
1. Discuss factors for selecting and purchasing aquatic equipment.
2. Define muscle terminology.
3. Identify the major muscle(s) responsible for primary movements in exercise.
4. Describe how gravity affects the muscle action and muscle use for primary exercise movements performed on land.
5. Explain how and why muscle action and use varies for submerged movement as compared to land movement. Give examples.
6. Determine the resistance direction and muscle action/ use for buoyant equipment.
7. Determine the resistance direction and muscle action/ use for weighted equipment.
8. Determine the resistance direction and muscle action/ use for drag equipment.
9. Determine the resistance direction and muscle action/ use for rubberized equipment.
10. Describe the purpose and use of flotation equipment.

Key Questions:
1. What factors should you consider when making an investment in aquatic equipment?
2. What muscles are responsible for primary movements in exercise?
3. How does gravity affect the muscle being used and the type of muscle action?
4. How do the water's viscosity and drag affect the muscle use equation when submerged?
5. When using buoyant equipment, in which direction is the movement resisted and in which direction is the movement assisted?
6. How does using weighted equipment in the water differ from using weighted equipment on land?
7. What is "drag coefficient"? What affects the intensity of drag equipment?
8. Is using rubberized equipment in the pool any different from using it on land?
9. How does the type and size of flotation equipment affect positioning in the water?

Selecting and Purchasing Aquatic Fitness Equipment

Fortunately for aquatic fitness professionals, there is a growing variety of fitness equipment available for use in aquatic training. Some of this equipment is used in land fitness and can be brought into the aquatic environment, and some equipment is developed specifically for use in the water. Following is a partial list of the general types of equipment utilized in the aquatic environment.

• Webbed gloves
• Foam hand bars
• Plastic paddles
• Foam noodles (pictured below)
• Foam belts for around the waist
• Foam cuffs for on the arms or ankles
• Fins hand held, or attached on the ankles or wrists
• Plastic hand held drag equipment
• Plastic drag equipment attached to the legs
• Drag parachutes
• Rubber balls
• Water walkers
• Various hand held weighted dumbbells
• Foam kick boards
• Foam wafers or boards
• Rubber tubing and bands
• Floats
• Aquatic spinning bikes
• Aquatic deck attached resistance training equipment
• Aquatic ergometers such as treadmills, bikes, and ski machines

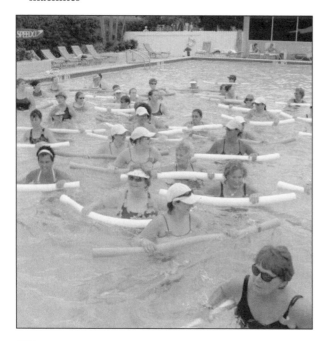

Fitness equipment brings variety and additional training opportunities to your fitness class. Before you decide to invest in equipment, there are several factors to consider in order to prevent purchasing equipment that will not work at your pool, with your population, or hold up in the aquatic environment. Consider these factors BEFORE you invest in and use equipment in your aquatic programs.

1. **What will the equipment be used for?** Do you need equipment to aid in stretching, build muscular strength, or for neutral buoyancy? Consider what you will specifically use the equipment for before you purchase. Is the equipment made for one specific exercise, or are there several exercises that can be performed with a single piece of equipment? Can the equipment be used in several types of class formats? Be sure that the equipment selected can be used to achieve the goal of the intended training.

2. **Who will use the equipment?** Consider what type of population you train, and if the chosen equipment will be safe and effective for that group to use. Can it be gripped comfortably? Can it easily be put on and removed? Can it be moved and manipulated by your population? Will the intensity level created by the equipment be appropriate for your students?

3. **Can you easily store and transport the equipment?** Do you have a well ventilated place near the pool where the equipment can be stored? Many pools have limited deck and storage areas. Some equipment is bulky or must be hung to dry. Can you lock the equipment up, to prevent someone from misusing or abusing the equipment? Can you easily transport the equipment to the pool area? Many equipment suppliers sell bags, racks, cabinets, or bins to store and lock away aquatic equipment. Consider the price of storage when purchasing equipment.

4. **Is the equipment durable and relatively maintenance free?** How long will the equipment last and do you need to buy replacement parts? What is the cost of the equipment as related to the estimated life of the product? Will you have additional revenue to replace or buy parts for the equipment? Is there a warrantee that comes with the equipment?

5. **Can you test the equipment before you purchase?** It is always a good idea to try before you buy. Testing the equipment may reveal

advantages or disadvantages for using that particular equipment for training in your class or at your facility.

6. **Can the equipment be used safely and effectively in your pool environment?** Can the equipment be used with your pool slope, pool bottom, and participant working space? Adding equipment requires more space per student. If you have a small pool, you may have to reduce the number of students you allow in the class with equipment. Is your pool and air temperature appropriate for equipment use? Is there adequate traction to use the equipment?

7. **Will the equipment bring additional students to your class?** Will the equipment pay for itself by providing additional revenue by recruiting participants, or through increased retention to your aquatic fitness programs? Will the equipment have a positive financial impact?

There may be additional considerations for your facility to purchase equipment including budget and equipment availability. It is always a prudent decision to buy from a reputable equipment manufacturer as opposed to making or adapting your own equipment. There may be liability issues associated with homemade or altered equipment. You can use the following aquatic equipment purchase guide to help you make good choices.

Aquatic Equipment Purchase Guide
1. What is the objective of the class or exercise the equipment will be used for?
2. Does the equipment being considered assist the objective?
3. What is the average fitness level of the class or individual?
4. Will the equipment be appropriate for the targeted population?
5. Is the equipment essential for developing a new program?
6. Is the equipment essential for the expansion of an existing program?
7. Is the equipment vital to the retention of existing members?
8. List all of the potential uses for the equipment.
9. What is the cost of the equipment? Are there shipping costs and taxes?

---

10. What is your estimated rate of return on the purchase? (For example: How many memberships will you need to generate to pay for the equipment?)
11. What is your estimated time frame for breaking even?
12. Is there adequate storage and a means of transporting the equipment?
13. What is the estimated life of the equipment? When will it have to be replaced?
14. What is your cost per month or year for replacement or repair?
15. Are you able to try the equipment before buying it?
16. What effect (positive, negative, or neutral) do the following pool conditions have on the performance of the equipment?
   • Pool space
   • Pool depth
   • Pool slope
   • Pool bottom/ surface
   • Water temperature
   • Air temperature
   • Deck space/ maneuverability

Primary Movement and Muscle Actions

It is very important to understand muscle action when considering equipment. It is difficult enough to learn and understand concentric and eccentric muscle action with different types of equipment on land. In the water, you need to understand the effects of gravity, buoyancy, the water's viscosity and drag resistance, as well as understand equipment that is unique to the aquatic environment. It is quite a challenge, and may take awhile to master.

Terminology and Definitions

Before tackling muscle actions with equipment, it is important to clarify muscle actions and review terminology in various environments without equipment. Table 7-1 provides a review, definitions, and explanations for muscle terminology.

Table 7-1

Muscle Terminology

AGONIST:

The prime mover or the muscle primarily responsible for the movement. The muscle that is actively contracting.

ANTAGONIST:

The muscle that opposes the prime mover. Often it yields or relaxes to allow the agonist to contract.

SYNERGIST:

The muscles that assist the prime movers. Secondary muscles or movers.

CONCENTRIC MUSCLE ACTION:

The principle action of a muscle. A muscle generating force while shortening. Dynamic (moving) action. The actin and myosin filaments slide over each other, shortening the muscle fiber.

STATIC MUSCLE ACTION:

Isometric action. A muscle acting to generate force without change in the muscle length. There is no change at the joint angle. The actin and myosin fibers form cross bridges and recycle producing force, but the force is too great to allow the filaments to slide over each other. Examples would include:

• Static contraction of the muscles in and around the pelvic girdle to maintain proper pelvic position and alignment while the legs move.
• Static contraction of the muscles around the scapulae to hold the shoulder blades down and back while the arms move.

ECCENTRIC MUSCLE ACTION:

A muscle generating force while lengthening. Dynamic (moving) action. The actin filaments are pulled farther away essentially stretching the sarcomere.

ASSISTED MOVEMENT:

Assisted movement refers to any part in the range of motion of an exercise movement that is facilitated by the forces of gravity or buoyancy, or by the properties or mechanics of an apparatus or particular piece of equipment. Assisted movement usually manifests as an eccentric contraction. The muscle is contracting and lengthening to control the facilitated movement.
Examples would include:

• The return movement toward the anchored point when using rubberized resistance equipment. (equipment assisted)
• Movement toward the ground or center of the earth (along the gravity vector) if using weighted equipment. (gravity assisted)
• Movement toward the surface of the water (along the buoyancy vector) when using buoyant equipment. (buoyancy assisted)

RESISTED MOVEMENT:

Resisted movement refers to any part in the range of motion of an exercise movement where additional resistive force is created by moving a load against the forces of gravity or buoyancy. The additional resistance force can also be created by the properties or mechanics of an apparatus or particular piece of equipment. Resisted movement usually manifests as a concentric contraction. The muscle is contracting and shortening to move the load.
Examples would include:

• Muscle action that pulls rubberized equipment away from its anchored point. (equipment resisted)
• Muscle action that lifts a weight upward from the ground or center of the earth along the gravity vector. (gravity resisted)
• Muscle action that pulls a piece of buoyant equipment downward toward the bottom of the pool along the buoyancy vector. (buoyancy resisted)

Pure Movement, Movement on Land, and Submerged Movement

Pure Movement

Understanding muscle action without any environmental effects is the first step in understanding equipment use. Use the muscle table in Chapter 1 and use the table in Appendix C to help you review basic muscle action. "**Pure movement**" is muscle action void of gravity, water, or equipment. If you were in outer space, there would be no environmental impact and your movement would be caused by the contraction of the muscle(s) that move that joint.

Example of Muscle Action in Pure Movement: Standing upright, flexion and extension of the arm at the elbow.

Flexion	Biceps brachii (see figure 7-1)	To bend the forearm up or move it out of anatomical position.
Extension	Triceps brachii (see figure 7-2)	To lower the forearm down or return it to anatomical position.

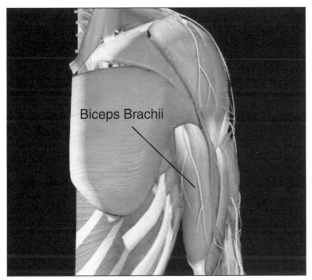

Figure 7-1 Location of Biceps Brachii Muscle

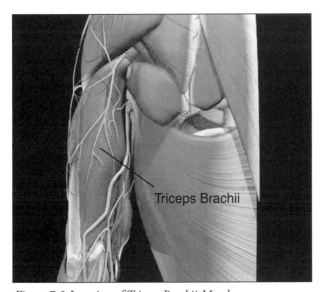

Figure 7-2 Location of Triceps Brachii Muscle

Movement on Land

Movement on land is affected by the pull of gravity. As mentioned previously, gravity is a vertical vector that pulls toward the center of the earth. Any movement performed <u>away</u> from the ground is <u>gravity resisted</u>. Any movement performed <u>toward</u> the ground is <u>gravity assisted</u>. Because gravity assists downward movement, you need to engage an eccentric muscle action to lower a limb or weight toward the earth with control. If you relaxed the muscle involved, the limb or weight would just fall downward, instead of being moved downward at a constant rate with control. See the table in Appendix C to review concentric and eccentric muscle action of primary movements performed on land.

Example of Muscle Action on Land in Gravity: Standing upright, flexion and extension of the arm at the elbow.

Flexion	Biceps brachii	Concentric muscle action
Extension	Biceps brachii	Eccentric muscle action

Submerged Movement

Submerged movement is affected by the environmental conditions imposed by the water. As mentioned in Chapter 6, the primary force affecting movement in the water is the water's viscosity/ resistance/ drag. Because the water surrounds you and affects movement in every direction, every movement in every plane is resisted in the water. Since it takes muscular contractions in both parts of the muscle pair to flex and then extend a limb, the muscle action is concentric for both parts of the muscle pair. See Appendix C to review submerged muscle actions.

**Example of Muscle Action in Submerged Movement:
Standing upright, flexion and extension of the arm at the elbow.**

Flexion	Biceps brachii	Concentric muscle action
Extension	Triceps brachii	Concentric muscle action

Types of Aquatic Equipment and Muscle Actions

After you find equipment to use with your clients, the next step is to learn how to use it properly. Proper use involves understanding the function, purpose, limitations, properties, safety factors, and biomechanics of the equipment. If you understand the properties and biomechanics of the equipment, you are on your way. Safe use and limitations easily follow.

Aquatic equipment falls into five general categories. These categories include buoyant, drag, weighted, rubberized, and flotation equipment. It is important to consider assisted and resisted movement, agonist and antagonist muscle relationships, type of muscle contractions, and the effect each type of equipment has on single and multiple joint movement.

Buoyant Equipment

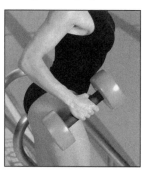

Buoyant equipment is relatively specific to the aquatic environment. This equipment is comprised of a material such as dense closed-cell foam, that floats in the water. Although light-weight on land, it can create a great deal of resistance in the water. It interacts with the forces of buoyancy. We know that the buoyancy vector is vertical, points upward, and buoyancy affects movement toward the surface and bottom of the pool. Any movement toward the bottom of the pool with a buoyant object is <u>buoyancy resisted</u> and is usually a concentric muscle action. This movement goes against the objects tendency to float or be supported by the water's buoyancy. Any movement toward the <u>surface</u> of the water is <u>buoyancy assisted</u> and is

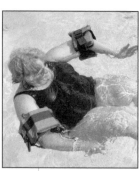

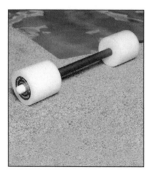

usually an eccentric muscle action. The muscle has to generate force as it lengthens to control the upward movement facilitated by buoyancy. See Appendix D to review muscle actions with buoyant equipment.

Example of Muscle Action in the Water with Buoyant Equipment: Standing upright, flexion and extension of the arm at the elbow.		
Flexion	Triceps brachii	Eccentric muscle action <u>assisted</u> by buoyancy
Extension	Triceps brachii	Concentric muscle action <u>resisted</u> by buoyancy

Weighted Equipment

Muscle action for weighted resistance in the water is very similar to land. Weighted equipment sinks in the water and is influenced by the forces of gravity. The gravity vector, like buoyancy, is vertical but points downward instead of upward. Although the effects of gravity are diluted in the water, as long as the weighted resistance is denser than water and sinks, it will be affected by gravity. The difference is that a 10-pound weight weighs less in the water than on land. Any movement performed <u>upward</u> against the forces of gravity are <u>gravity resisted</u> and usually creates concentric muscle action. Any movement performed <u>downward</u> is <u>assisted</u> by the forces of gravity and usually creates eccentric muscle action. When compared, buoyed and weighted muscle actions are the opposite of each other. See Appendix D to review muscle actions with weighted equipment.

Example of Muscle Action in the Water with Weighted Equipment: Standing upright, flexion and extension of the arm at the elbow.		
Flexion	Biceps brachii	Concentric muscle action <u>resisted</u> by gravity
Extension	Biceps brachii	Eccentric muscle action <u>assisted</u> by gravity

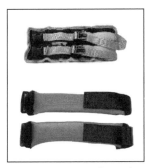

Weighted and buoyed equipment compliment each other well in programming. It is difficult to work the deltoids, abductors, iliopsoas, and erector spinae, for example, with buoyant equipment in the water unless you assume some awkward positions or risk the low back. Most movements for these muscle groups are buoyancy assisted and they primarily work as antagonists. Using weighted equipment works them without a problem. On the other hand, it is difficult to work the adductors, latissimus dorsi, abdomen, and gluteus maximus standing in the water with weights. Buoyed equipment works these groups easily. Once again, it is very important to plan your resistance programming in the water if you are going to use equipment. Use of weighted equipment should be carefully supervised and monitored if done at all in deep water.

Drag Equipment

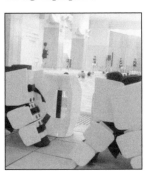

Drag equipment satisfies the muscle balance equation more simply than if using weighted or buoyed resistance. When you introduce a piece of drag equipment, you are just increasing the drag forces of the water. The muscle equation becomes the same as the equation for moving in the water without equipment, however the resistive force has been magnified. You are back to using primarily concentric contractions in any direction of movement. Drag equipment usually increases the surface area or turbulence to create additional resistance for muscle action. Because surface area is increased, drag equipment can be cumbersome and may actually reduce the potential for full range of motion. Your client needs to be careful not to bump the equipment against other body parts and create bruising. Regardless of these disadvantages, drag equipment is often preferred by trainers and clients alike. The movement and resistive forces feel most consistent with natural movement in the water. See Appendix D to review muscle actions with drag equipment.

Example of Muscle Action in the Water with Drag Equipment:
Standing upright, flexion and extension of the arm at the elbow.

Flexion	Biceps brachii	Concentric muscle action <u>resisted</u> by water
Extension	Triceps brachii	Concentric muscle action <u>resisted</u> by water

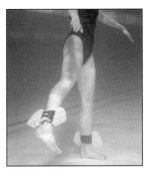

The important concept to note regarding the drag directional force vector is that drag always opposes the direction of movement. Unlike the forces of buoyancy and gravity which always have vertical force vectors, the force of drag can potentially be in any direction depending on the exercise movement. The amount of resistance created by a piece of drag equipment is based upon the frontal surface area or shape, the velocity or speed of the movement, the projected surface area, turbulence, and water density.

The "**drag coefficient**" of a piece of equipment varies with its shape. A square plate has a drag coefficient of 1.00; a circular plate, 1.15; a spherical cup facing forward, 1.40; a spherical cup facing rearward, 1.20; a cylindrical column facing forward, 2.30; and a cylindrical column facing rearward is 1.20. (see figure 7-3) These numerical drag coefficient values indicate the relative difficulty of the respective shape to be moved through the water (i.e., a cylinder facing forward would be harder to move than a spherical cup facing rearward). These relative values presume that all spheres have the same projected area.

The drag force varies linearly with and proportionately to the object's **projected area**. If you select a piece of equipment of twice the area of another, it shall provide twice the drag. Likewise, a piece of equipment that is three times the area of another will provide three times the drag.

Relative velocity, or the speed at which the object is moved though the water, is the most significant factor with regard to the drag force because of the

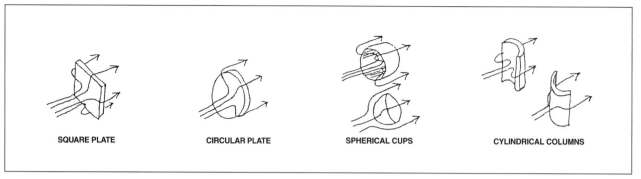

SQUARE PLATE   CIRCULAR PLATE   SPHERICAL CUPS   CYLINDRICAL COLUMNS

Figure 7-3 Drag Coefficient

"squared term." If you double the speed of the movement, the force increases by a factor of four. Likewise, if you triple the speed of the movement, the force increases by a factor of nine.

Since the speed of the movement is such a significant component of the total drag force, instructors will find it very difficult to dictate that an entire class participate in movements at the same velocity. In most cases, the student should be the one to determine his/her appropriate movement speed. Speed regulation dictated by music speed in beats per minute theoretically will only work with participants of equal fitness/ability levels and thus requires careful planning of movement patterns and transitions, as well as variations for different abilities.

Turbulence also affects the performance of a piece of drag equipment. Eddies, vacuums, and other water flow irregularities cause the drag force to increase tremendously. The mathematics required to illustrate turbulence effects are well beyond the scope of this text, but you should know that surface roughness, surface irregularities, surface profile, and holes/slots all contribute to turbulence.

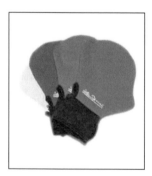

An example of one of the most popular pieces of drag equipment is aquatic webbed gloves. Aqua gloves are worn on the hands to increase the drag of the hands and arms through the water, thus increasing resistance and workload for the upper torso. Aqua gloves come in a variety of shapes, sizes and materials. The type of material from which the glove is constructed will affect its drag. More porous material such as lycra will allow more water to pass

through the glove and will not be as intense as a neoprene or rubber glove. You should choose the type of gloves best suited for your participants.

All equipment, whether it is weighted, buoyed, or rubberized, will increase drag forces to some degree because it creates a larger surface area than just your limbs or body. When you move weighted or buoyed equipment through the water, drag properties will add additional resistance. Although the drag contribution may be minimal, it is still something to consider.

Drag equipment can be used for whole body or cardiorespiratory exercise as well. Drag parachutes used on land for running can also be used in the water to create resistance. Usually a smaller parachute is used in the water. There are drag vests used in swimming that can easily be adapted for vertical exercise. If a client is very fit or in training for a particular endurance sport, you may want to consider drag resistance equipment to increase cardio-respiratory endurance.

Rubberized Equipment

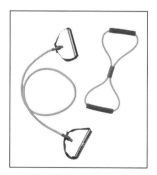

The muscle action created by rubberized equipment is virtually the same regardless of the environment. Any muscle action <u>away</u> <u>from</u> the anchored point is <u>resisted</u> and concentric. Any muscle action <u>toward</u> the anchored point is <u>assisted</u> and eccentric. Rubberized equipment is usually comprised of bands or tubes. The position of the anchor determines the muscle group being worked. In the example below, if you anchor or hold the band lower than the elbow, you work the biceps concentrically and eccentrically. If you anchor the band higher than the elbow, flexion and extension of the elbow would work the triceps eccentrically and concentrically. Many types of rubberized equipment have been created including bands and tubes with handles, straps, and ways to anchor the equipment with your own body or some outside source (door, pool ladder, partner.) Rubberized equipment is reasonably priced, compact, and easy to transport. See Appendix D to review muscle actions with rubberized equipment.

Example of Muscle Action in the Water with Rubberized Equipment:
Standing upright, flexion and extension of the arm at the elbow.

Anchored Low-below the elbow

| Flexion | Biceps brachii | Concentric muscle action <u>resisted</u> away from the anchored point |
| Extension | Biceps brachii | Eccentric muscle action <u>assisted</u> toward the anchored point |

Anchored High-above the elbow

| Flexion | Triceps brachii | Eccentric muscle action <u>assisted</u> toward the anchored point |
| Extension | Triceps brachii | Concentric muscle action <u>resisted</u> away from the anchored point |

Flotation Equipment

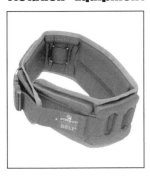

Flotation equipment is generally not used to increase resistance. Instead, it is primarily used to create neutral buoyancy. There are many types of flotation belts available for use in deep water. A client will want to use some type of neutral buoyancy to help maintain vertical alignment in deep water exercise. Neutral buoyancy holds the head above water so various muscle groups can be isolated and exercised. A client may want to use a flotation belt while using drag fins in the hands or on the ankles in the deep water. Flotation belts can also be used with buoyant leg cuffs and hand bars. Flotation equipment can be used for stretching and relaxation programs allowing free movement in deep or shallow water. Sometimes buoyed resistance equipment is used for flotation. An example would be using foam hand bars while in a supine position to do abdominal crunches. In this case, the hand bars would be used for maintaining neutral buoyancy more than for resistance.

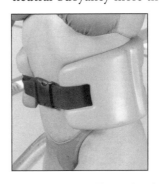

The type and size of flotation equipment can affect positioning in the water. If a belt with a large back piece is used on a client who has a lot of subcutaneous fat at the rear of the body, the added buoyancy may cause a pitch forward. This would make it very difficult for the client to maintain vertical alignment. The client may want to switch the large part of the belt to the front if possible to balance out the buoyancy. If a belt with movable cubes is used, have the client experiment with the cube placement around the body to find where the buoyancy is most comfortable and functional. Body composition, in particular fat deposits and muscle density, will affect the placement and use of flotation equipment. Be aware of how a belt will adjust so it can be large or small enough to fit a client.

Always have your client try out equipment and practice upright recovery in shallow water before going to the deep water. Have your client avoid jumping into the pool while wearing equipment. Instruct them to sit on the side of the pool, put the equipment on, and then slip into the pool from the side, or enter from steps, a ladder, or a ramp. Work with your client to insure safe use of equipment both in the pool and while on deck.

When working with a non-swimmer in deep water, the flotation equipment should be attached to the trunk of the body (belt or vest); also, the individual should be comfortable in water over his/her head and be able to regain vertical position.

Summary Table for Muscle Actions

Table 7-2 is a summary for muscle action for a standing arm curl. This table combines all of the information from the previous tables in this chapter to help you better see the entire muscle action picture. It is quite amazing that the exact same movement, flexion and extension at the elbow, causes different muscle use and muscle actions depending on the environment and type of equipment used. Although it may take time to completely understand muscle actions and equipment use in the water, it is imperative to learn this information so you know the result of each movement.

Table 7-2

Summary Table for Muscle Actions

Environment/Equipment	Muscle	Muscle Action	Resisted or Assisted
Pure Movement Flexion Extension	Biceps brachii Triceps brachii		
Land-No Equipment Flexion Extension	Biceps brachii Biceps brachii	Concentric Eccentric	Gravity resisted Gravity assisted
Submerged-No Equipment Flexion Extension	Biceps brachii Triceps brachii	Concentric Concentric	Water resisted Water resisted
Buoyant Equipment Flexion Extension	Triceps brachii Triceps brachii	Eccentric Concentric	Buoyancy assisted Buoyancy resisted
Weighted Equipment Flexion Extension	Biceps brachii Biceps brachii	Concentric Eccentric	Gravity resisted Gravity assisted
Drag Equipment Flexion Extension	Biceps brachii Triceps brachii	Concentric Concentric	Water resisted Water resisted
Rubberized Equipment Anchored low Flexion Extension	Biceps brachii Biceps brachii	Concentric Eccentric	Rubber resisted Rubber assisted
Rubberized Equipment Anchored high Flexion Extension	Triceps brachii Triceps brachii	Eccentric Concentric	Rubber assisted Rubber resisted

Summary

1. There are many factors to consider when deciding to purchase aquatic fitness equipment. Use the Aquatic Equipment Purchase Guide to objectively evaluate the proposed equipment prior to approaching management with a purchase requisition or personally submitting a purchase order.

2. Also, become familiar with the aquatic environment and its unique properties so that you will use appropriate water-based (rather than land-based) equipment movements and activities for an effective workout, which will yield positive results and keep your students smiling and coming back for more.

3. Strive to learn and understand the properties and muscle action of aquatic fitness equipment so you understand the purpose and results of each movement performed.

Review Questions

1. List five factors to consider when selecting and purchasing aquatic equipment.
2. When the movement is facilitated by the properties of the equipment, it is considered to be _____ movement.
3. When performing a standing leg curl on land, knee flexion is a(n) _____ action of the hamstring muscles, and extension is a(n) _____ action of the hamstring muscles.
4. When performing a front kick in the water, hip flexion is a(n) _____ action of the iliopsoas muscles, and extension is a(n) _____ action of the gluteus maximus muscles.
5. With drag equipment, a lateral arm raise is (resisted or assisted) up and (assisted or resisted) down.
6. Describe how the anchor point affects muscle use when working with rubberized equipment.

See Appendix E for answers to review questions.

References

1. Kuethe, A and C. Chow. (1997). *Foundations in Aerodynamics.* 5th Edition. Indianapolis, IN. John Wiley and Sons Publishers.

2. Lindle, J. (2002). *Aquatic Personal Trainer Manual.* 2nd Edition. Nokomis, FL. Aquatic Exercise Association.

3. Sova, R. (2000). *AQUATICS: The Complete Reference Guide for Aquatic Fitness Professionals.* 2nd Edition. Pt. Washington, WI. DSL, Ltd.

4. Wholers, B., K. Shreeves, B. Shuster, D. Richardson and J. De La Torre. (1991). *PADI Adventures in Diving: Advanced Training for Open Water Divers.* Revised Edition. Rancho Santa Margarita, CA. PADI Americas.

Select Images provided by:
Hillman, S. (2004). *Complete 3D Human Anatomy.* London, UK. Primal Pictures, Ltd. Website: www.primalpictures.com

Equipment Photos provided by:
HYDRO-FIT®
www.hydrofit.com

HYDRO-TONE®
www.hydrotone.com

SPONGEX/AQUA CELL™
www.spongexcorp.com

SPRI PRODUCTS®
www.spriproducts.com

SPRINT AQUATICS®
www.sprintaquatics.com

THERA-BAND®
www.fwonline.com

WATER GEAR®
www.watergear.com

Chapter 8: Aquatic Choreography

INTRODUCTION

Aquatic fitness leaders, whether working in a group setting or training one-on-one, will benefit from understanding how to incorporate the unique properties of water to provide a safe, effective, and enjoyable workout through creative choreography. This chapter will discuss choreography definitions, styles of choreography, and various impact alternatives for aquatic fitness programs. Music options and suggested tempo for shallow water aerobic activity will be provided. Deep water exercise will be discussed briefly in this chapter, with more detail in Chapter 16.

Unit Objectives

After completing Chapter 8, you should be able to:
1. Define basic choreography terms.
2. Demonstrate base moves for aquatic choreography for the lower and upper torso.
3. Identify and differentiate between the common choreography styles used in aquatic exercise.
4. Understand and be able to differentiate between various impact options for aquatic exercise including Levels I, II, and III, grounded/anchored, and propelled/elevated. Describe water specific movements.
5. Demonstrate five basic ways to vary arm use and arm patterns in aquatic exercise.
6. List the pros and cons of using music in your aquatic workout.
7. Describe appropriate use and demonstrate execution of movement in the aquatic environment including land tempo, water tempo, and 1/2 water tempo movement.
8. Demonstrate safe and effective toning exercises for major muscle groups. (Appendix A & B)
9. Demonstrate safe and effective stretching exercises for major muscle groups. (Appendix A & B)

Key Questions:
1. How can you vary the way you present your base moves to your class to add variety and broaden the learning experience?
2. Can you present a variety of impact options to your class to accommodate all levels of participants?
3. What are options for using the upper torso safely in aquatic exercise?
4. How can the use of land, water, and 1/2 water tempo movements add variety and aid safe transitions in your aquatic choreography?

Common Choreography Definitions and Terms

Although the term "choreography" may bring to mind a variety of images, it simply means the arrangement or written notation of a series of movements. Well-planned choreography can make every aquatic class or workout exciting; at the same time it will provide a balanced workout that promotes safety and effectiveness. Below are some common terms and their definitions that will allow an easier understanding of aquatic choreography.

Component or Move

The smallest part or segment in choreography. A knee lift, kick, or jumping jack would be considered a "move" or basic component of choreography.

Pattern or Combination

A pattern or combination is two or more moves linked together to form some type of repeatable sequence in choreography.

Choreography Styles or Types

Different ways of linking together moves or patterns either in sequencing, number of repetitions, or both.

Beats

Regular pulsations having an even rhythm. Beats can be found in music, created by a metronome or other device, or created by the instructor.

Tempo

The rate of speed at which the beats occur.

Water Tempo

An appropriate rate of speed used in the aquatic environment to allow for slower reaction time and full range of motion in water choreography. Recommended water tempo is between 125 and 150 beats per minute, utilized half time for a typical shallow water aerobic class. Slower and/or slightly faster tempos may be utilized depending upon type of movements, program format, level of participants, and resistance equipment usage.

Transition

A transition occurs when there is a change from one move to another move. Changing from a knee lift to a leg curl would be a transition. A transition also occurs when changing from one pattern to another.

Directional transitions occur when the line of travel is changed within a combination or pattern. Leaping four times to the right, turning, and leaping four times to the left would constitute a directional transition.

Alignment and Form

Alignment is the positioning of the body during exercise and transitions. Proper posture and body positioning (form) promotes better muscle isolation and reduces the risk of injury. You should prepare choreography for your class which promotes and enhances proper alignment and form in your students. General alignment and form factors to consider and watch for in your students include:

Upright posture during movement. Avoid bending forward from the spine or waist when doing knee lifts, kicks, inner thighs, etc. Keep the shoulders down and back, chest lifted, abdominals engaged, and the back of the neck long to maintain good alignment.

Try to "place" the limbs instead of "fling" them. Avoid "snapping" the knees, elbows, shoulders or hips.

Avoid excessive twisting of the knees in relation to the foot. The knees should remain over the toes. When doing twisting movements, twist from the waist keeping the hips and legs stationary, or twist from the hip (hip rotation) keeping the knees over the feet.

When lunging, have the support knee over or behind the heel to avoid placing stress on the knee.

When performing a leg curl, bring the heel up behind to slightly above knee height. Bringing the heel to the seat, or over flexing, places a lot of stress on the knees. Keep the knees side by side and slightly apart. Allowing the knee to come forward to curl the leg, works the hip flexors instead of isolating the hamstrings.

Cue

A cue is a signal to class participants. It is the act of communicating information to instigate action through verbal and/or non-verbal signals.

Base Moves in Aquatic Choreography

Movement variations begin with base moves or components. Base moves are the smallest part or segment in choreography. Base moves can be varied to create intensity and variety. Traveling with a knee lift or a front kick would be an example of how to vary a base move and create more intensity through increasing inertia. Components can also be combined with other base moves to create patterns or combinations in choreography.

An experienced instructor becomes more accomplished at creating safe, effective, and efficient workouts. Fostering a deep understanding of the physical laws and properties of water allows the instructor to add variety, balance, and uniqueness in a water workout without sacrificing safety or effectiveness. If an exercise session in the water is choreographed like a workout on land, a lot of what the water has to offer will be missed. The water is a unique environment offering unique movement opportunities.

Below are common aquatic choreography base moves for the legs and arms. Please refer to Appendix A for a description and pictures of several of these moves.

Base Shallow Water Moves for the Lower Body:

JOG (Land on alternating feet)	JUMP (Land on both feet)	HOP (Land repeatedly on one foot)
• Narrow • Wide • In In Out Out • Out Out In In • Knee Lifts • Kicks • Hamstring Curls • Inner Thigh Lifts • Side Leg Raise (Pendulum) • Rocking Horse • Leaps • Mamba • Cha Cha • Crossing Jog (Grapevine) • Side Steps	• Narrow • Wide • Jumping Jacks • Cross Country Skis • Moguls • Twist • Cheerleader Jump • Tuck Jump • Frog Jump • Heel Clicks	• Knee Swings • Kick Swings • Jazz Kicks • Can-can Kicks • 1/2 Water Tempo "Doubles" for alternating feet • Knee/Kick back

Base Shallow Water for the Upper Body:

Movement from the **Shoulder**:	Movement from the **Elbow/Forearm**:
• Abduction (Frontal and Transverse Planes) • Adduction (Frontal and Transverse Planes) • Flexion • Extension • Hyperextension • Rotation • Circumduction	• Flexion • Extension • Supination • Pronation

Choreography Styles or Types

Choreography styles or types are different ways of linking together base moves or patterns either in sequencing, number of repetitions, or both. Just as in land-based exercise, aquatic fitness programs utilize a variety of styles or types of choreography to effectively create a safe, effective, and enjoyable workout. Although many instructors tend to use only one or two styles of choreography, trying a new type of choreography will add variety and fun to your class as well as advance your leadership skills.

Below are the most common styles of choreography which work well for water exercise. The individual moves are described in Appendix A.

Linear Progression or Freestyle Choreography

Linear progression is a style of choreography where a series of moves are performed without a predictable pattern (hence the term "freestyle"). The instructor will generally continue through a long list of moves until the class is finished, with or without repeating any given component. Even though a set combination is not planned, it is still imperative that the instructor understands how to transition safely and effectively into each new movement. Cueing and transitions are discussed in Chapter 9.

Even though this choreography has no repeatable patterns, it is still planned and executed to deliver a balanced work out.

Example:
8 rocking horse right, 8 rocking horse left
16 jogs with knees high
8 leg curls bounce center
8 cross country ski bounce center
16 jumping jacks
16 pendulums
etc.

Pyramid Choreography

In pyramid choreography, the number of repetitions for each move in a combination is gradually decreased and/or increased. The instructor may use 16 repetitions each of four different moves, then repeat those same moves in 8's (8 repetitions each), then 4's, and then 2's. It is also possible to reverse back to the original pattern by repeating the combination in a series of 4's, 8's and finally 16 repetitions.

This style works well for teaching a more complex combination that would be confusing if initially shown in the final format. By building a broad base of repetitions for each movement, the participants can "learn" the pattern with correct technique. Then, with a gradual decrease in the number of repetitions while maintaining the sequence, the workout becomes more challenging – both physically and mentally.

Example:
16 kicks to the front
16 side leg lifts
16 kicks to the back
8 bounces in place
8 tuck jumps

next…
8 kicks to the front
8 side leg lifts
8 kicks to the back
4 bounces in place
4 tuck jumps

next…
4 kicks to the front
4 side leg lifts
4 kicks to the back
2 bounces in place
2 tuck jumps

finally…
2 kicks to the front
2 side leg lifts
2 kicks to the back
1 bounce in place
1 tuck jump

Add-On Choreography

Add-on choreography is a way of building patterns gradually while providing positive reinforcement through repetition as the sequence is learned. It is sometimes called the "memory" or "building block" method. After one move is established ("A"), another move is taught ("B") and then added on to the first ("A-B"). More moves usually follow, one at a time, to develop a simple or sometimes intricate combination.

This style allows the participants to "work out while learning"; it is not necessary to disrupt the flow of the class while teaching the combination.

Example:
Teach and practice "A"…
8 jogs forward with heels high
8 jogs backward with knees high

then teach and practice "B"…
cross country ski 3 bounce center

put together "A-B" and practice…
8 jogs forward with heels high
8 jogs backward with knees high
4 sets of cross country ski 3 bounce center

then teach and practice "C"…
jazz kick (or football punt)

put together "A-B-C" and practice…
8 jogs forward with heels high
8 jogs backward with knees high
4 sets of cross country ski 3 bounce center
16 jazz kicks (or football punt)

Pure Repetition or Patterned Choreography

In this type of choreography, a set pattern of moves is taught in its final form initially. Students learn by repeating the total combination over and over. The number of repetitions needed to learn the pattern depends on its complexity. This style will work well with less intricate patterns and/or with more advanced participants.

Often pure repetition is utilized when the instructor choreographs a specific routine to each different song. In this case the pattern may also include slight variations to accommodate the music (i.e., always performing a portion of the combination during the chorus).

Example:
4 leaps to the right
7 rocking horses right, and turn to the front
8 pendulums
4 leaps to the left
7 rocking horses left, and turn to the front
8 pendulums

repeat pattern over and over

Layer Technique

The layer technique begins with a pattern that can be repeated; the pattern first can be taught via pure repetition, add-on, or pyramid choreography. When participants are comfortable with the pattern, changes are gradually superimposed; moves are replaced with other moves one at a time in the pattern. The pattern can be "peeled back" or "unlayered" to the original pattern if desired.

Example (*denotes the change):
begin with…
4 wide steps right, 4 wide steps left
4 sets jumping jacks in 3's
8 ankle touches to the front
4 front kick bounce center

change to…
4 wide steps right, 4 wide steps left
4 sets jumping jacks in 3's
8 ankle touches to the front
*2 sets of knee swing 3 bounce center

change to…
4 wide steps right, 4 wide steps left
4 sets jumping jacks in 3's
*8 leg curls
2 sets of knee swing 3 bounce center

change to…
4 wide steps right, 4 wide steps left
*8 jumping jacks with ankle cross
8 leg curls
2 sets of knee swing 3 bounce center

finally end with…
*8 slides to the right, 8 slides to the left
8 jumping jacks with ankle cross
8 leg curls
2 sets of knee swing 3 bounce center

As an instructor, you are not limited to the five styles of choreography discussed; other styles or methods may also be utilized. However, the styles shown above are relatively simple and work well in the water. Often instructors become proficient and comfortable using one style of choreography. By stepping out of your comfort zone and introducing a variety of choreography styles to your class, you may be reaching and motivating a greater number of students with the learning process. People have different learning styles or preferences. Teaching freestyle choreography may appeal to some students because of its non-repeating style. It may, however, be unappealing to a student who likes order and patterns. Building block choreography may appeal to the part-whole learner because of its introduction of one element at a time. On the other hand, it may be frustrating to the whole-part learner who would prefer seeing the entire pattern first.

It is impossible to cater to each student individually in a group setting. You can, however, touch the preferred learning style of most of your students for at least part of the class by using various choreography styles. This may draw a larger population to your class as well as provide both familiarity and challenge to all students. Varying your choreography can add to your student's overall feelings of satisfaction and enjoyment. By simply incorporating different styles of choreography into aquatic fitness programs, old moves feel new and fresh. Instructors can expand their skill by introducing new methods of choreography as well as new movements and combinations. Participants will enjoy the change!

Impact Options for Aquatic Exercise

Water is an excellent medium for exercise because of the reduced gravitational forces experienced by the body when partially submerged. This provides a lower impact alternative to land-based programming. Even within the aquatic realm, we can modify the impact forces created by the workout. It is important as an instructor to keep this in mind as our students will often adapt to increasing the intensity of their workout, but may not physically be able to increase the impact. Many participants choose the water specifically for a lower impact exercise alternative.

Obviously the depth of water will directly affect the amount of impact transferred through the musculoskeletal system. Moving deeper in the water decreases the impact for a given exercise. Exercising without touching the pool bottom, as in deep water exercise, will actually create a non-impact workout.

How we perform a given movement will also influence the amount of force with which we strike the pool bottom. Compare the difference in strike forces of walking and jogging on land. Many movements can be performed in the water either with a bounding (jogging) or a non-bounding (walking) style. [Note: It is difficult to perform non-bounding moves if exercising in armpit depth or greater.] Incorporating both techniques allows for greater variety in your choreography and at the same time allows for students to choose the option which works best for their own ability level. We can take the bounding moves a step further and make them "plyometric" in nature by pushing forcefully off the pool bottom to propel the body up and out of the water. The intensity and impact will both increase.

Following are basic impact variations typically used in aquatic choreography.

Impact Level Variations

Choreography designed in various levels of impact will offer additional movement opportunities for your students. Level I, II, and III movements are impact variations unique to the water and can be successfully performed because of the buoyant properties of the water. Level II and III movements should be performed in water which is chest to armpit depth to allow for freedom of movement of the legs and arms without the risk of striking the feet or toes on the pool bottom. In water that is too shallow, Level II movement would involve excessive hip and knee flexion while range of motion would be hindered in Level III movements.

Level I movements are performed in an upright position with water level at waist to armpit depth. Impact is most commonly used in Level I movement. A bounding jumping jack, kick, knee lift, or leg curl would all be examples of Level I movement. Level I movements, or regular rebound, utilizes acceleration to push students up out of the water increasing intensity and impact. Most Level I movements can also be performed with less impact, for example marching instead of jogging. (see section on Grounded/Anchored Movement)

Level II movement is performed by flexing at the hips and knees to submerge the body to shoulder depth while executing the move. Impact is virtually eliminated although contact is still made with the pool bottom. Shoulders remain at the water's surface as opposed to the body moving up and down as in Level I. Many instructors and students have the misconception that Level II movement is less intense than Level I movement because it lacks impact. Level II movements challenge the muscular system to exert energy due to the absence of momentum - unlike performing Level I or rebounding moves. By flexing at the hips and knees, leg levers are altered in a way that can create more drag forces. By eliminating vertical force, more horizontal force can and should be created by increasing range of motion. Level II encourages the participant to increase intensity by creating more horizontal force against the water's resistance as opposed to vertical force. Participants need to be properly instructed and encouraged to create this force in order to reap the benefits of Level II movement while enjoying the variety it creates. There is a slight upward shift in the upper torso workload due to the arm levers being submerged deeper under water.

Level III movements are performed without touching the pool bottom. The body is submerged to the shoulders as in Level II, while the participant is encouraged to perform the movement without having their feet strike or touch the bottom. Impact is completely eliminated and workload is shifted more to the upper body (keeping the body buoyant) and the torso (stabilization and alignment) as the movement is executed. Jumping jacks and cross country skis are common movements performed at Level III. The challenge of Level III movement is determined in part by body size and density. A more dense (muscular, lean) participant will need to expend more energy to remain afloat as compared to a more buoyant participant. All participants should be encouraged to exert force against the water's horizontal forces and use full range of motion to maintain intensity. Participants who are not comfortable with taking their feet off the bottom of the pool can be encouraged to perform the movement at Level I or II instead.

One additional option in impact is to combine Level II and Level III. The shoulders remain submerged while for part of the move you touch down (Level II), and another part you remain suspended (Level III). For example, a jumping jack can be performed on all three levels. It can also be performed as a combination: Level II touching down on the "out" movement and Level III remaining tucked on the "in" movement. This could be cued "Jack touch OUT, tuck and hold IN" or more simply "Jack and Tuck" once the participant is in Level II. A cross country ski, bounce center could be done the same way; touching when the legs are apart front to back and suspended (tuck) as the legs switch positions.

Grounded/Anchored Movement

Just as on land, impact can be a problem for some participants in the water. At times, instructors may desire a low impact way to add variety to their programs. **Grounded** or **anchored movements** are finding their way into more and more class formats providing viable movement variation.

Grounded movements vary somewhat from Level II movements both in body position and weight transfer. Grounded moves do not require the shoulders to be at the water's surface so body can remain in an upright position. Grounded movements are performed with one foot in contact with the pool bottom at all times. A Level II jumping jack would be performed with both legs leaving the pool bottom to move out and in. A grounded jumping jack would be performed as a 1/2- jack (or side step squat) in the water with the right leg moving out and in, then the left leg moving out and in. The 1/2- jack can be performed by alternating right and left legs or by performing a number of repetitions with the right before switching to the left. A grounded cross country ski would be performed by moving the right leg front and back for several repetitions, and then switching to the left. A variation of a grounded cross country ski would be a one legged front or back lunge, stepping front and together, or back and together.

One-footed moves (or alternating lead leg movements) can also be grounded or performed at Level II. The difference lies in weight transfer. In a Level II knee lift, weight is transferred with a quick touch on the pool bottom of the right and left foot. In a grounded knee lift, one foot is left firmly planted. An alternating knee lift in a grounded position becomes a "march." Repeating 4 or 8 repetitions of the movement on the right before switching to do 4 or 8 repetitions on the left is a method often used to create intensity in grounded movement.

In addition to the benefit of creating variety and a low impact option for participants, most grounded movements are easily demonstrated or taught by the instructor from deck. For the most part, participants mimic the movement in the same manner it is performed on deck. With a little creativity, an instructor could offer an entire grounded class or incorporate grounded movements into almost any shallow water format. Instructing participants to effectively use the drag forces of water would insure an intense workout without having both feet leave the pool bottom.

Propelled/ Elevated Movement

Plyometric, or jump training, is a form of dynamic-action land resistance training that became popular during the late 1970's and early 1980's. The term "stretch-shortening cycle exercise" often replaces the term "plyometrics" and describes this type of resistance exercise more accurately. (3) The primary goal of plyometric training is to improve jump ability by using the stretch reflex to facilitate recruitment of additional muscle motor units. Training techniques utilize jumps and tuck jumps in place, jumping on and off a box, and jumping while wearing weight belts. Stretch-shortening exercise can be performed for the upper body, for example, by using a medicine ball. Positive changes in motor performance tests were seen to be greater with concurrent strength and plyometric training than with either training type alone. There appears to be value in adding plyometric training to a program when gains in motor performance and force output are desired.

As an injury prevention method, it is generally recommended that an individual be able to perform a back squat with at least 1.5 to 2 times body weight before doing plyometric training. Plyometric training is considered an advanced training strategy. (3)

Utilizing water can add a new dimension to jump training. Reduced gravity provides for reduced motor unit recruitment via the stretch reflex, therefore making the movement less "plyometric." However, jumping in the water can enable the participant to recruit more motor units via the water's drag, surface tension, viscosity and resistance properties. The advantages of water jump training are reduced impact and built-in increased resistance in all directions of submerged movement. Plyometric training on land, due to its high impact nature, can increase risk of injury to weight bearing musculoskeletal structures. The water's resistance creates additional workload and allows for increased motor recruitment with decreased impact.

Research indicates favorable results from aquatic plyometric training programs. A study conducted at Ohio State determined that "an appropriately designed aquatic plyometric training program is effective in enhancing power, force, and velocity in physically active women." (9) Another study conducted in 2001 (1) found a significant difference in both water and land plyometric training protocols. Both programs improved vertical jump and there was no difference found between the two training programs.

High jumps in the water can be utilized in a typical group class as well as in sports specific training.

Performing movements in chest deep water, combined with lower impact options for less fit students, would reduce risk of injury for most participants. Utilizing the laws of inertia, acceleration, and action/reaction to propel movements upward, forward, or backwards can add variety to movement and increase intensity. Strict adherence to safety including appropriate water depth, appropriateness for the class population, and low impact alternatives should always be considered before adding elevated movement to your class format.

In addition, power or tuck jumps utilize acceleration to increase intensity. However the focus of this type of movement is not to propel the body upwards out of the water (as in propelled or plyometric-type training). Instead, with power or tuck jumps the emphasis is to pull the knees forcefully toward the chest (tucking the knees toward the body) and then push the legs forcefully away and toward the pool bottom to increase the muscular effort. These elevated options can be performed in Level I, Level II, or deep, and add a viable option in program design.

Movement	Propelled/Elevated Options
Bounce Two-footed jump in place	• Tuck jump (knees together) • Frog Jump (knees apart) • Tuck jump forward and back (jump over the "log") • Tuck jump right and left (ski mogul) • Jump and turn (1/4, 1/2, and full turns)
Jumping Jack	• Knee tuck jumping jack (tuck in, tuck out, or both) • Cheerleader (jump and split legs apart to the side- abduction- and land with heels together) • Heel Clicks (start in abduction, jump and click heels while suspended, land with feet apart)

	• Heel crosses (start in abduction, jump and cross heels while suspended, land with feet apart)
Cross Country Ski	• Knee tuck cross country ski • Jump and split front to back, land with feet together

Water Specific Movements

One of the best parts of being an aquatic fitness instructor is to lead your class in **water specific movements**! These movements can be performed in the water (making life fun and interesting), but are impossible to perform or considered high risk on land. Water specific movements often involve taking both feet off the pool bottom at the same time, give a class that "aqua flavor," and make the class a unique experience. Many propelled or elevated movements are also considered water specific.

With a little ingenuity, water specific movements can be combined with traditional movements to create unique patterns that challenge balance, reaction time, coordination, and the mind, without the fear of falling or being hurt. Consider combining the following water specific movements with traditional moves to create challenging patterns or invent some water specific moves of your own. Remember to always test the move before using it. Check it for form and safety, and prepare alternative movements for those who may not want to try water specific moves.

"Kelly Kick"

Kick forward right, left, right. Hold the right leg up in the air and jump over the lifted right leg with the left foot, to end facing the opposite direction with the right leg still lifted, but now behind the body (hip extended).

"Quick Kick"

Jump and quick kick the right leg and left leg before landing. (Front or side)

"Double Leg Kick"

Tuck the knees to the chest, straighten both legs forward, tuck, and lower the legs to the bottom again.

Tuck the knees and straighten both legs to the right (or left) side, tuck and come down.

"Catch-up Kick"

Kick the right leg front (or side) and hold it in the up position. Lift the left leg kicking it up to touch the lifted straight leg and then lowering the left leg again. You are quickly kicking the "standing" leg up to meet the lifted leg and then returning down. Can be performed right or left.

"Tuck and Heel Jump"

Jump and tuck the knees to the chest. Jump and curl both legs behind. This is the equivalent to doing a double knee lift and then a double leg curl.

"Jump and Turn"

Add 1/4, 1/2, or full turns to your movements.

Arm Patterns in Aquatic Exercise

It's easy to overlook arm patterns as a simple way to add variety to movements. Often an instructor gets "stuck" using the same arm patterns with the same leg movements. Participants will find it very challenging both mentally and physically if an arm pattern is changed. It can also add entertainment to the class!

There are five basic ways to add variety using arm movements. The first is to change a specific arm move that is combined with a specific leg move. For example, a typical jumping jack arm movement would be arm abduction and adduction as the legs are abducting and adducting. To add variety, try combining a jumping jack with arm movements in the transverse plane (parallel with the ground such as chest press and elbow pull back) or the sagittal plane (movements done front to back such as pushing front and back.) You can also vary the movement in the frontal plane by crossing the arms forward, back, alternating a front/back cross, or doing a T-jack starting with the arms out to the sides and adducting then abducting.

A second way to add variety in arms is to utilize arm combinations or patterns. The leg movement may stay the same for eight counts, but the arm movement may vary every four counts or for the whole eight counts as in the examples below.

JUMPING JACK WITH ARM PATTERN

Water Tempo	1	2	3	4	5	6	7	8
LEGS	Out	In	Out	In	Out	In	Out	In
ARMS	Abduct	Transverse Adduct	Transverse Abduct	Adduct	Abduct	Transverse Adduct	Transverse Abduct	Adduct

FRONT KICK WITH ARM PATTERN

Water Tempo	1	2	3	4	5	6	7	8
LEGS	Right	Left	Right	Left	Right	Left	Right	Left
ARMS	Push L forward and R back	Push R forward and L back	Push both arms front	Pull both elbows back squeezing shoulder blades	Adduct behind	Abduct and pull elbows in to sides	Adduct behind	Abduct and pull elbows in to sides

A third way to add variation is to use the arms above the water's surface. Arm movements should avoid combining movement in and out of the water (except for some swimming strokes) and should typically stay all in the water or all out of the water for the combination or pattern. If you need to make the transition from water to air or back, consider using short levers to avoid stress on the shoulder and elbow joints. Most instructors use arms out of the water sparingly because arm movement overhead can create instability in the low back if the abdominal muscles are not properly contracted to stabilize the trunk. An instructor may want to consider using arms overhead with stationary movements for safety.

The advantage to using arms out of the water is to incorporate overhead range of motion. The disadvantage is not utilizing the water's resistance. As long as the water depth is adequate, most instructors do arm movements in the water for the majority of their class to utilize the resistance of the water to create upper torso endurance. Arm movements performed safely out of the water can add fun to class by incorporating a clap overhead with a jumping jack or reaching the arms overhead to perform a cheerleader jump.

A fourth option for arm involvement is to keep the arms in a neutral position. Neutral arm movements neither assist nor resist leg movements. Usually a neutral arm is simply held above the water's surface. Holding the arms out of the water helps to train stabilizer muscles such as the abdominals and back. Taking the arms out of the water and crossing them on the chest during water walking may create more work for the trunk muscles while moving through water, a more dynamic environment than air. With the arms out of the water, there would be no arms available to aid the trunk muscles with stability, and the trunk muscles would have to work harder. The difference in resistance for the upper limbs out of the water and the lower limbs in the water forces the body to develop its kinesthetic awareness and challenge the core (torso) musculature to stabilize. You would be trading off upper torso limb training for more intense torso core training.

It is important to inform your students that there will be a dramatic difference between moving body parts out of the water versus in the water. You may also want to note that this difference may feel awkward and take some time to get used to. Safety for the delicate lumbar and cervical spine areas is important. Arms above the head does not mean arms "behind" the head. The arms above the head refers to arms up and slightly forward as if reaching out from the eyebrows or forehead. This reduces the temptation for an instructor or a student to hyperextend the back or neck when the arms are above the head. Arms above the head is a natural position. People reach up all the time, whether to grab a box of cereal or wave good-bye to a friend. This range of motion is necessary for functional development, yet the focus should not be to keep the arms over the head for extended periods. This would put stress on the shoulder girdle and on the deltoids. Once again, consider your students' needs and abilities when making your decision to incorporate neutral arm movements in your choreography.

NOTE:

There often is a mistaken belief that arms out of the water and over head are actually more strenuous because they create an elevated heart rate. In actuality, the use of arms over head stimulates the "pressor response." Numerous studies suggest that arms lifted above the head make the heart work harder to pump the blood against gravity. Arm movement in general does not create the same energy expenditure as the larger muscles in the hips and thighs. Therefore, the increased heart rate created by the use of arms overhead and the stimulation of the pressor response does not typically create a proportional increase in energy expenditure. The exerciser does not necessarily burn more calories or increase the cardiovascular response because of the elevated heart rate in this position. The bottom line is that while the heart rate may go up because the arms are elevated, prolonged elevation does not *proportionately* increase oxygen consumption, fat burning, or improve cardiovascular fitness.

When creating movement variations that utilize a variety of arm patterns, it is important to consider the properties of water. Moving a limb through water, as compared to air, increases resistance through the increased viscosity of the water. It is difficult to utilize the arms in the water without involving many of the large trunk muscles as well. This is why a workout in the pool can be more strenuous than a traditional land aerobic workout for the upper torso and can add to

energy expenditure. A simple jumping jack arm (abduction and adduction) on land involves a concentric and eccentric contraction of the deltoid muscles. In the water the same movement uses both the deltoids and latissimus dorsi, working both parts of the muscle pair. This paired muscle work aids in the development of muscle balance.

Additionally, is it important to acknowledge that arms in the water assist with balance and stability. As a fifth option, you can have the arms merely float (or rest) in the water during activity, making it is easier for a water exercise participant to maintain proper body position and alignment. This can help individuals who have difficulty with maintaining balance and require extra assistance during exercise. However, for fit individuals, "floating" the arms can be used to avoid using the postural muscles and allow the participant to "slack off" during exercise. The core muscles such as the abdominals and back may not be used as much to support and stabilize the body when the arms merely float. Consider the individual needs of your participants and create arm movements to provide a challenge that is appropriate.

In designing your choreography, common sense must rule with arm movements. Arms can be used to assist movement, impede movement, assist with balance, or create a more challenging trunk workout. Arms can be used in or out of the water. Use arms to create variety in choreography, but remember that any arm movement repeated for a long period in one position may actually push the limits of safety. Practice variety and moderation. Be creative with your arms but be safe.

SUMMARY OF ARM USE OPTIONS IN AQUATIC EXERCISE:	
1. Change "typical" arm and leg patterns.	• Combine a jumping jack leg with transverse abduction and adduction. • Combine cross country ski legs with biceps and triceps curls.
2. Create arm combinations or patterns.	• Keep the legs the same for 16 counts, but change the arms in a 4 or 8 count pattern.

3. Use the arms above the water's surface.	• Clap overhead with a jumping jack. • Extend the arms overhead in a "V" with a cheerleader jump.
4. Hold the arms in a neutral position out of the water.	• The arms neither assist nor impede. They remain in neutral position above the water and allow for greater torso musculature involvement. • Example: Cross the arms on the chest while water walking.
5. Float the arms on the surface of the water.	• The arms are used to help with balance and stability.

Music

Music can be used for motivation, maintaining cadence, and achieving a desired intensity. Although music is not required for aquatic fitness programming, an instructor may want to take advantage of the positive reinforcement that music can provide. According to the article "The Effects of Music on Exercise" (6), music can provide many benefits to exercise. Participants perceived better performance when music was a part of their fitness program, although actual performance may or may not show improvement. Music can positively affect the mental attitude of students during exercise; proper music selection is important. In addition, music can evoke pleasant association with the fitness program.

In situations where the acoustics are extremely poor, adding music might create an environment in which it is more difficult to learn and teach. For example, special population groups with limited hearing capabilities may find that music prohibits them from effectively understanding the instructor's verbal cues. Instrumental music selections and emphasis on non-verbal cueing techniques may help to offset these potential drawbacks to music use within an aquatic fitness class. Instrumental selections may be preferred to lessen acoustical problems; vocal cues will not "compete" with the

lyrics. This type of music appeals to programs that are intergenerational (i.e., students of all ages). Other considerations are the music preference of students, ability levels of the class, and the actual pool environment. The depth and slope of the pool will affect the speed of movement as well as the complexity of your choreography.

When utilizing music, AEA suggests approximately 125 – 150 beats per minute (bpm) at half tempo for traditional shallow water aerobics activities. Some instructors choose to utilize alternative music tempos, but choreography must be appropriate. Half tempo simply means counting every other beat. Music of this tempo will be motivating and allow for full range of motion and long lever movements. This speed of execution also enables participants to fully benefit from the water's unique properties.

Execution of Movement

We incorporate three methods of movement when exercising in the pool: land tempo, water tempo, and 1/2 water tempo. Using these three methods assures that proper intensity is maintained during the aerobic portion of the workout and allows for full range of motion in movements. These three tempos provide variations for each movement. A knee lift can be performed at land tempo, water tempo, 1/2 water tempo doubling the knee, or 1/2 water tempo with a bounce center. The tempos can also be combined to add additional variety. An example of a combined tempo knee lift would be to perform 4 water tempo knee lifts followed by 2 knee bounce centers.

Land Tempo (LT)

Recommendation: 125 to 140 bpm used at tempo. When using land tempo movement, you may not want to exceed 140 bpm because of the resulting reduction in range of motion.

Cued: Often cued as "double time" or "land speed."

Some instructors will increase intensity simply by increasing speed. Although this is effective, the quality of movement in the aquatic environment starts to deteriorate as tempo increases. Land tempo movement is the same speed of movement used on land. Impact or movement occurs at each beat. Excessive use of land tempo in the water is not recommended. A muscle is worked most effectively through its full range of motion. Land tempo reduces range of motion considerably, even less than on land, reducing the muscular conditioning effectiveness of the exercise. One of the finer qualities of the aquatic environment is the resistance provided by the water for movement in all directions. Faster speed of movement reduces the exerciser's ability to push against the water's resistance in all directions of movement, reducing water's natural quality of providing muscle balance. In addition, land tempo should be used prudently to avoid increasing risk of injury due to poor alignment or fast transitions.

It is not suggested, however, that land tempo be completely avoided in aquatic programming. Well-placed land tempo movements can add variety and fun to aquatic choreography. Land tempo should be considered in the aquatic environment keeping the following recommendations in mind:

- Land tempo should be used sparingly and should not constitute more than 10-15% of your programming.
- Consider the use of one footed and short levered moves for land tempo. Long levered movements can cause additional joint stress at faster tempos.
- Do not perform movements that combine environments. Keep the movement all under the water, or all above the water.
- Consider using land tempo movements in place. Traveling with fast movement may increase injury risk.

- Be sure that land tempo movements do not sacrifice alignment or joint integrity.
- Combine land tempo movements with water and 1/2 water tempo movements in such a way that allows for slower, safer transitions in neutral alignment.

Water Tempo (WT)

Recommendation: 125-150 bpm used at 1/2 tempo. (67-75 bpm with a metronome.)

Cued: Often cued "singles" or "water tempo."

Water tempo is defined as "an appropriate rate of speed used in the aquatic environment to allow for slower reaction time and full range of motion in water choreography." (12) It is recommended that the land tempo of 125-150 beats per minute be used at 1/2 tempo. This would equate to a tempo of 67 to 75 beats per minute on a metronome.

As stated in the definition, water tempo allows for full range of motion, balanced muscular conditioning, and additional time for safe transitions. The majority of your aquatic programming exercises should be comprised of water tempo movements combined with 1/2 water tempo movements. Water tempo allows full range of motion for long levered movements. When the tempo approaches the higher end of this recommended range, it may become necessary to use shorter levered movements to maintain full range of motion.

LAND TEMPO (LT) MOVEMENTS
**8 LAND Tempo Beats

MOVE	Beat 1	Beat 2	Beat 3	Beat 4	Beat 5	Beat 6	Beat 7	Beat 8
Jumping Jack	Out	In	Out	In	Out	In	Out	In
Cross Country Ski	Right	Left	Right	Left	Right	Left	Right	Left
Knee Lift	Right	Left	Right	Left	Right	Left	Right	Left
Leg Curl	Right	Left	Right	Left	Right	Left	Right	Left

WATER TEMPO (WT) MOVEMENTS **8 LAND Tempo Beats								
MOVEMENT	Beat 1	Beat 2	Beat 3	Beat 4	Beat 5	Beat 6	Beat 7	Beat 8
Jumping Jack	Out		In		Out		In	
Cross Country Ski	Right		Left		Right		Left	
Knee Lift	Right		Left		Right		Left	
Leg Curl	Right		Left		Right		Left	

1/2 Water Tempo (1/2W)

Recommendation: 125-150 bpm used at 1/2 tempo with a bounce added every other water beat.

Cued: Often cued "doubles," "bounce center," or "1/2 water."

One-half water tempo is simply performing water tempo movements with a bounce every other water beat. This bounce is often, but not always, performed high impact in the water. One-half water tempo adds variety to aquatic exercises and the bounce center (BC) can be used to transition from one move to another in neutral alignment. It allows for "more concentrated muscular force in all directions of movement and encourages a greater range of motion" due to the reduction in joint speed. (2)

There are several options for placement of the bounce depending on the move. For a jumping jack, the move would be performed jump out, bounce at the out position, jump in, bounce at the in position. (Cued as a "double jack.") A cross country ski could be performed by jumping the feet apart front to back, bouncing in this position, jumping and switching the feet front to back, and bouncing in this position. (Cued as a "double ski.") It can also be performed 1/2 water tempo by jumping the feet apart front to back, jumping and bringing the feet together to bounce center, jumping with the opposite feet front to back, and then jumping to land with the feet together again. (Cued as a "ski bounce center.") A knee lift, and most other "one footed" moves, can be performed 1/2 water tempo by lifting the right and bouncing one time with the right knee lifted, switching to the left knee lifted, and bouncing with the left knee remaining lifted. (Cued as a "double knee lift.") It can also be performed by lifting the right knee, bouncing center with both feet, lifting the left knee, and bouncing center with both feet. (Cued as a "knee bounce center.")

For additional variety in 1/2 water tempo, the bounce can be performed before the movement. For example, students can "bounce center, ski" or "bounce center, knee lift." When planning transitions with the bounce center first, you may be left in a leg up or leg forward position to start the next move. However, when the bounce is second as previously described, or on the even count, the move sequence ends in a neutrally aligned position (bounce center or BC) allowing for transition to just about any move. This makes 1/2 water tempo a valuable tool for creating smooth transitions and flow in your choreography. Transitions will be discussed further in Chapter 9.

1/2 WATER TEMPO MOVEMENTS
**8 LAND Tempo Beats

MOVE ↓	Beat 1	Beat 2	Beat 3	Beat 4	Beat 5	Beat 6	Beat 7	Beat 8
Jumping Jack	Out		Bounce Out		In		Bounce In	
Cross Country Ski (Double Ski)	Right		Bounce Right		Left		Bounce Left	
Cross Country Ski (Ski Bounce Center)	Right		Bounce Center		Left		Bounce Center	
Knee Lift (Double Knee)	Right		Bounce R up		Left		Bounce L up	
Knee Lift (Knee Bounce Center)	Right		Bounce Center		Left		Bounce Center	

Below are a few examples of combined tempo movements. The more experience you gain as an instructor, the easier these concepts become. Whether you teach from deck or in the pool, effective use of cueing, technique demonstration, impact options, and tempo variations help to create an effective class.

LAND TEMPO (LT) MOVEMENTS
COMBINED WITH WATER TEMPO (WT) AND 1/2 WATER TEMPO (1/2 W) MOVEMENTS
**16 LAND Tempo Beats

COMBINED MOVES ↓	Beat 1	Beat 2	Beat 3	Beat 4	Beat 5	Beat 6	Beat 7	Beat 8	Beat 9	Beat 10	Beat 11	Beat 12	Beat 13	Beat 14	Beat 15	Beat 16
4 WT Knee lifts (KL) with 8 LT Leg curls (LC)	R KL		L KL		R KL		L KL		R LC	L LC	R LC	L LC	R LC	L LC	R LC	L LC
4 LT Jumping Jacks (JJ) with 2 1/2W Cross Country Skis (CC)	O JJ	I JJ	O JJ	I JJ	O JJ	I JJ	O JJ	I JJ	R CC		BC		L CC		BC	

COMBINED TEMPO MOVEMENTS CONTINUED...
**16 WATER Tempo Beats

MOVES ↓	Beat 1	Beat 2	Beat 3	Beat 4	Beat 5	Beat 6	Beat 7	Beat 8	Beat 9	Beat 10	Beat 11	Beat 12	Beat 13	Beat 14	Beat 15	Beat 16
2 1/2W Cross Country Ski (CC)/ 4 LT Jumping Jacks (JJ)/ 8 WT Leg Curls (LC)	R CC	BC	L CC	BC	O/I JJ	O/I JJ	O/I JJ	O/I JJ	R LC	L LC	R LC	L LC	R LC	L LC	R LC	L LC
2 WT with 1 1/2W Jumping Jack (JJ)/ 6 WT Cross Country Ski with 1 1/2W Ski Bounce Center (CC)	O JJ	I JJ	O JJ	O JJ	I JJ	O JJ	I JJ	I JJ	R CC	L CC	R CC	L CC	R CC	L CC	R CC	BC

COMBINED WATER TEMPO MOVEMENTS CONTINUED...
**16 WATER Tempo Beats

MOVES ↓	Beat 1	Beat 2	Beat 3/4	Beat 5	Beat 6	Beat 7/8	Beat 9	Beat 10	Beat 11	Beat 12	Beat 13	Beat 14	Beat 15	Beat 16
2 WT Inner Thighs (IT) with 3 LT Inner Thighs (IT)/4 1/2W Kick Bounce Center (K)	R IT	L IT	RLR IT	L IT	R IT	LRL IT	R K	BC	L K	BC	R K	BC	L K	BC

Summary

1. It is important to know and understand basic choreography definitions and terms common to group fitness instruction.

2. There are Base Moves generic to aquatic choreography.

3. Although aquatic fitness choreography falls into various styles or types, the end result should be the same- a well-designed, safe, and effective program that helps students meet their personal exercise goals.

4. There are various impact level options available for aquatic choreography including Level I, II, and III, grounded or anchored movement and propelled or elevated movement. Water specific movement can be incorporated as well.

5. Arm patterns are often combined with leg patterns to provide toning for the upper torso and to increase energy expenditure. There are five primary ways to use the arms in aquatic choreography.

6. Music, an optional component of any fitness program, can provide a positive impact upon participants and your programming.

7. Water is an exercise medium with unique properties. To be most effective, the instructor should realize the principles that govern the aquatic environment and design exercise movements accordingly. Utilizing primarily water tempo and 1/2 water tempo movements in your choreography will allow you to provide effective exercise through full range of motion.

Review Questions

1. What is the difference between beats and tempo?
2. Which choreography style replaces moves with other moves one at a time in the original pattern or sequence?
3. What tempo does the following chart represent (see chart at bottom of page)?

See Appendix E for answers to review questions.

Chart for Review Question 3

Beat ➜ 8 <u>LAND</u> Tempo Beats	1	2	3	4	5	6	7	8
Front Kick	R		L		R		L	

References

1. Cesarin, T., C. Mattacola and M. Sitler. (2001). Efficacy of Six Weeks of Water Training on Vertical Jump Height. *Journal of Athletic Training.* April-June. 36:2, pp. S-57

2. Denomme, L. and J. See (2006). *AEA Instructor Skills.* 2nd Edition. Nokomis, FL. Aquatic Exercise Association.

3. Fleck, S. and W. Kraemer. (2003). *Designing Resistance Training Programs.* 3rd. Edition. Champaign, IL. Human Kinetics Publishers.

4. Howley, T and D. Franks. (2003). *Health Fitness Instructor's Handbook.* 4th Edition. Champaign, IL. Human Kinetics Publishers.

5. Kinder, T. and J. See. (1992). *Aqua Aerobics, A Scientific Approach.* Peosta, IA. Eddie Bowers Publishers.

6. Kravitz, L. (1994). The Effects of Music in Exercise. *IDEA Today Magazine.* San Diego, CA. IDEA Health and Fitness Association. 12:9, pp. 56-61.

7. Lindle, J. (2002). *Turn Up the Heat.* Instructor Training Workshop. West Harrison, IN. Fitness Learning Systems, Inc.

8. Lindle, J. (2002). *Waved Water Choreography.* Instructor Training Workshop. West Harrison, IN. Fitness Learning Systems, Inc.

9. Robinson, L., S. Devor, M. Merrick and J. Buckworth. (2004). The Effects of Land vs. Aquatic Plyometrics on Power, Torque, Velocity and Muscle Soreness in Women. *Journal of Strength & Conditioning Research.* Vol. 18. p. 84-91.

10. See, J. (2002). *Get Decked.* Instructor Training Workshop. Nokomis, FL. Innovative Aquatics.

11. See, J. (1997). *Successful Strategies.* Instructor Training Workshop. Nokomis, FL. Innovative Aquatics.

12. See, J. (1998). *Teaching with a Full Deck.* Instructor Training Workshop. Nokomis, FL. Innovative Aquatics.

13. Sova, R. (2000). *AQUATICS: The Complete Reference Guide for Aquatic Fitness Professionals.* 2nd Edition. Pt. Washington, WI. DSL, Ltd.

14. Wilmoth, S. (1986). *Leading Aerobics Dance Exercise.* Champaign, IL. Human Kinetics Publishers.

Chapter 9: Aquatic Exercise Programming and Leadership

INTRODUCTION

This chapter discusses the basic

recommendations for developing the

components of an aquatic fitness

program. Various class formatting

options will be considered.

Instructor techniques will be covered

with a focus on safety and

effectiveness. High-risk aquatic

exercise movements and

qualifications for group fitness

leadership will be discussed.

Unit Objectives

After completing Chapter 9, you should be able to:
1. Demonstrate an understanding of the basic components of an aquatic fitness class and be able to use these components to design a safe and effective class.
2. Describe the differences in aquatic program formatting.
3. Understand proper form and alignment when teaching aquatic exercise.
4. Demonstrate verbal, visual, and tactile cueing techniques.
5. Give examples of basic, intermediate, and advanced transitions.
6. Describe the pros and cons of teaching from on the deck and in the pool. Understand the importance of weight transfer and proper cadence when teaching from the deck. Describe various ways to demonstrate moves from deck.
7. Understand why it is important for aquatic programming to promote muscle balance.
8. Describe why some movements are considered high risk or ineffective for an aquatic fitness program.
9. Describe professional behavior and attire for an aquatic fitness instructor.

Key Questions
1. What are the three components inherent in an aquatic fitness work out?
2. What are the primary differences in aquatic class formats?
3. Why is it important for an instructor to teach with proper form and alignment?
4. What is the difference between verbal, visual, and tactile cueing?
5. What would be an example of a basic, intermediate, and advanced transition?
6. Is using high impact from deck to teach class the only option for an aquatic instructor?
7. What movements in aquatic fitness are considered high risk or ineffective?
8. What qualities are employers looking for when hiring aquatic instructors?

Class Components

Whether the aquatic exercise class is in shallow or deep water, strength or aerobic in nature, designed for kids, baby boomers or older adults, the basic program format is similar. The components of a training session as dictated by the American College of Sports Medicine's recommendations should include a warm up, endurance phase, optional activities, and a cool down. (1) The purpose of class formatting is to ease the body into an exercise state and then gradually return it to resting state. Each component serves a physiological purpose to minimize risk and enhance the training process.

A seasoned instructor will use a variety of methods to create interesting program formats while maintaining the key elements of each training component. Change is good. Most clients enjoy variety in class format, from music to movement. When a facility offers variety in programming formats it allows clients to cross train. Program variation usually targets specific fitness components such as cardiorespiratory endurance, muscular fitness, or flexibility. Some class formats provide training for all three fitness components while others may specifically target just one. Regardless of the class format, it is important to remember the purpose for each training component and follow general recommendations for the fitness industry.

Warm Up Component

According to the ACSM (1), the warm up serves the following purposes:
• facilitates the transition from rest to exercise,
• stretches postural muscles,
• augments blood flow,
• increases metabolic rate,
• increases connective tissue extensibility,
• improves joint range of motion and function, and
• enhances muscular performance.

The warm up component consists of three parts. These parts can be performed distinctly in three sections ranging from 3-5 minutes each, or can be combined into one flowing experience that takes 9-15 minutes. You have options for variety even within the warm up component!

The first part of the warm up component is acclimation to the environment. This is important regardless of the mode of exercise. When you go from

indoors to cold temperatures or hot humid temperatures outside, it is important to spend time acclimating before starting strenuous exercise. Students need to get in the water and adjust to the water's temperature. In water fitness, this is often referred to as the "**thermal warm up**." The thermal warm up can include rhythmic movements such as water walking the length of the pool, or a sequence of marching in place or jogging, combined with varying arm movements such as reaching forward, side to side, up, down, and across the body. If exercising in cooler water such as 80-84 degrees Fahrenheit, the thermal warm up may need to be lengthened in duration by 5 to 10 minutes to assure that adequate body heat is generated before progressing to the pre-stretch. The primary goal of the thermal warm up is acclimation to the water.

The second part of the warm up is the **pre-stretch**. One important aspect of the pre-stretch is to generate body heat by moving body parts that are not being statically stretched. You can maintain an elevated body temperature by jogging in place while performing static stretches for the upper body. Likewise, you can hop on one leg while stretching hamstrings of the opposite leg. It is critical to maintain core temperature while statically stretching. Static stretching is typically of moderate intensity, and may primarily have an acute affect as opposed to the long term benefit of stretching during a cool down.

Depending upon the temperature of the water, you may choose not to include a pre-stretch at all, or at least to modify it by using a dynamic stretch instead of a static stretch. Some instructors prefer dynamic or "active" stretching as opposed to static stretching because it is easier to maintain core temperature. If you are in appropriate water temperature, you can choose between a static or dynamic stretch. If you are in cooler water, you should include dynamic stretching only. Dynamic stretches are incorporated into whole body movement. Instead of holding the stretch for 5-10 seconds, as described above, use slow, large range of motion movements to stretch the muscles (i.e. slow horizontal shoulder abduction, adduction to stretch pectorals and rhomboids; slow kicks front to stretch hamstrings, slow kicks back with knee flexed to stretch hip flexors and quadriceps). Whichever method is chosen, it is imperative to keep the core temperature elevated and the limbs warm. Good judgment needs to be used on the part of the instructor considering class members and environmental conditions. Whenever possible, the pre-stretch is a nice component to include, but is one that can be safely omitted if the risks outweigh the benefits.

The third part of the warm up is often called the **cardiorespiratory warm up**. The primary purpose is to gradually elevate heart rate and oxygen consumption in preparation for more strenuous exercise. It is a means of "easing" the body into exercise. The cardiorespiratory warm up allows the body to perform more efficiently during strenuous exercise and makes the transition much more comfortable.

Some instructors will use the cardiorespiratory warm up as a "preview" of coming attractions. New choreography can be taught at a slower pace. This might also be a time to include a social element such as partnered water walking or other formation work. Children would enjoy games that are moderately active such as follow the leader or pretending to be different animals. In a sports training class, basic locomotor movements such as hopping, jumping, galloping, leaping, and skipping done in multiple directions creates an effective and fun warm up that prepares the body for more strenuous programming. Whatever is chosen, however, major muscle groups must be prepared for the action to follow.

If the combination of water and air temperature is not favorable for properly warming the body and preparing it for exercise, class may need to be canceled. If you are in an outdoor pool with a water temperature of 78 degrees F, no sun, and cooler air temperatures with a breeze, it may be impossible to complete a successful warm up. If participants are uncomfortable and unable to warm up, the class may become a negative experience. Communicating and posting policies for class cancellation can help to ward off confusion about when conditions are unfavorable for class. No one likes to cancel class, but if environmental conditions are unfavorable it is a wise choice for safety reasons. Be aware of water and air temperature so you can make an appropriate decision to modify your program format or cancel class if conditions dictate.

Conditioning Phase

The conditioning phase of a class format consists of the primary exercise mode. Generally it is cardiorespiratory in nature, but not always. The conditioning phase may also focus on muscular fitness or flexibility, or all three components.

Cardiorespiratory Endurance Training

For cardiorespiratory endurance training, formatting can vary depending on the mode and type of training. Cardiorespiratory training can be done in a continuous, interval, or circuit class format. Each format challenges the cardiorespiratory and metabolic systems differently. To review these differences, please refer to Chapter 4. The Aquatic Exercise Association recommends water temperatures of 83 to 86 degrees Fahrenheit (29-30 degrees Celsius) for most cardiorespiratory endurance training class formats. This allows optimal response to exercise and you can avoid physiological chilling responses (caused by cooler water temperatures) and the need for the heart to work harder to cool the body (caused by warmer water temperatures.)

Movements can range from simple isolated movements to complex combinations and patterns. Of course, you want to consider your class population. Target the use of large muscles, and perform movements at an intensity to promote oxygen consumption. ACSM recommends 20 to 60 minutes performed in your target heart rate range. The length of this component will depend on the ability, purpose, time frame, and intensity of the class. You can review ACSM guidelines and monitoring intensity in Chapter 4.

IDEAS FOR CARDIORESPIRATORY ENDURANCE TRAINING CLASS FORMATS:	
Dance Aerobics	
Water Striding or Jogging	These programs can be taught in continuous, interval, or circuit formats.
Deep Water Training	
Kick Boxing	
Boot Camp	
Sport Specific Training	
Aquatic Step	
Formats can be developed for special populations including arthritis, perinatal, older adults, larger adults, children, or cardiac rehabilitation.	

Some examples for cardiorespiratory exercise might include: jumping jacks in place, jogging forward with breast stroke arms; cross country ski elevating out of the water; straight leg kicks moving forward. Many formats can be chosen from sport movement and aqua boot camp to dance choreography or kick boxing. Effective use of the physical laws will create a workout that utilizes the principles of water most effectively.

Muscular Fitness Training

The endurance component may target muscular fitness training as opposed to cardiorespiratory endurance. Muscular fitness training includes specific exercises - performed with or without equipment - to target upper body, lower body, or trunk musculature. The intention is to isolate muscles or muscle groups to improve muscular endurance and/or strength.

Water temperature must be appropriate for a muscular conditioning class. If the water is too cold, participants will chill because they are not generating as much heat isolating muscles as would be generated with total body movement. Generally, water temperatures of 83-86 degrees F (29-30 degrees C) are recommended for muscular conditioning. If you are incorporating more total body movement with the muscle isolations, you can use the lower end of this range. If you plan to do a lot of muscle isolation with little total body movement, then you may want to consider the upper end of this range. For muscle isolations, you may be able to use water temperatures above 86 degrees F (30 degrees C). It is not a bad idea to incorporate at least a few total body movement segments during class to insure that body temperature remains in a comfortable range.

Remember the principle of progressive overload when beginning a muscular training program. Do more repetitions with less resistance to promote endurance gains, and use higher resistance to fatigue with fewer repetitions to promote muscular strength gains. Muscular fitness conditioning stations can be alternated with cardiorespiratory stations in a circuit workout. You can also create a class format that uses only muscular fitness conditioning stations. Some instructors incorporate muscle isolation with full body movement as an active rest component in an interval work/rest cycle. Just as with cardiorespiratory training, there are several format options for muscular fitness training as well.

IDEAS FOR MUSCULAR FITNESS TRAINING CLASS FORMATS:

Muscular conditioning program incorporating muscle isolation activities as the primary component of class.

Combining muscular conditioning with cardiorespiratory circuit stations.

Using muscular conditioning for the recovery cycle in an interval class.

Targeting muscular endurance with moderate resistance and more repetitions.

Targeting muscular strength with more intense resistance equipment working to voluntary fatigue.

Targeting core musculature with the water's resistance and/or added equipment. Incorporate stationary isometric, isotonic, and dynamic isometric muscle contractions to enhance posture and energy.

Incorporate muscular toning into a continuous training format. After the cardiorespiratory cool down, do muscle isolation exercises before the final stretch.

Use an aquatic step as a tool to teach a muscular fitness class.

Incorporate muscular fitness into a kick boxing or boot camp class.

Muscular Flexibility/ Range of Motion Training

A third option for the endurance phase of a class format is to target muscular flexibility and range of motion. You must still consider the importance of the thermal warm up and progressive overload when choosing this type of class format. Because of the slower nature of movement in these programs, water temperature will need to be a little warmer. Recommendations for water temperature are between 85 and 88 degrees F or 30-31 degrees C. Enhanced flexibility and range of motion are the primary goals of this class. It is easy to forget the importance of range of motion in a fitness regimen and the role of flexibility as a primary component of fitness.

Yoga and Tai Chi programs have become very popular in land fitness. Many exercisers want this option for variety and to augment more vigorous cardiorespiratory and muscular fitness training. These programs also meet the needs of participants who just want physical activity or lower intensity exercise. These class formats open the door to less active individuals wanting physical activity in a group class environment and expand your clientele.

Aquatic exercisers have reflected this trend with the popularity of Tai Chi, Ai Chi, Yoga, and stretching/relaxation programs in the water. Water adds a new dimension to range of motion and relaxation class formatting. As long as the water is warm and comfortable, buoyancy offers assisted stretching and the component of floating to enhance relaxation. Water provides constant kinesthetic feedback. Many facilities with warm water pools offer these class formats. Vigorous cardiorespiratory formats would lead to the risk of heat related illness while a slower paced range of motion class is ideal. Remember to add full body movement or dynamic stretching segments to keep body temperature elevated.

IDEAS FOR MUSCULAR FLEXIBILITY AND RANGE OF MOTION TRAINING CLASS FORMATS:
Adapted Tai Chi programs
Ai Chi programs
Adapted Yoga Poses incorporated into class
Extended Final Stretch segment to focus on flexibility
Use of Buoyant, Weighted, and Flotation equipment to enhance range of motion
"Weightless" Deep Water range of motion programs
Arthritis/ Fibromyalgia programs

Cool Down Component

According to the ACSM (1), a cool down serves the following purposes:
- To provide gradual recovery from the endurance phase of exercise.
- Permits appropriate circulatory adjustments.
- Permits the heart rate and blood pressure to return to near resting levels.

- Enhances venous return reducing the potential for post exercise hypotension and dizziness.
- Facilitates the dissipation of body heat.
- Promotes more rapid removal of lactic acid.
- Promotes flexibility in the post stretch.

In most aquatic fitness programs, the cool down consists of two parts: the **cardiorespiratory cool down** and the **post stretch**. In the cardiorespiratory cool down, slow, lower intensity, controlled movement is used to help the body recover to near resting values. Walking, low impact movements, or movements of lower intensity are often incorporated into the cardiorespiratory cool down. The cooling effect of the water will often assist with recovery, depending of course on the temperature of the water. The body's ability to conduct heat to the water speeds up the cooling process.

Many instructors will introduce an "**optional activities**" segment in class right after or in place of the cardiorespiratory cool down. Optional activities may include toning exercises after a cardiorespiratory class, or skill work after a cardiovascular sports specific class. The optional activities segment of class may also focus exclusively on abdominal or core work. If included, it usually lasts anywhere from 5 – 15 minutes depending on total class length.

The post stretch consists of stretching exercises to return muscles to a pre-exercise length. Exercise is a series of muscle contractions, or shortening of the muscle tissue. It is important to stretch after exercise to retain and promote flexibility. Water temperature will dictate a static or dynamic post stretch.

Just as for warm up, class format will dictate the cool down as well. If muscular flexibility training was the primary endurance component of class, the cardiorespiratory cool down and possibly the post stretch will be omitted. Often a muscular flexibility class will conclude with a relaxation or centering exercise as opposed to a structured cool down. A post stretch should always be considered after a muscular fitness class. It is important to return muscles to their resting length or beyond if additional flexibility is desired.

Program Format Variations

Other deviations from the general recommendations for class components may be found in programs that have specialized formats. We will discuss the most common formats, any component variations, and the factors that make the workout unique.

Circuit Training

Circuit training is often referred to as station training. The stations can be cardiorespiratory, muscular fitness, flexibility, or any combination. The circuit format can be group led, where everyone in the class is doing each station at the same time. The instructor is teaching each station and each person in class does the same moves and uses the same equipment at the same time. The circuit can be self led, with individuals or small groups rotating around the class from station to station. A circuit class can also be a combination of group and self led. The instructor may alternate leading the class in a cardiorespiratory station, and then have participants move in small groups to various equipment stations. Circuit training is very versatile and is only limited by your imagination.

Interval Training

The aerobic segment of class is composed of a series of work cycles that include high intensity and low intensity segments. The typical bell heart rate curve for intensity level is replaced with fluctuating cycles. Work cycle ratios (high intensity: low intensity) vary with the level and abilities of the students, anywhere from 1:3 to 3:1 usually measured in minutes. With advanced students, the intensity may move into anaerobic training for short duration segments. For deconditioned participants or certain disease states, the intensity may oscillate above and below the lower aerobic threshold. An interval format is especially suited for well-conditioned participants. It is also recommended for sports specific training as similar conditions are encountered during many athletic activities.

Aquatic Dance Exercise

Some aquatic programs are geared to more highly developed choreography sequences and may incorporate dance-oriented movements. The class components remain similar; the difference is found in the level of complexity in choreography, which challenges the participants both physically and mentally. In this type of training, it is helpful to teach segments of the combinations during the warm up to prepare the students for what is ahead. This also prevents unwanted decreases in intensity levels during the cardiorespiratory segment of class.

Deep Water Fitness

This format provides a non-impact exercise option; most other aquatic programs are low or reduced impact. Ideally this class is conducted in the diving well of the pool as it allows for unrestricted, full range of motion movements for students of all heights. The class components will follow a similar course, but the program is designed so that participants do not touch the pool bottom throughout the workout. Deep water exercise can be extremely intense and appeal to very fit individuals, but it can also be utilized for rehabilitation and special population programming since there is no stress impact incurred. Movements must be performed in opposition to develop balance and control. Different types of flotation equipment are available to incorporate into this class setting to allow for neutral buoyancy. Some equipment is more appropriate than others depending upon your students' levels and needs. The final stretch may be performed in a buoyant position or in contact with the pool wall for stabilization. For additional information, see Chapter 16.

Aquatic Step

Step training is a fitness program that incorporates a step (bench, platform) to step up and down from during a portion of the class. It can be performed safely and effectively in a pool environment. Water depth must be appropriate, the pool slope should be gradual to prevent the steps from moving excessively, and adequate space is required depending upon the size of the step utilized. A good indication of appropriate water depth is to have water level at the elbows when the students stand on the bench. This relates to approximately chest depth when standing on the pool bottom. Typically, aquatic programs utilize the step during the aerobic and/or muscle conditioning segments. The step is an excellent tool to be used in a circuit class at a few stations, especially if your facility only has a minimum number of benches.

Striding (Water Walk and Jog)

Striding can be incorporated simply as a warm up and/or cool down for other class programs, or the entire class format may be designed around striding patterns. The choreography is typically simple, making it easy to follow and easy to instruct. Striding programs can encourage social interaction among participants. With simple modifications of intensity and impact, this format can be designed for all levels of students.

Muscular Conditioning

This type of training focuses on muscular strength and/or endurance as well as stretching activities for flexibility. It may be incorporated as a segment of another program or as an independent class format. Muscular conditioning programs often incorporate additional equipment to promote added resistance for continued overload to the muscular system. The key is to isolate specific muscle groups and to utilize precision and control during all movements. Warmer water is beneficial as the amount of full body movement is limited.

Aquatic Kick Boxing

Fitness Kick Boxing is an interval workout that utilizes changes in speed and resistance to create effective training cycles. Aquatic Kick Boxing transfers these training techniques and movement patterns (kicks, punches and blocks) into the water for a high intensity, highly resistive, yet lower impact exercise option. By utilizing the unique properties of the water, in particular buoyancy and drag forces, an optimum cross training program can be created for group exercise participants as well as personal training clients.

Aquatic Tai Chi

Tai Chi, with its flowing and graceful movement patterns, transfers well into an aquatic environment, as long as the water and air temperatures are appropriately warm. Benefits of Aquatic Tai Chi include balance, coordination, agility, flexibility and mental focus.

Ai Chi

Ai Chi was created in Japan by Mr. Jun Konno in the early 1990's. This simple aquatic exercise and relaxation program utilizes a combination of deep breathing and slow, broad movements of the arms, legs and torso. The flowing continuous patterns of Ai Chi are facilitated by warm water and air temperatures.

Aquatic Yoga and Pilates

Many instructors are adapting yoga poses and Pilates movements for use in the pool. Water and air temperature must be appropriate to prevent chilling. Focus is on breathing techniques, core strength, and flexibility.

Pre and Post Natal

Aquatic programs are ideal for women during pregnancy and postpartum because of the lessened amount of impact stress during aerobic activity, the cool and comfortable environment, and the continuous resistance created by the water. Water programs may allow women to continue their fitness program throughout pregnancy when land-based workouts become unsafe or uncomfortable. Another option that has become popular is parent-child programs.

In a perinatal class, the focus should be on maintaining the current level of fitness rather than striving to make significant improvements. The warm up and cool down should be longer and should have more gradual changes in intensity. Choreography should be kept simple and allow for postural imbalances, and proper nutrition and hydration should be encouraged. A physician's approval is recommended for all perinatal participants. Caution students to monitor intensity, limit stretching activities to pre-pregnancy range of motion, and to avoid becoming overheated during exercise. For additional information, see Chapter 12.

Arthritis Programs

The Arthritis Foundation has developed an aquatic certification program for instructors wishing to lead specialized arthritis programs. Other instructors choose to "mainstream" participants with minor arthritic conditions into general programs. Remember that either way, the initial focus of students with arthritis is to regain and maintain range of motion and functional skills. Some students may also desire to improve aerobic capacity, develop muscular strength, and/or alter body composition, but these goals must be achieved without compromising safety. Follow the 2-hour pain rule. If the participant experiences pain/soreness for more than 2 hours after a workout, the work intensity or duration was too demanding.

Warm water is more comfortable and allows for lower intensity activities without becoming chilled. The warm up is critical and should be longer than typical fitness programs. Limit the number of repetitions performed per muscle group, and try to submerge the afflicted joint during movement. Focus on all muscle groups and fine motor skills such as movements in the fingers, wrists, ankles and feet. Safe access into the pool and locker rooms must also be considered. For additional information, see Chapter 12.

Instructor Form and Alignment

"A good example is the best teacher," and as an aquatic fitness instructor, your teaching form provides the example. By demonstrating proper alignment as you lead the class, you encourage the participants to do the same. Maintain correct body alignment, good posture, precise and controlled movements, and proper tempo at all times—whether you are in the pool or on the deck. Correct body alignment allows for the ears to be centered over the shoulders, the shoulders over the hips, and the hips over the ankles from a side view. The chest should be "open" and the rib cage lifted, abdominal muscles pulled inward and upward, and the shoulders back yet relaxed. Avoid hyperextension—in particular the spine, knees and elbows—during exercise demonstration.

Continuously monitor participants for correct alignment and form as well. Specific form cues should be incorporated to reinforce the desired position and/or alert participants to the improper position of the body or limb. It is generally preferable to use positive rather than negative form cues such as:

"Keep abdominals tight and back aligned."

rather than

"Don't arch your back."

Motivational cues can also help to keep students performing the movements correctly. Encourage "good behavior" through positive reinforcements. Remember to always incorporate both verbal and visual cueing to have the best effect. Cueing is discussed in more detail below.

The Art of Cueing

As mentioned previously, cueing is a specialized form of communication. It is the act of communicating information to instigate action. When an instructor uses cueing techniques effectively, a class seems to flow and the student is relatively unaware of how movements develop from one to another. The sequences just seem to fit together. Learning how to use different **types** of cueing and various **delivery** methods is a difficult skill for an instructor to accomplish. It takes practice and experience. Mastery may not be achieved until after years of teaching.

Cues are used to serve several purposes. Below is a list of the different types of cues.

1. **Form and safety cues** address proper posture, safe joint action, appropriate levels of force and intensity, breathing techniques and muscle focus.

2. **Motivational** cues encourage students to act in a positive manner, both mentally and physically. Students should feel positive about their bodies' capabilities and be eager to challenge themselves within safe boundaries and without the stress of competition.

3. **Transitional** cues inform students that a change is about to take place and explains how to make that change safely and effectively. Timing is very important so that transitional cues are delivered early enough to educate but not so early that the timing of execution is confusing. These transitional cues are also discussed in the transition section of this chapter.

   • **Directional** cues communicate the desired direction you want your students to travel or the direction you would like for them to move their bodies. Examples would include move forward, backward, sideward, or move up, back, up and back as in a rocking horse.

   • **Numerical** cues communicate the desired repetitions of each movement or the number of remaining moves before a change.

   • **Movement** or **Step** cues tell students the basic movement that is being performed, i.e., jumping jacks, rocking horse, jog, etc.

   • **Footwork** cues are more detailed movement cues that usually describe more specifically how the lower body should be used. Usually footwork cues are expressed as "right" and "left."

   • **Rhythmic** cues express the musical counts used during movement. Tempo changes and complex counts are considered rhythm cues, i.e., land tempo, water tempo, half water tempo, cha-cha (1,2, 3 & 4), single-single-double.

4. **Relaxation** cues are not only for the cool down and stretch but also valuable during aerobic and muscular training in order to elicit the perception of a comfortable exercise environment while still challenging students. Like motivational cues, relaxation cues are perceived mentally and physically. An example would be "relax your shoulders."

5. **Imagery** cues can be used during intense movement to help students take a "mental break" from the work, possibly allowing for a higher intensity for a longer period of time. They can also be used to facilitate relaxation and stretching.

6. **Feedback** cues are used to maintain an open line of communication between instructor and participants. Inquiring about students' level of fatigue, understanding of described movement, alignment, muscle focus, etc. provides the instructor with valuable information for modifying the daily class plan and class goals.

After considering the type of cue, next consider how you will **deliver** the cue. There are three primary ways to deliver your cue: visual, verbal, and touch (tactile).

Verbal/Audible Cueing

Verbal/audible cueing is the most common type of cue used by instructors. These include any cue that is absorbed by hearing such as spoken words (vocal), whistles, claps, musical changes, bells, etc. Make the most of each word spoken when using vocal cues. Use your voice sparingly to avoid vocal chord damage.

Vocal cueing is most effective when it is:
• given early enough to allow for reaction time,
• limited to one to three carefully chosen words,
• iterated at a rate that can be easily understood by your students, and
• varies in tone.

When you are counting a combination for students, consider counting backwards such as "8, 7, 6, 5, 4, 3, 2, 1." On the last two counts, the instructor should tell the students "where they want to be." Since "3" rhymes with "where they want to be," this is a good memory trigger for a new instructor. By leaving the last two counts for a directional cue, this gives the students forewarning that the combination is about to change or progress. Some instructors do this by counting forward, saving count 7 and 8 for the verbal cue. It may also wake students up from a choreography "stupor," and put them on notice to pay attention for something new about to happen. Transitions that involve changes in movement planes, especially those incorporating long levers, may require you to cue earlier, perhaps on the fifth or sixth count. Keep in mind that the added resistance of the water slows down reaction time.

Visual Cueing

Visual cues may not be used as often by an instructor, but are actually the type of cue that most students notice. There are a higher percentage of visual learners as compared to auditory or tactile learners. In addition, pool acoustics are notoriously poor making it difficult for students to understand the instructor's spoken words. With this in mind, visual cueing is an important skill to learn.

Visual cues include any cue that is absorbed by seeing such as hand signals, eye contact, facial expressions, posture, physical demonstration, and body language. As you use visual cues, watch your class for reactions. If you receive the action you desire from your students, then your visual cue was effective and successful. Video taping to evaluate your visual cueing is a great way to improve your technique.

Tactile Cueing

Touch or tactile cues are not used as often as auditory and visual cueing. The tactile learner learns best by doing. A tactile person practices the movement and masters an awareness of how that movement feels in his/her body. Helping these students with touch to improve alignment and execution can increase the movement's effectiveness and facilitate the learning process. An instructor or personal trainer should always ask permission to touch so clients are not offended or startled. Remember that "manipulation" or forcing a client's body into a movement or position is different than touch, and can lead to some serious implications for the fitness professional. Learn to use touch appropriately and effectively.

EXAMPLES OF VERBAL & VISUAL CUEING TECHNIQUES:

Movement	Verbal Cue	Visual Hand Cue
Walk	"Walk"	Two finger wag
Jog	"Jog"	Whole hand wag
Knee Lift	"Knees"	Thumbs up
Heels Up	"Heels"	Thumbs point over shoulders
Rocking Horse	"Rock"	Wave side, palm front then down
Jumping Jack	"Jack"	Hands together, arch hands up and out, up and in to show jump out and in.

Step Slide	"Slide"	Slide level hands open and closed
Straight Leg Kicks	"Kick"	Use extended arm to "kick" in desired direction
Karate Kicks	"Karate"	Punch with arms straight forward from the shoulder
Jog 3 & Turn	"3 and turn"	Wag fingers three times and then move the hand in a circle
Side Leg Raise	"Pendulum"	Raise one arm to the side and back down, the other arm to the side and back down
Power Moves	"Power"	Make a fist with one hand

Additional Cueing Tips

Strongly consider using all three methods of delivery to reach a wide range of clients. This concept appeals to all learning styles and reaches more of your students. You will actually need to plan and practice cue execution. After designing choreography, practice the movement and plan out the audible, visual, and touch cues that will be used during class. Write down words to be used, when to incorporate claps/whistles, body movement and arm/hand signals, facial expression, posture, etc. Practice delivering cues before participants need them. Cueing with the rhythm of the music sometimes helps with this timing.

For most instructors the skill of cueing does not come naturally. With practice, cueing becomes easier and eventually becomes second nature. Develop good cueing skills from the start to avoid the need to go back and break old habits that might not be very effective. If you are coming to the water from teaching land, you will find that cueing in the water is a little different. Because tempo is so different in the water, it may take additional practice to learn effective water cueing techniques.

If you develop a pattern that you use often, consider making cueing easier by "naming" the pattern. You can actually name an entire combination of 32 counts and only have to cue the pattern with one word. For example, jump forward 8 counts, leap right for 8 counts, jump back for 8 counts, and leap left for 8 counts. Since this movement pattern creates a box, made up of four, 8-count movements, the instructor could name the entire 32-count pattern "Box." This one syllable word reflects the entire combination and saves the instructor's voice. Teach the pattern elements and directions and then gradually reduce the cue to one word.

Also, do not be afraid to use directional cues as step cues. For example, you may always want to say "Go" when you want your students to jog forward. Say "Back" when they jog backwards. Just try to stay consistent. Additionally, it may be advisable if the entire aquatic exercise staff begins to use the same verbal and visual cues. This would make it easier on the students and substitute instructors. The participants could always follow any instructor and using standard cueing techniques would not impair creativity.

Another great cueing technique is merely telling your students to "watch me." If you are not sure how to cue something, or the change is difficult to articulate, a simple reference to the fact that a change is coming may be enough to cue your students for the next step. Additionally, if you have had the same students for some time, they may be able to immediately pick-up on what you are doing.

Sometimes it is easier to have students follow from behind when teaching a more complicated foot pattern. You can look over your shoulder to check on the students, maintain visual contact, and to show them you still care. When you are pretty sure the students are following the pattern, you can turn around to face them again and mirror image them. If an additional lifeguard is not on duty while you are instructing, you will want to turn your back on your students only for short periods of time for safety reasons.

After the class has the entire combination using both the verbal and the visual cueing techniques described in this chapter, then the instructor can start to challenge the students intellectually. See if the students can perform the movements with just the verbal cues. Then see if the students can perform the movement pattern with just the visual cues. Then see if the students have paid enough attention to perform the entire combination without any visual or verbal prompting from the instructor.

Once choreography and cues are designed, practice presenting all of this information in front of a mirror or in front of fellow instructors. Analyze the use of eye contact, body language, precision/control and energy/enthusiasm. Eye contact is necessary to create trust, confidence, and sincerity between instructor and student. Also, eye contact is valuable for giving feedback and other specific cueing information. General body language communicates the instructor's attitude about fitness, self, class format and class participants. Leaning on one hip and slouching says that the instructor is not interested in leading class or in the progress of class participants. Practice positive body language in the mirror every day, including smiling, posture, laughing, focus, and concentration.

Sharpen demonstration skills by distinguishing beginning and ending movement points, using "finished" hands, maintaining desired posture and alignment, and marking transitions with verbal and visual cues. A combination of all of these skills will communicate desired movement, but additional energy and enthusiasm for teaching will electrify programs and motivate participants to adhere to a long-term exercise program. Harness the needed enthusiasm by establishing a pre-class ritual that creates a positive mind set. Some instructors meditate in the car before entering the fitness facility, some listen to a particular song, and others may recite a favorite quote before starting class.

Cueing Style

Cueing **style** is very personal and develops over time. Some instructors find the drill sergeant, command-based style effective while others find suggestive cueing gets results. Depending on the personality of class participants, a blending of styles usually creates an effective level of communication. If a class is generally meek and thrives on strong leadership, a command-based style may prevail. On the other hand, a class of aggressive, strong-willed, independent students may be offended by commands. Experimenting with various styles will quickly identify the cueing styles appropriate for each class. A versatile instructor will be able to customize cueing styles to match the needs of each class.

Smooth Transitions to Create Flow

Smooth transitions from one movement to another are critical in designing a well-balanced and enjoyable workout. The performance of movements, as well as the reaction time for changing movements, is slower when exercising in the water. Although this allows additional lag time to prepare for the next exercise or combination, it also means that transitional cues must be given earlier than in a land-based routine. While cueing on the seventh beat on an 8-count phrase may prepare the students in land exercise, completing the cue by the fifth or sixth beat of an 8-count phrase may be needed for a smooth transition in the water. Aquatic fitness instruction requires different skills than land-based programming, including cueing technique.

Various types of transitional cues can be given for any movement. For example, to cue a "Rocking Horse 7 and Up", you can incorporate any of the following:

- Directional — cueing for the direction the body is moving.
  "Up, back, up, back, up, back, up and turn"
- Numerical — cueing the number of repetitions before change.
  "1,2,3,4,5,6,7, and up" or "8,7,6,5,3,2, and up"
- Footwork — cueing as to which foot the weight should be on.
  "Right, left, right, left, right, left, right, right"
- Movement or Step — cueing to describe the actual move.
  "Rock, rock, rock, rock, rock, rock, rock, kick"
- Rhythmic — cueing to describe the tempo of the step, depending upon whether it is water tempo or water half tempo. You might cue a "single" rocking horse versus a "double" rocking horse.

A mixture of the above types of transitional cues may actually be more effective than relying upon a single method. Novice instructors may find it easier to use a "neutral move" or "holding pattern" between various movements when developing choreography. This would involve returning to a simple "neutral" move such as a jog or bounce in the shallow water before making a transition to another move. This allows more time for both the instructor and the students to prepare for each component of the sequence.

Be especially cautious on transitions where direction of travel is altered or when moving the limbs from one plane to another. These types of transitions may temporarily take the body out of normal alignment and cause added stress. All transitions should feel fluid, allowing change from one move to another or one direction to another without interrupting the energy of the class.

GENERAL RULE OF THUMB FOR TRANSITIONS:

Jump or Bounce (feet together/two-footed) transitions to any other base move in all planes. This makes 1/2 water tempo with the bounce center easy to use for transitions from plane to plane or move to move.

Jog (alternating lead/one-footed) transitions to any other alternating lead base move in the same plane.

Hop (same lead/one-footed) transitions to any other same or alternating lead base move in the same plane.

The water's buoyancy allows students to perform transitions that may be awkward or risky on land. Even with the water's buoyancy, risk of injury increases when the body is out of alignment.

Transitions fall into 3 primary categories: Basic, Intermediate, and Advanced. Your class population, the goal of your class, and the format of your class will help to determine which type of transitions you choose to use.

A **basic transition** is a transition where the next move begins where the previous move ended, or it passes through neutral alignment. An alternating knee lift ends on the 8th count with the right foot on the ground and the left knee lifted. This move would easily transition into any other one footed move, for example a front kick, leg curl, or inner thigh. (see Appendix A

for descriptions of cardiorespiratory movements) This transition would require you to continue with an alternating leg movement, to be a transition that flows. You could easily maintain neutral alignment, with minimal coordination and core strength as you pass through the transition. A basic transition usually passes from a one footed move to a one footed move, or a two footed move to a two footed move and is performed generally in the same plane. For example, a knee lift to a front kick is a transition that occurs from a one footed move to a one footed move, and both movements are in the sagittal plane.

If you have a population that requires basic transitions, and you want to transition from a one footed move to a two footed move (for example- a knee lift to a cross country ski), you may want to consider passing through neutral alignment. The knee lift ends with the right foot down and the left knee lifted on the last beat in an 8 count. Instead of transitioning directly from a knee lift (one footed move), to a cross country ski (two footed move), you could add a bounce center or a 1/2 water tempo knee lift (knee lift, bounce center) to make the transition. This would pass the one footed movement (knee lift) through neutral alignment or a bounce center before going to the two footed movement (cross country ski). This type of transition is simpler to cue and easy for all levels of participants to perform with good form.

An **intermediate transition** requires a little more coordination and core strength to pass through the transition and still maintain safe alignment. This type of transition would be safe for more fit or experienced participants without musculoskeletal or medical conditions. An intermediate transition requires additional cueing skills and choreography planning in order to maintain the flow in class.

If we use the example of the knee lift to the cross country ski, an intermediate transition in this case

Knee lift to a cross country ski- Basic Transition								
Water Tempo Beat ➔	1	2	3	4	5	6	7	8
Knee Lift	R knee	BC	L knee	BC	R knee	BC	L knee	BC
Water Tempo Beat ➔	9	10	11	12	13	14	15	16
Cross Country Ski	R ski	L ski	R ski	L ski	R ski	L ski	R ski	L ski

Knee lift to a cross country ski- Intermediate Transition

Water Tempo Beat ➜	1	2	3	4	5	6	7	8
Knee Lift	R knee	L knee	R knee	L knee	R knee	L knee	R knee	L knee
Water Tempo Beat ➜	9	10	11	12	13	14	15	16
Cross Country Ski	L ski	R ski	L ski	R ski	L ski	R ski	L ski	R ski

Knee lift to a cross country ski- Advanced Transition

Water Tempo Beat ➜	1	2	3	4	5	6	7	8
Knee Lift	R knee	L knee	R knee	L knee	R knee	L knee	R knee	L knee
Water Tempo Beat ➜	9	10	11	12	13	14	15	16
Cross Country Ski- Level III	R ski suspended	L ski suspended	R ski suspended	L ski suspended	R ski suspended	L ski suspended	R ski suspended	L ski suspended

would not pass through neutral alignment. You would end the 8 count of knee lifts with the right foot down and the left knee lifted. By tightening the core, you could safely transition directly into a LEFT foot forward cross country ski by jumping and placing the left foot forward and the right foot back. You could also choose to jump and switch feet in mid water landing with the right foot forward and the left foot back. You want your students to perform the transition with erect posture, avoiding bending or twisting the torso. The student should strive to maintain neutral alignment from the hips upward and use the arms to aid balance if needed.

An **advanced transition** can be considered in choreography designed for fit students or trained athletes. This transition requires additional core strength and coordination to pass through the transition safely. Many times the body does not maintain neutral alignment and the torso may be bent or twisted.

Consider the transition from the knee lift to the cross country ski again. The knee lift ends with the left knee lifted. An experienced fit student could safely make a transition to a Level III cross country ski

with the left foot or the right foot forward. This would require the body to pitch forward slightly and the upper torso to become more involved as the body passes into a suspended movement. The abdominal muscles would need to remain contracted to protect the lumbar spine, and this transition would require a little more coordination.

Transitions in aquatic exercise should be dictated by the population of the class, goal of the class, and the skill of the instructor to deliver quality transitional cues. For new instructors, it may be easier to plan basic transitions that pass through neutral alignment. This gives participants an opportunity to safely catch up if you cue late or forget to cue. A more experienced instructor can start to incorporate intermediate and advanced transitions if appropriate for the class population. If you are just starting as an instructor, keep your transitions simple and safe. Consider using a neutral move such as bounce center in shallow water, or a 1/2 water tempo movement that bounces center to make transitions. This will allow you to develop your cueing skills with simple and safe transitions that facilitate flow and professionalism in your class.

Examples of Basic, Intermediate, and Advanced Transitions.

Movement	Basic	Intermediate	Advanced
Knee lift to a cross country ski (one footed move to a two footed move)	Knee lift bounce center to a cross country ski	Knee lift to a left foot forward cross country ski	Knee lift to a Level III cross country ski
Rocking horse to a jumping jack (one footed move to a two footed move- plane change)	Rock 3 bounce center, to a jumping jack	Rocking horse ending right/front foot up, to a jumping jack	Rocking horse ending right/front foot up, to a tuck knee jumping jack
Cross country ski to a jumping jack (plane change)	Cross country ski bounce center, to a jumping jack	Cross country ski ending left foot forward, to a jumping jack	Tuck knee cross country ski ending left foot forward, to a tuck knee jumping jack, Level I or II
Twist to a jumping jack (plane change)	Twist bounce center, to a jumping jack	Twist ending left, to a jumping jack facing forward	Twist ending left, to a Level II jumping jack facing forward

Methods for Safe and Effective Instruction

There are three options for instructor positioning to teach an aquatic fitness class. The instructor can teach the class
- from on the pool deck
- from in the pool, and
- by going back and forth between the deck and pool.

There are advantages, disadvantages, and safety concerns for all three of these methods. This section outlines the pros and cons of each teaching position, includes tips for each method, and alerts you to safety concerns.

Teaching From the Pool Deck
Advantages:
- You are highly visible to the students.
- You can use your whole body, upper and lower torso, to provide visual cues.
- Often, but not always, you can be heard better from this position.
- You can see what your students are doing. You have better visibility of your class. This is especially important if you are expected to be the lifeguard as well.
- Some movements, due to their complexity, can only be explained and demonstrated from deck where the student can see what your whole body is doing.
- Complex choreography is better explained and demonstrated from deck.
- New students can usually follow deck instruction best because the instructor is more visible.
- It is easier to change or adjust your music.
- Recommended by AEA for most situations.

Disadvantages:
- You are exposed to the elements. (heat, humidity, sun, wind, chill)
- You increase your risk for overuse injury due to slipping or impact.
- Your students may be in prolonged neck extension looking up at you on deck.
- The tempo and execution of movements (air and gravity) must be altered to approximate water conditions (viscosity and buoyancy).
- It is difficult to demonstrate water specific movement from land.

Conveying Movement Execution and Weight Transfer From Deck

Safe and effective demonstration of impact options for various moves and combinations is one of the toughest challenges an instructor faces when teaching from deck. On deck, the instructor needs to portray Level I, II, and III, propelled/elevated, and water specific movements at an appropriate tempo with gravity and without buoyancy. Needless to say, this requires creative thinking and movement, as well as the assistance of props such as chairs, stools, ladders, and whatever else you can invent.

Full (High) Impact

Many water movements can be portrayed on land as they are performed in the water by simply adjusting tempo. Jumping jacks, cross country skis, jogs, knee lifts, kicks, turns, leaps, and rocks can all be demonstrated with full impact on deck. Full impact most approximates the actual mechanics of the movement as it is to be performed in the water. If you want your students to perform a jumping jack in the water, you simply perform jumping jacks on land at appropriate water tempo.

If only deck demonstration were this simple. Most pool decks are made of an unforgiving surface such as concrete or tile, and may be slippery or wet. Instructors who teach using full impact increase their risk for overuse and acute injuries. Most instructors have resorted to the use of low or no impact demonstrations to save wear and tear on their musculoskeletal system. You can reduce slipping and impact stress by wearing a supportive pair of shoes and using a non-skid, cushioned mat on deck. Often full impact is used to demonstrate the first few repetitions of a movement or to motivate. For the most part, it is used sparingly.

Reduced (Low) Impact

Reduced impact (keeping one foot in contact with the ground) saves wear and tear on the musculoskeletal system but challenges the instructor with proper demonstration of weight transfer for 1-footed moves. In addition, students have to be taught to use both legs and impact despite the instructor's use of one leg and low impact on deck. Some instructors hold up signs saying "both feet" or "jump" to help with this problem. Others point out students with proper mechanics for students to imitate or use nonverbal cues to motivate their students.

Low impact at water and 1/2 water tempo can challenge an instructor's balance skills. The use of a pole or chair for support can help with balance during some of the more difficult transitions. Maintaining a wide base of support (feet at shoulder's width or slightly wider) and lowering your center of gravity a few inches (slight squatted position) improves stability and balance and makes many movements easier to perform at slower tempos on land.

Proper weight transfer demonstration on deck for 1-footed moves can better imitate water full impact weight transfer by quickly shifting or slightly exaggerating the shift of weight from one foot to the next during low impact movement. Using a high knee march to demonstrate knee lifts may encourage students to march in the pool as well. Plantar flexing at the ankle and rolling from the ball of the foot to the heel to quickly "shift weight" from one foot to the next gives more of the appearance of "jumping" from foot to foot to perform a knee lift. This technique may better motivate your students to add impact to the movement in the pool.

Use of low impact also makes it easy to teach a multi-level class. Students who can use impact and higher intensity levels are encouraged to do so. Students who need lower impact and/or intensity can perform the movements using low impact in the water. The advanced student can do a jumping jack with full impact or elevations in the water, while the student needing low impact/low intensity can do 1/2 jacks, and a student needing low impact/high intensity can do 1/2 jacks with tucked knees at the same time. Low impact demonstration is often the preferred method of deck instruction for most movements and combinations due to its versatility and safety.

Non-Impact

Some instructors, by necessity or choice, teach from deck with non-impact instructional techniques. This requires the instructor to become more skilled at verbal and nonverbal cueing techniques to motivate students and guide them through transitions and move changes.

In one method of non-impact deck instruction, the instructor supports the weight of his/her body on the arms by using the rails of a pool ladder, two sturdy chairs, or by some other means. The feet are lifted from the ground to perform the leg movement without impact. This method is often employed by deep water instructors to imitate suspension of the body in deep water. Although very effective, suspending the body from the arms for long periods of time can be hard on the shoulder, elbow, and wrist joints. To reduce the risk of injury, the moves can be shown for a few repetitions and then demonstration can shift to another method.

Another method of non-impact deck instruction utilizes a chair or stool. The instructor sits on the edge of the chair and imitates water movements by flexing at the hips and utilizing both legs. This method requires strong abdominal muscles to support the low back, and strong hip flexor muscles. Although chairs are readily accessible, they may not be as versatile as a stool. With a 32" or 36" stool, the instructor can demonstrate moves with less hip flexion. A more extended leg may give students a better idea of how the move should be performed in a standing position. Since the stool has no back or arms, it is easier to demonstrate turning or movements requiring directional change. Many instructors find that several water specific and elevated moves can be taught quite effectively from a chair or stool. Although the mechanics demonstrated on deck are not identical to what is desired in the water, the movements can be taught from a chair or stool with additional verbal and visual cueing for students to achieve the correct movement in the water.

One very effective and widely used method of non-impact instruction from the deck involves "the use of arms as legs." Instructors verbally cue "my arms are your legs" and some instructors even place shoes on their hands to further drive home the visualization. Using your arms to demonstrate the out/in movement of a jumping jack or the front/back movement of a cross country ski works quite well. It is also very easy to convey proper tempo and weight transfer without balance or impact issues. Tempo combinations such as two water tempo and one 1/2 water tempo jack (single, single, double or out, in, out, out) are easily conveyed. Combining use of the arms with verbal and non-verbal cueing can effectively convey most movements with minimal wear and tear on the instructor's body.

Well-inflected and timed verbal cueing can also be very effective in conveying water movements from deck. Often an instructor will use a high impact or low impact means of demonstration for a few moves, then shift the demonstration to an all verbal cue once the students have "caught on." Using the cue "out, in,

out, turn" can verbally convey the desire to have students do a jumping jack and then jump out and do a 1/2 turn in a 4-count sequence. Although verbal cueing can save wear and tear on the musculoskeletal system, voice injury can become a risk. The instructor should take all necessary precautions to reduce risk of voice injury as outlined in Chapter 11.

The most effective way to demonstrate desired water movements from deck is to combine high impact, low impact, non-impact, verbal, and non-verbal methods. Shifting from one method to another, or combining methods, reduces the risk of impact, upper torso, and voice injury by not overusing one part of the body. In addition, using several methods allows you to choose the most effective way to demonstrate each move, be it suspended, elevated, or at Level II. Combining deck impact options allows the use of a variety of teaching methods and techniques to provide higher quality instruction for students.

Conveying Appropriate Tempo From Deck

Tempo needs to be adjusted in the aquatic environment due to water's viscosity, drag, and resistance properties. Execution of movement and water tempo are discussed in Chapter 8.

Teaching From In the Pool
Advantages:
- You are not exposed to the elements and have the benefit of the cooling effect of the water.
- You benefit from the cushioning effect of the water and reduced impact stress.
- You can circulate around your class giving one-on-one feedback and contact. You can utilize touch training when appropriate.
- You can "feel" the movement in the water as the student's do. This enables you to better motivate and more precisely adjust intensity for many movements.
- It is easier to demonstrate with proper tempo and weight transfer from in the water.
- It allows you to "connect" with your class.

Disadvantages:
- It is very difficult for students to see what you are doing. If you have a large class or several new students, teaching from in the pool can be very challenging.

- You are virtually eliminating visual cueing with the lower torso. Since the majority of students are visual learners, some may get very frustrated when they cannot "see" what they are supposed to do.
- It may be more difficult for students to hear or understand you.
- Some movements are impossible to explain or demonstrate from in the pool.
- From a safety standpoint, you want to teach from on the deck if there is no lifeguard available so you can easily recognize a water rescue situation.

Some instructors cannot easily teach from deck due to physical limitations. An instructor who has chronic back pain, arthritis flare-ups, or is in the later stages of pregnancy may prefer to teach from in the water. Many water instructors have their roots in water fitness class participation. They were enthusiastic and dedicated participants who were recruited and encouraged to learn to instruct. These individuals may have been in water fitness programs because of physical limitations that restricted exercise on land, and therefore improper teaching from the deck could pose health problems.

It is possible to be an effective instructor from in the water. Adjustments will need to be made to cueing and choreography based on class participants. If you have a large number of students who are new to the water or your class, you will need to be skilled at verbal cueing, use simplified choreography, and circulate through the class to help new students. If you have a group that has been with you for several programs, you may be able to introduce more advanced moves, choreography, and patterns. If they have a firm grasp of basic choreography elements, you can build on those moves and challenge your class with more complicated choreography. Teaching complicated choreography is more difficult, and sometimes impossible to teach from in the pool.

Some instructors teach first from the deck and then enter the pool to repeat a pattern in the water. When teaching from in the pool, consider the following tips:

- More importance is placed on verbal cueing including the use of voice inflection and the ability to explain the same move in several different ways. Because the instructor is in the pool circulating, at times facing away from some students, a submersible microphone is highly recommended. You should speak slowly and use concise 2-3 word phrases to cue. Since you will not have the visibility of the lower body to visually cue, skill in verbal cueing becomes very important.

- Change your positioning in the pool throughout class. You can use a circle format with you in the middle or along side students in the circle. Some instructors remain in the middle and have their students form groups on their right and left. If you have a large class, you may need to have them form 2 or three circles around you. Position newer students on the inside circle so they can see you best.
- Maintain eye contact as much as possible with students. Sometimes student facial expressions can cue you in to who is having difficulty. Eye contact also opens the door to verbal communication. Give students the opportunity to ask for help often. Phrases like "Who can I help?" or "Does anyone need assistance?" can encourage students to ask for help when they don't understand.
- Use the buddy system. If you have a large class with new students, ask seasoned participants to "buddy up" with the newer students. They can help by explaining and demonstrating moves. You can offer "class ambassadors" a break in their class fees for helping with new students.
- If you have a shallow area close to where you are teaching, you can go to the shallower water to demonstrate moves. This way the class may be able to see more clearly what you are doing and take cues for form and alignment. Remember safety factors since impact increases in shallower water.
- Teach elements first, then simple combinations, and progress to more complex combinations and patterns. Building block choreography works well. Also consider teaching a combination stationary before adding the element of travel. Develop patterns with travel elements that move different students to or around you so you can "visit" with everyone.
- Circulate around the pool checking on all students offering one-on-one assistance, demonstrations, and explanations. Wear dark colored tights so students can easily see what your legs are doing under water.
- Show leg movements with your fingers, arms and hands. Most instructors find this modified means of visual cueing very helpful. You can lift just your hands or fingers for a knee lift front, and lift your whole arm for a front kick. Moving your hands in and out is a great visual demonstration for a jumping jack both in the water and on the deck. Demonstrate arm movements above the water's surface and then do the movement submerged. Consistency is the key with this kind of cueing. Use

the same hand signals consistently for each move. Combine these modified visual cues with verbal cueing for greater success.

- Use props to help with instruction. Put shoes on your hands to demonstrate a movement right above the water's surface or on the pool deck. Hold a noodle above the surface of the water and have students do a football jog in a squat position, or level two movements under the noodle. Have cue cards at different places around the pool deck to hold up for visual aid.

- When teaching deep water exercise from in the pool, face your students and mirror image their movement. Be very careful of voice injury. You can seriously injure your voice when projecting at water level in neck deep water.

Teaching From On the Deck and In the Pool

Most instructors will agree that the best method for teaching aquatic fitness is to be both in the pool and on the deck. This method combines the *advantages* of both deck and pool teaching and reduces the *disadvantages* of both methods.

There are safety concerns for an instructor who goes back and forth between the pool and deck. Be sure that you can safely exit and enter the pool. If your pool DOES NOT have easy access, you may choose to teach the first half of class from the deck to familiarize the students with all of the moves. Then you may choose to get in the pool for the second half of the class and use those moves to create combinations, patterns, and add travel. This minimizes the number of times you have to get in and out of the pool.

A good pair of water shoes is also essential. You want a pair that will cushion impact, reduce slipping, and allow you to go safely from deck to pool. Good shoes are a wise investment in your health.

If you have physical limitations that hinder your ability to teach from deck, consider options that will allow you to be on deck and instruct safely. For example, teaching from a chair or stool and using your arms as your legs will virtually reduce impact. Using a deck mat for cushioning and better footing, combined with the use of low impact movement may allow a pregnant instructor to demonstrate some moves from deck safely.

You will need to learn how to teach **effectively** from both places if you plan to teach from both locations. Teaching from deck requires a different set of skills than teaching from in the water. You will need to learn tempo, movement execution, and weight transfer from deck as well as cueing and choreography techniques for instructing from in the water. The extra effort will pay off when you learn as many teaching styles and techniques as possible. It will enable you to possess the skills to be in the best position possible to teach any particular segment of your class. It will enable you to reach a greater number of students as well.

Knowing how to teach from the deck and in the pool will expand your choreography and programming options. You can introduce and teach just about any movement. If it is better taught from deck, you can be there. If it is better taught from in the pool, you can teach it from in the water. Your marketability as an instructor expands as your teaching skills expand, allowing you to teach a greater variety of program formats.

"Leading" the Workout

There is a difference between "leading the workout" and "getting a workout". While there is no question that certain physical and psychological benefits are obtained whenever an instructor teaches, there is a HUGE difference between teaching to the group's level of fitness and the instructor's level. Always remember that the class belongs to the student. It is important for an instructor to reserve enough time and energy for a personal workout. Avoid using your class as your workout.

Your first and foremost role as an instructor is to provide an educational experience for your students. As previously discussed, this involves providing a safe, effective, enjoyable experience. This is what your students are paying for. They are not paying for your workout. You should consider going to someone else's class or developing a personal workout routine to increase your own level of fitness. This is an excellent way for the instructor to role model the benefits of variability or cross-training. Just as the principles of specificity apply to students, teaching the same programs at a similar level can apply to instructors as well. It simply does not provide a balanced workout. An instructor needs to "get in shape" to teach in order to avoid acute and overuse injury. Leading the workout means the instructor is not matching the student repetition for repetition, but rather is watching and correcting students by pacing the deck or moving among the participants.

A class can most effectively be taught to the mid-range ability of that particular group. In other words, pick the level where the majority of students seem to fall (beginner, intermediate, or advanced) and teach to that range while offering modifications to increase or decrease intensity to address everyone. This may not necessarily be your personal ability range.

As much as it would be nice to assume that everyone reads class descriptions and comes to the class that meets their needs and abilities, it is common knowledge that many programs are "zoo programs." This occurs when students of all sizes, shapes, and abilities gather together because the day and time are right. This creates a challenge for an instructor. It can be effectively managed by understanding and applying the principles of the water and expanding your teaching techniques.

AEA Standards and Guidelines for Deck Instruction

AEA recognizes deck instruction as the preferred method of leading aquatic fitness in most situations. Deck instruction provides the highest level of safety for the participants by allowing better observation and quicker response to emergency situations. Deck instruction also provides greater visibility- of the instructor to the participant and the participant to the instructor. AEA recommends that the instructor/trainer remain on deck when there is no additional lifeguard on duty, there are new participants in the program, or when new movements are being demonstrated.

The safety of the instructor does not have to be compromised if proper precautions are taken. Suggestions for safe deck instruction include:

- Avoid high impact movement demonstration.
- Utilize a chair for low impact demonstrations and balance needs.
- Wear proper footwear for deck instruction.
- When available, use a teaching mat to reduce impact stress.
- Wear appropriate clothing for the environment in which you work.
- Drink sufficient water to stay hydrated and protect your voice.
- Use a microphone when available or incorporate non-verbal cues.
- Position the music source where it provides the least interference with the instructor's vocal cueing.
- Use caution when utilizing any electrical source – including sound systems – near a pool due to potential hazard of electrical shock.
- Install grounded outlets around pool areas to reduce potential hazard of electrical shock.
- Lead the workout rather than participate in the workout

Muscle Balance

An important key to a safe and effective fitness program is to develop and maintain proper muscle balance. The human body typically works in muscle pairs to perform movement. Unfortunately common daily lifestyles have led to imbalances within these muscle pairs that can cause improper body alignment, poor posture, and chronic injuries. All fitness programs should be designed to help bring the muscle pairs back into balance through well-planned choreography, careful cueing, and adequate time spent on the final stretch.

The water provides resistance in all direction of submerged movement, but we can place the focus on one direction. Therefore, it is beneficial for the instructor to give good verbal and visual cues to encourage students to place more force in the direction of movement that will strengthen the weaker muscle of the pair. For example, when performing an arm cross in front of the body, focus the force on the return movement (pulling the arms back and squeezing the shoulder blades together) to strengthen the posterior deltoids, trapezius, and rhomboids. If we focus on the pull forward, we are placing the emphasis on the pectoralis and anterior deltoid muscles; these muscles already tend to be tight from daily activity and poor postural habits.

Another consideration is to stretch the muscles that you strengthen during a given workout. Too often we get in a hurry and skip over one of the most important components of our physical fitness program — flexibility. A strong muscle can be just as easily injured as a weak muscle if it is not flexible. Perform static stretches for all major muscle groups worked, and also consider adding stretches that lengthen muscles that are shortened from sitting, walking, stress, or common daily activities.

High-Risk and Ineffective Movements

As a general rule, there are very few contraindicated movements for aquatic fitness programs. But there are several high-risk movements that should be carefully evaluated before incorporating them into an exercise program. Almost every movement can be beneficial in the appropriate setting with the appropriate population (i.e. the "hurdler's stretch" is acceptable for track and field athletes who run hurdles). However, there are many moves that are so specialized in their benefits that they should be considered high risk for inclusion in general population fitness programs. Again the example of the "hurdler's stretch" – it would be considered high risk for a land-based aerobic class because of the potential for injury and the availability for a safer option. Ask yourself "Is there another movement that is just as effective but safer?"

Following are some movement considerations that should be carefully evaluated for safety and effectiveness. If you choose to include these movements in your program, additional options should be presented and demonstrated as well. New movements should be evaluated as far as safety and effectiveness prior to the actual class setting. Avoid experimenting with new movements during class time.

Very Fast Movements ("Land Tempo"/"Double Time")

Many instructors will intersperse land tempo or faster movements in choreography to add variety and sometimes intensity. If fast movement is used, consider short levers (such as knee lifts and leg curls) and performing the movements in place as opposed to traveling. It is acceptable to utilize speed to provide variety, but remember that range of motion is compromised and often the water's benefits are minimized. It is not acceptable to teach all or even the majority of a class at land tempo. It is more effective to increase intensity by utilizing the laws and principles of the water as opposed to just increasing speed.

When incorporating fast speed movements, allow students to self-modify the cadence as needed and use fast movements sparingly. Some instructors will use limited repetitions of land tempo exercises to add variety to choreography, but still teach the majority of class at water and 1/2 water tempo.

Extended Use of Arms Overhead

Movement of the arms over head is desirable for the shoulder joint and should be included at least in the stretching portion of each work out. Extended use of the arms overhead with fast ballistic movements however, can lead to fatigue of the deltoid muscles, shoulder elevation, and possible shoulder injury. Instructors sometimes extensively use arm movements over head in both land and water exercise to elevate heart rates. This can lead to a false perception of aerobic intensity due to the need of the heart to provide blood to the arms against gravity overhead as noted in Chapter 8. You will see an elevation in heart rate, but not a comparable elevation in oxygen consumption.

Also, with the arms above the water's surface, the participants have a tendency to look toward their hands increasing possible compression of the cervical vertebrae. With overuse of the arms out of the water, students will miss the benefits that water can provide through added resistance in all directions of movement and decreased gravitational pull. Variety through limited overhead movement can be fun, but should never compromise safety or be used for extended periods of time.

Very High-Impact Exercises

Plyometric jumps, which propel the body upward and out of the water, can be very useful for developing power in an athletic population, but should be used with caution for the general population. If you choose to include some of these moves in your class for more fit students, be sure you are at appropriate water depth to minimize impact stress when landing and cue for proper alignment. Give lower impact alternatives that provide similar results for less fit students.

Promoting Muscle Imbalance

Program designs that create or increase existing muscle imbalance should be reevaluated. Striding programs that only travel forward through the water, muscle conditioning programs that neglect flexibility, and aerobic programs that focus on hip flexion and forward movement of the arms will contribute to poor posture and increase potential for injury. Plan your program and your choreography carefully.

Any movement that leads to poor alignment should be eliminated or modified. Whether it is a specific exercise or a transition between moves, maintain proper alignment.

Prone Flutter Kicks

Prone flutter kicks, whether performed holding onto the wall or with a kick board or other flotation equipment, can lead to hyperextension of the lumbar and/or cervical vertebrae. Many aquatic fitness participants are non-swimmers and therefore are not comfortable working in a prone position with the face near or in the water. If prone flutter kicks are incorporated, suggest angling the kicks below the water's surface and to relax the head and neck. Provide options for those that are not comfortable with the movement, i.e., vertical flutter kicks in deep water with flotation equipment or standing leg swings.

Wall-Hanging Exercises

Exercises that require the participant to hang for extended periods of time with his/her back against the wall can be very stressful to the shoulder or wrist/finger joints. If the student rests the elbows on the pool deck, the shoulder joint is commonly in an elevated position and the rotator cuff muscles can become impinged. A certain level of strength would be required in the lower trapezius and latissimus muscles to hold the shoulder girdle down and in place.

Grasping the edge of the pool can strain the hands, wrists, and fingers in the attempt to maintain the position. Most wall-hanging exercises can be performed in a vertical position in deep water (with flotation at the torso) or modified to be performed in a standing position. If you choose to incorporate wall-hanging exercises, limit the position to one or two minutes before returning to standing. Include options for those unable to exercise in this position.

Hip Flexion Versus Abdominal Conditioning

Since many aquatic fitness participants are interested in strengthening/ toning the abdominals, instructors strive to provide a variety of abdominal exercise options. Unfortunately, many of the exercises included do not incorporate the abdominal muscles except as stabilizers/assistors; the primary movement comes instead from the iliopsoas, or hip flexors. Since the iliopsoas passes through the pelvic girdle, the participant may "feel" a tightening in the lower abdominal area when these muscles are contracted. In reality, the shortened iliopsoas can cause stress to the lower back if the abdominals are not strong enough to stabilize the pelvis. The abdominal muscles are NOT actively contracting to produce the movement and therefore the benefits are minimal.

The rectus abdominus contracts to produce spinal flexion, NOT hip flexion. Movements that flex the hip joint such as double-leg raises or bicycles do not flex the spine and therefore do not actively contract the abdominal muscles. Make sure that abdominal exercises are technically correct or desired results will not be achieved and the low back may be compromised.

Hyperflexion of the Knee

Quadriceps stretches that over flex the knee joint, such as pulling the heel to the buttocks, tend to overstretch the ligaments that provide stability in the knee. Show the proper way to do the stretch by holding the heel away from the buttocks, pointing the knee downward, and tilting the pelvis in a posterior direction. This stretch can also be performed by lifting, but not holding, the foot; by placing the foot on the wall behind you, contracting the buttocks and tilting the pelvis; and by dropping the knee toward the pool bottom while standing in stride position, contracting the buttocks and tilting the pelvis. Avoid over flexion of the elbow and wrist joints as well.

Spinal Integrity

Full neck circles are considered high risk for most participants and should be used sparingly if at all in a fitness program. Typically it is safe to tilt the head toward the shoulder (lateral flexion) or the chest (forward flexion), and to turn the head to look over either shoulder (rotation). Avoid letting the head fall toward the back (hyperextension) as this compresses the cervical vertebrae and can cause damage, especially when performed in a repetitive motion such as a circling movement. Cervical hyperextension should be performed in a slow controlled manner. Stress to the cervical vertebrae can also occur if students must tilt the head back for an extended time period to view the instructor on deck. This situation may result if the water level is significantly lower than deck level or if the students are exercising very close to the pool edge from which the instructor leads the class.

Avoid movements (aerobic activities, muscle conditioning exercises, and stretches) which would cause the participant to arch, or hyperextend, the lower back especially in a repetitive movement with added resistance. For additional safety, spinal and hip flexion, where the torso is brought toward the legs in a standing position, should always be supported, i.e., placing the hands on the thighs or the wall.

Professional Behavior and Attire

What makes a great instructor? Numerous qualities in combination create an individual that is capable of leading a safe, effective, and enjoyable aquatic fitness class. Strive to present yourself as an exercise professional in your appearance, attitude, and behavior.

Wearing proper attire for teaching aquatic fitness reflects your professional image. Instructors should dress for exercise as opposed to sun bathing or swimming. Supportive clothing that allows you to remain modest while teaching and entering and exiting the pool portrays professionalism and sets the tone that you are here to teach an exercise class. Proper aquatic attire includes the following:
- Supportive, non slip aquatic exercise shoes.
- Supportive bra for women and an athletic support for men.
- Chlorine resistive exercise clothes that may include unitards, a supportive bathing suit, tights or bike shorts worn over or under the suit to provide modesty, shorts worn over a bathing suit, shorts style swim trunks for men, or any other combination of acceptable, professional aquatic fitness attire.
- You may want to wear contrasting tight colors so your legs can be easily seen.
- If teaching outdoors, a hat, sunglasses and sunscreen.

Arrive early enough to class to be able to properly set up, prepare for your class, and greet participants. For consideration of other instructors, properly clean up and put away after your class. Follow facility procedures for taking time off or recruiting substitute teachers if you are ill or can't teach a class. Know and understand posted emergency procedures and follow facility procedures for processing class registrants.

Qualifications that employers look for in an aquatic fitness instructor include the following:
- Education and knowledge. Employers may want you to have a professional certification or equivalent. You should be able to demonstrate a reasonable understanding of the principles of water, exercise principles, choreography and cueing, and have a willingness to continue learning.
- Experience. Many employers seek instructors with teaching experience. If you do not have experience, many employers recruit instructors to serve in a mentoring or training program to receive practical experience before teaching.
- Energy and enthusiasm. Employers are looking for instructors that are excited about teaching and portray that excitement to students.
- Motivation. As an instructor you need to be self motivated as well as be able to motivate others. A motivated and motivating instructor retains and recruits participants for programs.
- Good interpersonal skills. To be a group fitness instructor, you need to have a friendly, compassionate personality.
- Adaptability. The aquatic environment is seldom stable. You need to be able to adapt to environmental and facility changes.
- Responsible. Employers want instructors that consistently show up and teach a good class.
- Sincere. You need to show that you care and are there to serve the clientele.

Becoming an outstanding instructor is a continuous process. To become an outstanding instructor, you need to be open to learning and improving not just for yourself, but for the participants who look to you and your skills to help them reach their fitness goals.

Summary

1. This chapter gave general recommendations for class formatting with allowances for environmental considerations, schedule variations, and student goals and abilities.

2. A sampling of possible program options were discussed. Water can truly provide something for everyone – deconditioned or elite athlete, strength training or range of motion, high-intensity aerobic or low-intensity "socialization."

3. Creativity is encouraged as long as the three principles of safety, effectiveness, and enjoyment are met.

4. Although deck instruction skills are highly recommended, it is realized that certain circumstances do require the instructor to be in the water with the students. Be comfortable with teaching both from on deck and in the pool so that you are prepared.

5. Learning to be a versatile exercise instructor increases your capability of reaching more individuals through your programs.

6. Continually evaluate your programs from all angles; recognize high-risk movements and be able to provide alternatives when required.

7. A great aquatic fitness instructor never reaches a state of equilibrium but fluctuates between learning and teaching!

Review Questions

1. Name three primary options available for the endurance component of an aquatic work out.
2. What is the difference between aquatic dance exercise and striding?
3. Give an example of a footwork cue.
4. Which type of cueing (verbal, visual, or tactile) is best to use at all times?
5. Which type of transition requires the greatest degree of core strength and coordination to safely execute?
6. Name three options for demonstrating or teaching movements from deck.
7. Why are prone flutter kicks considered a high risk movement for most class populations?
8. List four qualifications employers may look for in an aquatic instructor.

See Appendix E for answers to review questions.

References

1. American College of Sports Medicine. (2006). *Guidelines for Exercise Testing and Prescription.* 7th Edition. Baltimore, MD. Lippincott, Williams & Wilkins.

2. American Council on Exercise. (2000). *Group Fitness Instructor Manual.* San Diego, CA. American Council on Exercise.

3. Denomme, L. and J. See. (2006). *AEA Instructor Skills.* 2nd Edition. Nokomis, FL. Aquatic Exercise Association.

4. Howley, T and D. Franks. (2003). *Health Fitness Instructor's Handbook.* 4th Edition. Champaign, IL. Human Kinetics Publishers.

5. Sova, R. (2000). *AQUATICS: The Complete Reference Guide for Aquatic Fitness Professionals.* 2nd Edition. Pt. Washington, WI. DSL, Ltd.

6. Van Roden, J. and L. Gladwin. (2002). *Fitness: Theory & Practice.* 4th Edition. Sherman Oaks, CA. Aerobic & Fitness Association of America.

7. Wilmoth, S. (1986). *Leading Aerobics Dance Exercise.* Champaign, IL. Human Kinetics Publishers.

Chapter 10: Health Risk Appraisal and Physical Screening

INTRODUCTION

This chapter discusses the appropriateness and methods for health risk appraisal and physical screening. Whether you are required and properly trained to be involved in this process or not, it is important for the fitness professional to understand the mechanics and importance of the process. Following are basic guidelines for health risk appraisal and physical screening. For more detailed information, please consult the resources at the end of this chapter.

Unit Objectives

After completing Chapter 10, you should be able to:
1. Understand the basic process for health history, health risk appraisal, and physician's consent for a fitness participant.
2. Understand the appropriate use of physical screening for a fitness participant.
3. Describe commonly assessed physical parameters and commonly used assessments.

Key Questions:
1. What is the primary purpose of a preparticipation health history questionnaire?
2. What medical conditions typically require a physician's consent prior to participation in an exercise program?
3. Is it ethical for anyone to perform physical screening assessments or is training and practice required?
4. What are common assessments used for cardiorespiratory endurance, muscular fitness, and flexibility?

Physical activity reduces risk of disease, clears the mind, and improves quality of life. Most adults can participate safely in physical activity or physical fitness programs. Many facilities or programs require that the participant fill out a health history form and sometimes receive physician's consent before participating in an exercise program. Not all facilities require a health appraisal and risk assessment for every client that participates in a group fitness class. Facilities that have a higher exposure to liability (such as a hospital based facility) or offer special population programs generally require a health history and physician's consent for each participant. Community facilities, fitness chains, or privately owned facilities may only require a signed informed consent and waiver of liability as opposed to a health risk assessment. A typical informed consent/ waiver of liability states that the participant knows of no reason why he or she cannot safely participate in an exercise program and recommends physician consultation if there is any doubt. This allows the participant to take responsibility for his or her own health and medical conditions. Some facilities require a health risk appraisal and possible physician's consent, but do not require or perform physical assessments. It should be noted that the requirements for health risk appraisal and physical screening may vary from facility to facility and even from program to program within a facility. For example, a full health risk appraisal and physical screening may be required for a personal training client at a facility, but not for a group fitness participant.

Know and always follow your facility's procedures for initial processing of fitness participants, whether it is a health risk appraisal or signing an informed consent and waiver of liability. If you are an independent contractor responsible for your own policies and procedures, be sure to check with a lawyer in your area to determine which process you should use. More about the business and legal aspects for fitness professionals is discussed in Chapter 15.

Whether your facility requirements are to perform a health risk appraisal and physical screening or not, it is important as a fitness professional to understand the process. You need to stay alert to clients who may come into your programs needing additional screening or physician's consent. AEA recommends that anyone performing any type of health risk assessment or physical screening of fitness participants be appropriately trained and qualified to do so. Proper training and practice is required to become proficient at health risk appraisal, risk factor assessment, physical screening, and fitness assessment.

The risk assessment and physical screening process for a fitness participant consist of the following primary steps:
1. A complete health history.
2. A risk factor assessment for cardiovascular disease.
3. Physician's consent for cardiovascular disease risk if necessary, or for known cardiovascular, pulmonary, or metabolic disease.
4. Determination of orthopedic conditions, chronic disease, pregnancy, or other contraindications or risks for exercise.
5. Physician's consent or consultation for these conditions. You may need additional consent from the participant's specialist in addition to, or instead of, the primary care physician.
6. A physical screening.

Health History

A participant **health history** is usually conducted using a health history questionnaire, health history interview, or both. The purpose of a health history is to find out any past or present medical conditions that may affect the participant's ability to safely participate in a fitness program. These conditions may include past or present injuries, illnesses, or surgeries. A health history should also review and determine current risk including information about the individual's age, family history, gender, tobacco use, cholesterol, blood pressure, current physical activity level, diabetes, obesity, stress, and the use of medication and supplements. A proper health history form provides the information necessary to identify risk and determine if physician's consent is recommended.

Choose a form that is relatively quick and simple to fill out. Be sure it includes common health conditions and is thorough with risk assessment. A sample health history form is provided in this chapter. You can also refer to other professional resources for samples of health history forms. You may want to combine information from several forms to develop one to suit your clientele.

A health history form is not complete until it has been reviewed with the participant and all information is clear and fully understood. Reviewing the health history form with the participant is the best way to insure that you are receiving all of the information needed to make an adequate health risk assessment.

It is important to periodically reassess a client's health status. Annual reassessment is recommended unless a change in health status indicates a need for an immediate update. The information on these forms can increase the liability risk potential for the facility and fitness professional. Therefore, it is imperative to appropriately act on the information gathered in the health history form according to industry guidelines. (see figure 10-1, Sample Information and Health History Form)

Risk Factor Assessment

After the health history is completed, it is important to use industry guidelines and standards for determining the presence of, or risk for, cardiovascular, pulmonary, and metabolic disease. The American College of Sports Medicine suggests a preparticipation health screening and risk factor assessment for the following reasons:

- Identification and exclusion of individuals with medical contraindication to exercise.
- Identification of individuals at increased risk for disease because of age, symptoms, and/or risk factors who should undergo a medical evaluation and exercise testing before starting an exercise program.
- Identification of persons with clinically significant disease who should participate in a medically supervised exercise program.
- Identification of individuals with other special needs. (1)

Determine if a client has any risk factors or signs and symptoms suggestive of cardiovascular disease through a health history questionnaire and interview. The primary risk factors for cardiovascular disease include:

- Family History: Myocardial infarction, coronary revascularization, or sudden death before 55 years of age in father or other male first-degree relative (i.e., brother or son), or before 65 years of age in mother or other female first-degree relative (i.e., sister or daughter.)
- Cigarette Smoking: Current cigarette smoker or those who quit within the previous 6 months.
- Hypertension (High Blood Pressure): Systolic blood pressure of ≥ 140 mm Hg or diastolic ≥ 90 mm Hg, confirmed by measurements on at least 2 separate occasions, or on antihypertensive medication.

- Dyslipidemia (High Cholesterol): Total serum cholesterol of > 200 mg/dl (5.2 mmol/L), or high-density lipoprotein cholesterol <35 mg/dl (0.9 mmol/L), or on lipid-lowering medication.
- Impaired Fasting Glucose: Fasting blood glucose of ≥ 100 mg/dl (6.1 mmol/L) confirmed by measurements on at least 2 separate occasions.
- Obesity: Body Mass Index ≥ 30 kg/m², waist girth of > 102 cm. for men and > 88 cm. for women, or waist to hip ratio ≥ .95 for men and ≥ .86 for women. Body composition methods for determining obesity can be used as well.
- Sedentary Lifestyle: Persons not participating in a regular exercise program or meeting the minimal physical activity recommendations from the U.S. Surgeon General's report. (see Chapter 4) (1)

If you have elevated high density lipoprotein (HDL), the good cholesterol, it is considered a negative risk factor lowering your risk of cardiovascular disease. (1)

The signs and symptoms suggestive of cardiovascular disease are:

- Pain, discomfort (or other anginal equivalent) in the chest, neck, jaw, arms, or other areas that may be due to ischemia (lack of blood flow.)
- Shortness of breath at rest or with mild exertion.
- Dizziness or syncope (brief lack of consciousness.)
- Orthopnea (the need to sit up to breathe comfortably) or paroxysmal (sudden unexpected attack) nocturnal dypsnea (shortness of breath.)
- Ankle edema (swelling/water retention.)
- Palpitations or tachycardia (rapid heart beat.)
- Intermittent claudication (calf cramping.)
- Known heart murmur.
- Unusual fatigue or shortness of breath with usual activities. (1)

There should be questions on the health history form that determine if any of these risk factors or signs and symptoms are present in the participant. It is helpful to find a health history form that includes most of this information. Typically the client is interviewed to gather any additional information to clarify risk, for example the age of the relative with family history or if the participant has smoked in the past 6 months.

Information and Health History Form

Name _____ Date _____

Address (Street, City, State, Zip) _____

Home Phone ( ) _____ Cell Phone ( ) _____

Work Phone ( ) _____

Fax Number ( ) _____ Email _____

Employment (Company, Position) _____

Date of Birth _____ Age _____ Gender: _____ Male _____ Female

Person to Contact in Case of Emergency _____

Phone _____ Relationship _____

Do you now or have you had in the past:		
1. A history of heart problems in immediate family? (mother, father, sibling, grandparent) How old were they?	Yes	No
2. Cigarette smoking or other tobacco habit?	Yes	No
3. Elevated blood pressure or taking blood pressure medication?	Yes	No
4. High cholesterol, triglycerides, or on lipid lowering medications? What is your Total Cholesterol Level?	Yes	No
5. Diabetes or thyroid condition, impaired fasting glucose?	Yes	No
6. Any chronic illness or condition? Please Explain:	Yes	No
7. Difficulty with physical exercise?	Yes	No
8. Advice from medical professional not to exercise?	Yes	No
9. Recent surgery? (last 12 months) Please List:	Yes	No
10. Pregnancy (now or within last 3 months)?	Yes	No
11. History of allergy, breathing or lung problems?	Yes	No
12. Muscle, joint, or back disorder, or any previous injury still affecting you? Please Explain:	Yes	No
13. A heart condition or heart or vascular disease?	Yes	No
14. Do you have pain, discomfort, or other anginal equivalent in the chest, neck, jaw, arms, or other areas that may be due to lack of blood flow?	Yes	No
15. Shortness of breath at rest or with mild exertion?	Yes	No
16. Dizziness or fainting?	Yes	No
17. Troubled or rapid breathing at night or the need to sit up to breathe.	Yes	No
18. Ankle or leg swelling?	Yes	No
19. Rapid heart beating or palpitations?	Yes	No
20. Calf or leg cramping?	Yes	No
21. A known heart murmur?	Yes	No
22. Unusual fatigue or shortness of breath with usual activities?	Yes	No

What is your current level of activity? (Work and leisure pursuits) _____

_____

Are you currently participating in a regular exercise program? No Yes (please describe) _____

_____

Are you taking any medication, drugs, vitamins, herbs, or other supplements? If so, please list type, dose, and reason.

_____

_____

Current Weight_____ What do you feel is your ideal weight? _____

Are you seeing a Specialist or Therapist? _____ Phone ( ) _____

Office Location _____

Physician's Name _____ Phone ( ) _____

Office Location _____

Does your physician or specialist know you are participating in this program? _____

What are your personal fitness goals? What do you hope to accomplish through personal training? _____

_____

_____

_____

Figure 10-1 Sample Information and Health History Form

Physician's Consent

ACSM recommends placing the participant in one of three categories for risk stratification. (see table 10-1) The category will then determine if physician's consent is needed for moderate exercise, vigorous exercise, submaximal testing, and maximal testing. Use the following chart as a general guideline

Many fitness program participants take medications. Two common medications are beta blockers for hypertension and medications for colds and sinus/hay fever problems. Medication can affect an individual's resting and exercising heart rate. Some medications

will increase resting or exercise heart rate, some will decrease resting or exercise heart rate, and some will have no effect. It is suggested that a fitness professional be aware of how medication may alter a participant's heart rate. Check with the participant's physician, check a reputable resource that lists the effect of medication on heart rates, or consult a pharmacist. Some medications may make it impossible to safely achieve a target heart rate when exercising, and the participant may need to use perceived exertion as an alternate way to monitor intensity. (see figure 10-2, Sample Physician's Consent Form)

Table 10-1 American College of Sports Medicine

General Recommendations for Determining Physician's Consent		
Risk	**Criteria**	**Physician's Consent Recommended**
Low Risk	Younger individuals (Men < 45 years of age and women < 55 years of age) who are asymptomatic (0 signs or symptoms) and meet no more than one risk factor threshold.	Moderate Exercise: NO Vigorous Exercise: NO Submaximal Testing: NO Maximal Testing: NO
Moderate Risk	Older individuals (men ≥ 45 years of age and women ≥ 55 years of age) or those who meet the threshold for two or more risk factors.	Moderate Exercise: NO Vigorous Exercise: YES Submaximal Testing: NO Maximal Testing: YES
High Risk	Individuals with one or more signs/symptoms or known cardiovascular (cardiac, peripheral vascular, or cerebrovascular), pulmonary (COPD, asthma, interstitial lung disease, or cystic fibrosis), or metabolic disease (type 1 or 2 diabetes mellitus, thyroid disorders, renal or liver disease).	Moderate Exercise: YES Vigorous Exercise: YES Submaximal Testing: YES Maximal Testing: YES *Note: Moderate exercise is generally classified as under 60% HRR, and vigorous exercise is generally classified as 60% and above HRR.*

Additional Medical Concerns

After determining risk for cardiovascular disease and whether physician's consent is required, it may be necessary to screen the participant for additional medical concerns with regards to exercise limitations. Most fitness professionals who teach specialized programs for a particular condition, such as an arthritis class or a pre and post natal class, will require a physician's consent to participate in the class. For

specialized programs dealing with medical conditions or disease, physician's consent is a prudent practice.

If your facility conducts a full health screening and risk factor assessment, then determination and consideration of additional medical conditions that may require physician's consent before program participation is necessary. These concerns are considered in addition to cardiovascular disease risk. Examples of conditions that may require consent or consultation include pregnancy, orthopedic considerations such as injury or

Physician's Consent Form

I, _____ give permission to _____ to release my medical records and medical information to _____ for developing my fitness training program.

Signed_____ Date _____

Facility Name

Date _____

Dear Doctor / Medical Professional:

Your patient _____ wishes to start a fitness training program. The program will involve the following activities:

_____
_____
_____
_____
_____

If your patient is taking any medications that will affect their heart rate response to exercise, please indicate what effect it will cause (raise, lower, or has no effect on heart rate response):

Type of medication _____ Effect _____
Type of medication _____ Effect _____
Type of medication _____ Effect _____
Type of medication _____ Effect _____

Please identify any recommendations or restrictions that are appropriate for your patient in this exercise program:

_____
_____
_____
_____
_____

Thank You,

Fitness Professional, Facility Name, Phone Number, Fax, Email

_____ has my approval to begin an exercise program with the recommendations or restrictions I have indicated above.

Signed _____ Date _____ Phone _____

Figure 10-2 Sample Physician's Consent Form

recent surgery, arthritis, fibromyalgia, polio, multiple sclerosis, cancer, and other chronic diseases. These participants may be classified as low risk for cardiovascular disease, but still need physician's consent because of an existing condition, recent surgery or rehabilitation, or chronic disease.

> NOTE: The guidelines recommended above are generalized and somewhat simplified. If you are responsible for conducting heath risk appraisal, risk factor assessment, determination of physician's consent, and/or physical screening, it is recommended that you receive education and training beyond the scope of this certification. These processes are outlined in the ACSM's Guidelines for Testing and Exercise Prescription, and require training and practice for competency.

Physical Screening

In most settings, physical screening is <u>not</u> conducted for <u>group</u> fitness participants. Physical screening is used extensively in personal/ one-on-one training to establish a starting or reference point, determine strengths and deficiencies, define the scope of the program, and dictate an individualized program for the client. Even if your responsibilities as a fitness professional do not require you to perform physical assessment, understanding basic concepts about the screening process may help you recognize and accommodate participants who could benefit from individualized intervention. As with health appraisal and risk assessment, physical screening takes education, training, and practice in order to become proficient.

Physical screening is divided into two categories in this chapter. The first category is the health related components of screening and includes resting heart rate, blood pressure, and postural assessment. For health related fitness, blood cholesterol, blood sugar, and kidney and liver function may also be used to track improvements in health, but are not covered in this chapter. As mentioned in Chapter 4, some participants focus on the health related benefits of exercise as opposed to being concerned about improvements in physical fitness, and therefore are not

interested in fitness assessment or scores. In this case, metabolic or health related parameters of fitness may be used to set a reference point against which to monitor progress.

The second category is an overview of tools used to assess physical fitness. These tools test body composition, muscular fitness, cardiorespiratory fitness, and flexibility. Although there are many assessment tools available, only a list of commonly used assessment protocols are provided in this chapter. Testing protocols and norms are beyond the scope of this manual. It is recommended you receive additional education and training in order to administer physical assessments.

Health-Related Screening

Resting Heart Rate

Your resting heart rate can be used as an overall indicator of health and fitness. If your resting heart rate is high, it may be an indication of disease or poor physical conditioning. If your heart rate is low, your heart muscle is efficient and pumps more blood with each stroke. This may be an indication of good physical conditioning and good health.

It is easy to educate participants on how to take their resting and exercise heart rates. This will bring about greater awareness of health and help tune participants into their bodies. Remember that resting heart rate can be affected by medication, environmental conditions, stress, caffeine, nicotine, as well as other factors. A true resting heart rate is taken for three mornings, after you wake and before you rise, and averaged. This is a time when most people are unaffected by factors that could increase heart rate, and a more accurate reading can be obtained. Following is an explanation of how to take resting heart rate, terms for heart rate references, and reference norms for health.

1. Resting heart rate is best determined at the radial artery located at the lateral aspect of the palm side of the wrist, in line with the base of the thumb. (see figure 10-3)
2. The tip of the middle and index fingers should be used instead of the thumb. The thumb has a pulse of its own.
3. Start the stopwatch simultaneously with the pulse beat.

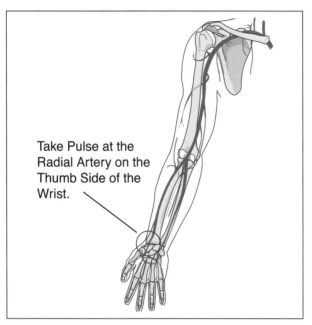

Take Pulse at the Radial Artery on the Thumb Side of the Wrist.

Figure 10-3 Radial Artery

4. Count the first beat as zero.
5. Continue counting for 30 seconds and then multiply by two to get the total heart beats per minute. *Adapted from Exercise Testing & Prescription (7)*

True Resting Heart Rate:
• Taken in the morning for three days (after waking but before rising) and then averaged.

Resting Heart Rate:
• Taken in the supine position after 30 minutes of rest. May be slightly higher than true resting heart rate due to caffeine use, medication, drug use, or stress. (see table 10-2)

Sitting Heart Rate:
• Taken after being seated for 30 minutes. May be slightly higher than a resting heart rate due to body position, medication, drug use, or stress.

Pre-exercise Heart Rate:
• Taken immediately before beginning exercise. It may be higher than resting or sitting heart rates due to the anticipatory effect of exercise which causes an elevation in heart rate.

Submaximal Exercise Heart Rate:
• This heart rate is taken during steady state submaximal exercise.

Maximum Heart Rate:
• The highest heart rate your body can physiologically achieve. It is the highest heart rate achieved during a maximal exercise test. It can also be <u>estimated</u> with the formula 220 – your age.

Blood Pressure

Blood pressure is the force that circulating blood exerts against the arterial walls. As the heart pumps blood into the closed circulatory system, a pressure wave is created. This pressure wave keeps blood circulating throughout the body. The high and low points of the pressure wave are measured with the aid of a sphygmomanometer (blood pressure cuff), which makes it possible to measure the amount of air pressure equal to the blood pressure in the artery. The systolic pressure is the high point of the pressure wave and represents the pressure created by the heart as it pumps blood to the body (contraction phase). This is the maximum pressure created by the heart during a complete cardiac cycle. The diastolic pressure is the low point of the pressure wave and represents the pressure in the arteries when the heart relaxes (filling phase). This is the minimum pressure that the arteries experience during a complete cardiac cycle.

Blood pressure is measured in millimeters of mercury (mm Hg). Blood in the arteries of the average adult exerts a pressure equal to that required to raise a

Table 10-2

Norms for Resting Heart Rate (beats / min)												
Age (yrs)	18-25		26-35		36-45		46-55		56-65		>65	
Gender	M	F	M	F	M	F	M	F	M	F	M	F
Excellent	49-55	54-60	49-54	54-59	50-56	54-59	50-57	54-60	51-56	54-59	50-55	54-59
Good	57-61	61-56	57-61	60-64	60-62	62-64	59-63	61-65	59-61	61-64	58-61	60-64
Above average	63-65	66-69	62-65	66-68	64-66	66-69	64-67	66-69	64-67	67-69	62-65	66-68
Average	67-69	70-73	66-70	69-71	68-70	70-72	68-71	70-73	68-71	71-73	66-69	70-72
Below average	71-73	74-78	72-74	72-76	73-76	74-78	73-76	74-77	72-75	75-77	70-73	73-76
Poor	76-81	80-84	77-81	78-82	77-82	79-82	79-83	78-84	76-81	79-81	75-81	75-79
Very poor	84-95	86-100	84-94	84-94	86-96	84-92	85-97	85-96	84-94	85-96	83-98	88-96

Source: Adapted from YMCA. Y'S Way to Fitness. 3rd edition.

column of mercury about 120 mm high during systole (systolic pressure) and 80 mm high during diastole (diastolic pressure). This is expressed as a blood pressure of 120 over 80 or 120/80 mm Hg. Blood pressure readings can vary greatly among individuals and also in an individual throughout the day.

Blood pressure measurements should be taken in a quiet, comfortable setting with the individual seated for approximately 10-15 minutes prior to the assessment, thus allowing relaxation and decreased anxiety. Blood pressure is measured with a stethoscope and a sphygmomanometer. The blood pressure cuff is wrapped around the arm over the brachial artery. Air is pumped into the cuff by means of a compressible bulb. This enables air pressure to be exerted against the outside of the artery. Air is added to the cuff until the air pressure exceeds the blood pressure within the artery and compresses the artery. At this time no pulse can be heard via the stethoscope which is placed over the brachial artery at the bend of the elbow. Slowly releasing the air in the cuff causes the air pressure to decrease until it equals the blood pressure within the artery. At this point the blood vessels open slightly, and a small amount of blood passes through the artery producing the first sound representing the systolic blood pressure. This is followed by increasingly louder sounds that suddenly change in intensity as the air pressure decreases. The sounds soon become more distant and then disappear altogether. The lowest reading at which sounds can be heard just before they disappear represents the diastolic blood pressure. This series of sounds heard while taking a blood pressure reading are known as "Korotkoff Sounds." (see figure 10-4)

If an inaccurate or abnormal reading was obtained, one or two minutes is allowed before repeating the blood pressure measurement so normal

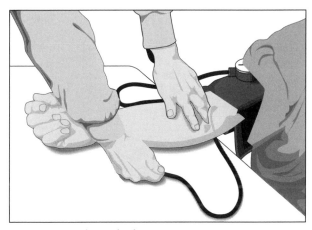

Figure 10-4 Taking Blood Pressure

circulation can return to the limb. If an abnormal reading is again obtained, the exam may be repeated on the opposite arm. If discrepancies between readings from arm to arm or abnormal readings occur, the individual should be referred to his/her physician for a medical consultation. Blood pressure should be measured in a standardized fashion using equipment that meets certification criteria. It is beyond the scope of this manual and certification to teach you how to take blood pressure. To learn how to take blood pressure, training and practice is required.

In May of 2003, new clinical practice guidelines were issued for the prevention, detection, and treatment of high blood pressure by the National Heart, Lung, and Blood Institute, a division of the National Institutes of Health (NIH). Table 10-3 outlines the new blood pressure categories and the corresponding pressures in mm Hg (mercury). More information regarding blood pressure measurement may be found in the American Heart Association's *Recommendations for Human Blood Pressure Determination by Sphygmomanometers*. *www.americanheart.org*.

Table 10-3 Blood Pressure

Pressure	Normal BP	Prehypertension	Stage I Hypertension	Stage II Hypertension
Systolic	< 120	120-139	140 -159	> 160
Diastolic	< 80	80-89	90 - 99	> 100

Postural Assessment

Posture is influenced by many factors including lifestyle, career demands, body type, muscle imbalances, and genetics. As a fitness professional you should understand the parameters of ideal posture and recognize postural deviations in your participants.

Remember, the role of the fitness professional is not to diagnose or correct anatomical abnormalities. The instructor can make the participant aware of his/her posture, emphasize proper body mechanics while teaching a fitness class, and avoid exercises that may exacerbate the condition.

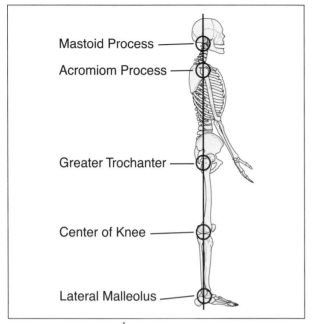

Figure 10-5 Bony Landmarks for Postural Assessment

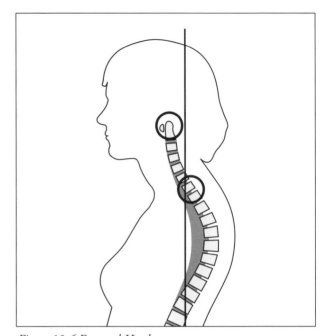

Figure 10-6 Forward Head

Figure 10-5 delineates bony landmarks that serve as a reference for the postural deviations listed below.

1. Forward Head: The mastoid process landmark is anterior to the lateral line of gravity. (see figure 10-6)
2. Kyphosis: An excessive increase in thoracic spine curve. The acromion process landmark is anterior to the lateral line of gravity. (refer to Chapter 3)
3. Lordosis: An excessive increase in the lumbar spine curve or an increase in the anterior pelvic tilt. The greater trochanter is posterior to the lateral line of gravity. (refer to Chapter 3)
4. Scoliosis: An "S" shaped curve of the spine. This is observed from the back of the individual, not the lateral line of gravity. (refer to Chapter 3)
5. Genu Recurvatum: Knee hyperextension. The knee landmark is posterior to the lateral line of gravity.

Physical Fitness Screening

Upon completion of the health history form, analysis of risk factors, resting heart rate, blood pressure, and postural assessment, the participant's physical fitness parameters may be assessed. The parameters of fitness, as outlined in Chapter 4, are appropriate body composition, flexibility, muscular strength and endurance, and cardiorespiratory endurance. The physical fitness assessment typically includes one assessment for cardiorespiratory endurance, an upper, lower, and core muscular fitness test, and may include several tests for flexibility. Fitness testing is not an absolutely necessary part of the health screening process for group fitness programs, yet has several advantages. It is not within the scope of this text to discuss in detail each of the physical fitness tests used for fitness assessment. Below is a brief description of some options for assessing each parameter of fitness and a table of commonly used assessments for each fitness component is included in each section.

Body Composition

Body composition assessment is an important aspect of the physical fitness evaluation. Body composition can be divided into two categories: (6) lean body mass which consists of muscles, bones, organs, internal fluids, etc., and (5) fat mass which is adipose tissue.

Many people refer to height/weight charts to determine proper body weight. Research indicates that in many cases this type of measurement is incorrect. The important factor is not body weight, but how much of the total body weight is fat. The term "percent body fat" refers to the amount of fat in the body and is expressed as a percentage of the total body weight. Table 10-4 lists general body fat percentage categories.

Table 10-4

General Body Fat Percentage Categories		
Classification	Women % fat	Men % Fat
Essential Fat	10-12%	2-4%
Athletes	14-20%	6-13%
Fitness	21-24%	14-17%
Acceptable	25-31%	18-25%
Obese	32% and higher	25% and higher

The most reliable and accurate method for determining body composition is by chemical analysis; however, it is necessary to destroy the organism to do this. There are several methods for estimating body composition that are not invasive. Table 10-5 lists commonly utilized body composition assessments.

Learning to assess body composition accurately using skinfold calipers requires training and a lot of practice. Often you will not have the equipment available to assess body composition using most of the methods mentioned in the table below. For field testing, circumference measurements are often used to estimate body fat, or Body Mass Index is utilized. If the technician is trained, skinfold calipers are often used to estimate body fat percentage.

Body Mass Index (BMI) is a crude index of total body fatness. It is commonly used as a measure of obesity in large population studies. There are a number of body mass indices, all of which were derived from body weight and height measurements. Below the Quetelet index is used, which is the ratio of body weight to height squared:

$$BMI \ (kg/m^2) = WT \ (in \ kg) \div HT^2 \ (in \ m)$$

The following example demonstrates this method of calculating the BMI. For example, a woman weighs 132-pounds (or 60 kilograms which is derived by dividing the weight in pounds by 2.2.) She measures 64 inches in height (or 1.6256 meters, which is derived by multiplying the height in inches by 0.0254.) Calculate her BMI as follows:

$$BMI = 60 \ kg \div (1.6256m^2) = 22.7 \ kg \ /m^2$$

A simpler formula that does not require a metric conversion is:

[Weight (in pounds) x 703] ÷ [Height (in inches) squared].

A BMI of 22.7 puts this woman in the normal classification for obesity as found in the table provided. Many studies have confirmed that the health risks associated with obesity start in the range of 25 - 30 kg/m². In actuality, the BMI is better suited as an indication of health risk to your clients than a true measure of body composition. This is an assessment that can be used to offer your client a broad picture of their health status. (table 10-6 summaries the risk of associated disease according to BMI and waist size chart)

Table 10-5

Methods for Body Composition Assessment		
Method	Advantages	Disadvantages
LABORATORY METHODS: Hydrostatic Weighing (Underwater Weighing)	• Considered most accurate at this point in time.	• Involves expensive equipment • Client may have difficulty going under water.
Dual Energy X-ray Absorptiometry (DXA)	• Relatively new method, considered highly reliable. • Safe, rapid, and accounts for individual differences in bone mineral content.	• Involves expensive equipment. • Further research needed.
Air Displacement Plethysmography	• Easy and simple- client sits in an egg shaped pod. • Measures body volume to estimate body density.	• Involves expensive equipment. • Further research needed, findings mixed.

continued on the next page

Method	Advantages	Disadvantages
FIELD METHODS: Skinfold Method	• Inexpensive, rapid, noninvasive, relatively accurate.	• Requires a high degree of technician skill. • Can be affected by skin compressibility, and caliper used. • Not as accurate for very obese clients.
Bioelectrical Impedance Method (BIA)	• Relatively inexpensive, rapid, noninvasive, relatively accurate. • Does not require a high degree of technician skill. • More comfortable/less intrusive. • Can be used for very obese individuals.	• Requires more expensive equipment than skinfold methods. • Accuracy can be affected by technician skill and water retention. • Equipment is less portable and requires a place for the client to lie down comfortably.
Near-Infrared Interactance Method (NIR) (Futrex)	• Easy, relatively inexpensive, rapid, noninvasive.	• Requires more expensive equipment than skinfold methods. • Still in the developmental stage. • Accuracy and validity questionable.
Anthropometric (Circumference) Method	• Very inexpensive, noninvasive. • Does not require a high degree of technician skill. • Can be more accurate than skinfold prediction equations for very obese clients	• Can be embarrassing. • Lower degree of overall accuracy.
Body Mass Index (BMI)	• Very inexpensive, noninvasive. • Does not require a high degree of technician skill. • Rapid and simple.	• Only provides a crude index of obesity.

Table 10-6

Risk of Associated Disease According to BMI and Waist Size			
BMI		Waist less than or equal to 40 in. (men) or 35 in. (women)	Waist greater than 40 in. (men) or 35 in. (women)
18.5 or less	Underweight	—	N/A
18.5 - 24.9	Normal	—	N/A
25.0 - 29.9	Overweight	Increased	High
30.0 - 34.9	Obese	High	Very High
35.0 - 39.9	Obese	Very High	Very High
40 or greater	Extremely Obese	Extremely High	Extremely High

Partnership for Healthy Weight Management. May 2000

Cardiorespiratory Fitness

Cardiorespiratory endurance assessment generally falls into one of two general categories: laboratory testing and field testing. Laboratory testing measures oxygen consumption while exercising on a bike, treadmill, or other ergometer The testing is quite involved and requires trained technicians and computerized equipment for measuring oxygen consumption. The testing can either be maximal testing or submaximal testing. In maximal testing, the subject exercises to exhaustion so maximal values for oxygen consumption and heart rate can be more directly attained. In submaximal testing, the subject exercises at one or more submaximal stages of exercise and that data is used to mathematically predict maximal values.

Field testing is simpler to administer and does not require a laboratory facility and expensive equipment. Scores obtained from field assessments primarily give the participant a generalized category for cardiorespiratory fitness. Some field tests actually use the data to mathematically estimate maximal oxygen consumption. Table 10-7 is a list of commonly administered cardiorespiratory endurance assessments.

Table 10-7

Cardiorespiratory Endurance Assessments	
Treadmill Submaximal Exercise Tests	Multistage or single stage walking, jogging or walk/jog protocols. Bruce and Balke protocols are most commonly used.
Treadmill Maximal Tests	Multistage, graded test, continuous or discontinuous walking, jogging, walk-jog protocols. Used for diagnostic and functional testing. Bruce and Balke protocols most commonly used.
Bicycle Ergometer Submaximal Exercise Tests	Multistage tests, continuous or discontinuous. YMCA, Astrand-Rhyming, and ACSM protocols are most commonly used.
Bicycle Ergometer Maximal Tests	Multistage, graded test, continuous or discontinuous. Used for diagnostic and functional testing. ACSM and Astrand commonly used.
Bench Stepping Submaximal Exercise Test	Some used to evaluate cardiorespiratory fitness, some to predict VO_2 max. Astand–Rhyming and Queens College step tests predict VO_2 max. The YMCA 3-minute bench test is most commonly used to evaluate cardiorespiratory fitness.
Distance Run Tests	Most common tests use distances of 1.0 or 1.5 miles. Nine or twelve minute tests measure distance in time. The 1.5-mile run/walk and 1.0 mile jog tests measure time for distance.
Walking Test	Rockport walking test measures time to complete one mile.
Swimming Test	Cooper 12-minute swimming test measures distance swam in 12 minutes, any stroke, rest allowed.
Cycling Test	Cooper 12-minute cycling test using a 3-geared bike at 10mph on a hard flat surface. Measures distance in time.

Muscular Fitness

Assessment of muscular fitness falls into two primary categories: assessment of muscular strength and assessment of muscular endurance. Occasionally, muscular power tests such as the vertical jump are used to test athletes, as power is an important aspect of athletic performance.

Specialized equipment found in therapy or sports medicine clinics is used for muscular strength testing. Since the testing is costly, it is not often used outside of therapy or sports applications. One repetition maximum (1RM) testing is also used to assess muscular strength. A set protocol and free weights are commonly used in 1RM testing. Since many participants do not have experience lifting heavy weight, 1RM testing is not commonly used for the average or deconditioned adult.

Most of the field tests used in general screening assess muscular endurance. Typical muscular endurance tests measure the number of repetitions of an exercise that can be performed in a specified period of time or to exhaustion. The curl-up and push-up tests are two commonly used tests due to their ease of administration. The participant uses their own body weight as resistance so no specialized or heavy equipment is needed. Table 10-8 lists typical protocols used for assessing muscular strength and endurance.

Table 10-8

Commonly Used Muscular Strength and Endurance Assessments			
One Repetition Max (1RM) Tests	Dynamic Strength Test	Variable resistance or constant resistance	Bench press, arm curl, latissimus pull, leg press, leg extension, leg curl.
YMCA Bench Press Test	Dynamic Endurance Test	Variable resistance	Lift a set weight at a set cadence until exhaustion.
Push-up Test	Endurance Test	Use own body weight	Timed test or perform push-ups until exhaustion.
Sit-up Test	Endurance Test	Use own body weight	Timed or until break cadence.
Curl-up Test	Endurance Test	Use own body weight	Timed or until break cadence.
Pull-up Test	Endurance Test	Use own body weight	Timed or until exhaustion.

Flexibility

Flexibility is typically measured in a static position. For example, in the standard sit and reach test, the participant bends forward in a sitting position and holds that position while the measurement is taken. Flexibility testing can be as simple as the "quick" flexibility tests described below, more involved such as the sit and reach test, or very technical such as the measurement of joint angles with a goniometer.

"Quick" Tests for Flexibility Assessment

Please Note: These are general descriptions. More information can be found in the two references found below. Do not allow your clients to stretch to the point of pain. Be sure they are warmed up before performing the assessments. The "normal" ranges of motion are suggested. Further evaluation can be made with a goniometer and/or referral to a physical therapist.

Shoulder Flexors ROM:
In a standing position, have the client reach and raise the arms forward and upward as far as possible. The humerus should be parallel to the ear.

Shoulder Rotators ROM:
In a standing position, have the client raise one arm overhead, bend the elbow, and reach down the back with the palm and fingers touching the back. At the same time, the client bends the other elbow and reaches upward from behind the back with the palm facing outward. The fingers should almost touch.

Hip-Flexor ROM:
Have the client lie supine on a table so that the knee joints of both legs are just beyond the edge of the table. Ask the client to maintain the pelvis in posterior tilt with the low back and sacrum flat on the table by bringing one thigh toward the chest. (Clasp both hands behind the knee and bring it towards the chest until the low back and sacrum are flat.) If the client can:

a. Touch the table with the back of the free thigh with the knee at 80 degrees of flexion, then the iliopsoas and rectus femoris are of normal length.

b. Only touch the table with the back of the free thigh if the knee is extended, then the iliopsoas is of normal length but the rectus femoris is tight (and possibly the tensor fasciae latae.)

Hamstring ROM:
Have the client lie supine on the floor with the legs extended and low back and sacrum flat on the floor. Place one of your hands on the client's thigh. Ask the client to relax the foot and maintain the knee in extension as you raise the leg as far as possible without the knee bending. The measurement at the hip should be at least 80 degrees of flexion, preferably 90.

RESOURCES:
- American College of Sports Medicine, ACSM's Resource Manual for Guidelines for Exercise Testing and Prescription, Williams and Wilkins, Baltimore, MD, 1998.
- Kendall, F., McCreary, E., and Provance, P., Muscles Testing and Function, Williams and Willkins, Baltimore, MD, 1993.

Aquatic Fitness Assessment Tests

To date, there are no aquatic fitness assessment tests with validated norms. A shallow water running test was evaluated at Ball State University. The purpose of the study was to assess the validity of a 500-yard run in the water to determine peak aerobic power and to compare it with the commonly used 1.5-mile run test. The researchers concluded that the 500-yard shallow water run test, especially when used with the descriptive measures of percent body fat and height, could provide a reasonable estimate of an individual's cardiorespiratory fitness classification. The resource for this study is: Kaminsky, Wehrli, Mahon, Robbins, Powers, and Whaley, Evaluation of a Shallow Water Running Test for the Estimation of Peak Aerobic Power, Medicine and Science in Sports and Exercise, May, 1993.

Although there has been research conducted (300 yd., and 500 yd. Shallow Run Test, Cisar et.al., San Jose State University and the study referenced above) validated norms have not been developed. It is believed by some exercise professionals that all fitness testing should be conducted on land because we function on land. The assessments would then reflect improvements in our ability to function in a gravity environment. Research now indicates that rehabilitation in the water does translate to an increased function on land.

It is possible to use non-researched tests in the water to measure possible health and fitness gains by measuring "change over time" criteria. Although these assessments are limited, and you cannot determine a fitness category or a norm percentile for your students, you can determine if they have made improvements by establishing a baseline score and then repeating the test. Hopefully you will see improvement in the scores. Below are a few suggestions for tests that you may want to experiment with. You can also develop your own "change over time" tests depending on your available resources and particular client population. Remember, to accurately measure change over time, the test should be as "controlled" as possible by performing the test in the same setting and in the exact same way.

1. <u>Cross Country Ski Submaximal Heart Rate Recovery Test:</u> The subject performs a cross country ski movement for three minutes at 140 beats per minute. A 15 second standing heart rate is taken immediately afterward.

2. <u>Flexibility Assessment:</u> Subject grabs the pool edge or ladder and walks the feet up until they are even with the hands. The instructor measures and records the degree of flexion at the knee joint.

3. <u>Upper Body Muscular Endurance Assessment:</u> The subject begins in the extended arm position and does push-ups at the pool side to 90-degree elbow flexion and back to extension. Instructions for standing push-ups instead of suspended push-ups are given for participants who may not be strong enough to support their body weight. The number of repetitions for one minute or until fatigue are counted and recorded.

4. <u>Lower Body Muscular Endurance Assessment:</u> The subject stands in waist-deep water. The subject performs one leg sit squat (to 90-degree knee flexion) and kicks for one minute or until

fatigue. The number of repetitions correctly performed are counted and recorded.

5. <u>Abdominal Muscular Endurance Assessment:</u> A supine position is assumed with buoyancy equipment held in the hands. The instructor holds the subject's crossed ankles while he or she performs flexion of the spine or curl-ups for one minute. The number of reps correctly performed are counted and recorded.

Interpretation of the Health Risk Appraisal and Physical Screening Process

Upon completion of the health risk appraisal process and the optional physical screening, the fitness professional should discuss the results of the assessment process with the individual. This should be done in a private setting that is comfortable and non-intimidating for the client.

As a fitness professional, you may be responsible for communicating whether a physician's consent is needed based on the health risk appraisal. You will not be discussing the results of physical screening unless you have been trained to administer the assessments.

A personal trainer, however, will use the health risk appraisal and physical assessment to recommend programs and exercises specific to the strengths and weaknesses of the individual, and set realistic goals to be obtained both long and short term. This process collects valuable information and allows the personal trainer to get to know the individual and open lines of communication. In some settings, a reassessment date is set approximately 12 weeks from the original fitness assessments. This reassessment/consultation will allow the individual to note the improvements that have been made in his or her fitness level and help the personal trainer to reevaluate and redesign the fitness program. This can be used as a motivation tool for the individual and the personal trainer.

Summary

1. It is important to understand and follow the procedures outlined by your facility to determine if health risk appraisal or physical screening is performed for fitness participants.

2. A health history form is used to gather information from a fitness participant.

3. There is a process to determine cardiovascular disease risk and whether a physician's consent is required. Follow industry guidelines as outlined by the American College of Sports Medicine. It is important to be properly trained for determining a risk stratification and following through on the recommendations made.

4. Beyond cardiovascular risk assessment, it may be necessary to require physician's consent for additional health considerations and chronic diseases.

5. Commonly assessed parameters for physical screening include resting heart rate, blood pressure, posture, body composition, cardiorespiratory endurance, muscular fitness, and flexibility. Be aware of common fitness assessment protocols used by trained technicians to assess baseline fitness levels for clients.

Review Questions

1. What are the 7 positive risk factors for cardiovascular disease?
2. A heart rate taken three mornings in a row, after you wake and before you rise is a _____ heart rate.
    a. true resting
    b. sitting
    c. sub maximal exercise
    d. maximum
3. Is the Rockport Walking test considered a laboratory or field test for cardiorespiratory fitness?
4. Name three assessments commonly used for measuring muscular endurance.

See Appendix E for answers to review questions.

References

1. American College of Sports Medicine. (2006). *Guidelines for Exercise Testing and Prescription.* 7th Edition. Baltimore, MD. Lippincott, Williams & Wilkins.

2. American Council on Exercise. (2000). *Group Fitness Instructor Manual.* San Diego, CA. American Council on Exercise.

3. Fitness and Amateur Sport. (1981). *Government of Canada: Canadian Standardized Test of Fitness Operations Manual.* 2nd Edition. Ottawa, Ontario, Canada. Fitness and Amateur Sport.

4. Golding, L and C. Myers. (1989). *Y's Way to Physical Fitness.* 3rd Edition. Champaign, IL. Human Kinetics Publishers.

5. Gross, W. (2000). *Some Weightloss Advertising Claims Hard to Swallow.* Federal Trade Commission, Partnership for Healthy Weight Management. www.consumer.gov/weightloss/press0500.htm

6. Heyward, V. (2002). *Advanced Fitness Assessment & Exercise Prescription.* 4th Edition. Champaign, IL. Human Kinetics Publishers.

7. Nieman, D. (2002). *Exercise Testing and Prescription with Power Web Bind-in Passcard.* 5th Edition. New York, NY. McGraw-Hill Publishers.

Select Images provided by:
Hillman, S. (2004). *Complete 3D Human Anatomy.* London, UK. Primal Pictures, Ltd. Website: www.primalpictures.com

Kumm, R. (2005). *LifeART Super Anatomy 1.* Baltimore, MD. Lippincott, Williams & Wilkins. Website: www.lifeart.com

Kumm, R. (2005). *LifeART Super Anatomy 7.* Baltimore, MD. Lippincott, Williams & Wilkins. Website: www.lifeart.com

Chapter 11: Emergencies, Injuries, and Instructor Wellness

INTRODUCTION

The information presented in this chapter is intended to help the aquatic fitness professional appreciate various medical emergencies and injuries that can occur at the poolside, as well as learn something about fitness professional wellness. Some injuries may be acute and others more chronic or overuse injuries. Recognize that these overuse injuries may occur in both clients as well as in instructors. In addition, realize that a fitness professional may be required to provide the initial first aid, initiate CPR, and even use an AED.

Unit Objectives

After completing Chapter 11, you should be able to:
1. Understand the difference between acute and chronic injuries.
2. Identify symptoms and treatment for common exercise injuries.
3. Demonstrate procedures for basic first aid including the RICE concept.
4. Adapt your first aid and CPR training to the water environment.
5. Demonstrate basic water safety concepts.
6. Identify a variety of emergency conditions and be aware of a recommended course of action for these situations.
7. Explain why emergency action plans are important.

Key Questions
1. What is the primary difference between an acute and chronic injury?
2. Is tendonitis considered an acute or chronic injury and what is the primary treatment for tendonitis?
3. What is the do-si-do position for administering rescue breathing in shallow water?
4. How do you identify a drowning victim and what is the instinctive drowning response?
5. What should you do if a water class participant has an epileptic seizure during your class in the water?
6. What action should you take if someone has a heart attack or stroke during your class?
7. How do you protect your voice from injury?

Acute Emergencies

Basic First Aid

Basic first aid of injuries can most often be managed by the RICE principle. **RICE** stands for **R**est, **I**ce, **C**ompression, and **E**levation. Resting after an injury allows the body to begin healing. Ice causes vasoconstriction of the blood vessels and therefore helps limit the amount of swelling allowed to the area. Ice also provides a numbing effect that will help to decrease pain. Compression and elevation of the injured part also help minimize swelling and pain caused by excessive swelling.

Some injuries that occur at the pool may be more serious than bumps, bruises or strains/sprains and may require calling for emergency help. These include hip/pelvic fractures, shoulder or kneecap dislocations, fractured ankles or wrists, neck injuries, and finally head injuries in participants taking blood thinning medications. Although the specifics of these more serious injuries are not discussed further in this chapter, it is mentioned now in the hope that fitness professionals will be prepared for whatever may happen at the pool.

Adapting Your First Aid and CPR Training to the Aquatic Environment

The American Red Cross safety courses teach you to CHECK, CALL, and then CARE for a victim of any emergency. The water emergency proceeds as follows:

1. **CHECK** before you help the victim:
   a. Is there an environmental danger such as electrical shock or a chlorine leak?
   b. What might have happened (heart attack, panic, slip into deep water unexpectedly, swallowed water)?
   c. What is the potential extent of injuries? (Does this require special handling of the spine or CPR?)
   d. How many victims are involved?
   e. Who can help you with the call, extraction if necessary, and clearing the pool?
2. **CALL** for help. As soon as there is recognition of a situation that requires back-up assistance, initiate the emergency action plan of that facility. Make the call to the local Emergency Medical Service (EMS) - '911' or other appropriate phone number. When dealing with an adult, make the call immediately.
3. **CARE** for the victim.

   a. In the case where you can quickly reach or throw to the victim, do it without hesitation. Reach an arm, leg, or pole, or throw a ring buoy. You can call for help as you do this.
   b. If you cannot make the rescue yourself, the lifeguard needs to be called as quickly as possible to the scene. You then back up the lifeguard by clearing the pool and supervising the other patrons. Bring the supplies the lifeguard needs and make sure the EMS call is made.
   c. Move victim to safety or remove victim from water. Give the proper care needed to help victim until EMS arrives and takes over.

How to Use a Spine Board for Water Removal

Should a victim need to be removed from the water, it is safest to use a spine board. Lifting a person from the water is not only difficult, but can be harmful to the person(s) trying to lift. The following presents an alternative technique for using the spine board for removal of a victim from the water. This technique is not always taught to lifeguards, but can be very effective. A prepared instructor can give directions to a class who has never done this before, and a combined effort can have the victim out of the pool within one minute. When a victim is unconscious, not breathing or does not have a pulse, you must get the victim out of the water as quickly as possible to begin the proper care. Remember that rescue breathing and CPR cannot be effectively performed in the water.

Here are the steps to this procedure:

1. Victim recognition. When a victim suddenly becomes unconscious, the instructor tells participants to immediately retrieve the spine board.
2. Emergency Medical Service (EMS) is called immediately.
3. The instructor enters the water and brings the victim's head above the water, tilting the head back to open the airway. This assumes that no spinal injury is suspected. If a spinal injury is suspected, a lifeguard should handle this situation implementing the skills he/she has been taught.
4. The initial assessment of breathing and circulation is made.
5. If the victim is unconscious, not breathing or does not have a pulse, the victim is placed on the spine board and the board is positioned perpendicular

to the side of the pool with the victim's head being closest to the pool wall. The victim is NOT strapped to the board.

6. Two individuals are placed on deck to help lift and guide the spine board and the victim from the water. These individuals grab the handholds of the spine board under the victim's armpits. When done correctly, the victim is supported at the shoulders while being lifted.

7. Several other individuals are instructed to push down on the foot of the spine board as the two individuals on deck lift and slide the spine board onto the deck of the pool. The movement of sinking the foot of the spine board causes it to "pop" out of the water, assisting those on deck who are lifting. This is true because most spine boards are buoyant.

8. In a deep water rescue, it is helpful for the instructor and participants to wear flotation belts to assist them with positioning and placing the person on the board. This allows them to concentrate on procedure as opposed to keeping afloat.

9. As soon as the removal is complete, a primary survey should be performed. Then rescue breathing or CPR is begun if needed and is continued until EMS arrives.

10. If needed and available, implement the use of an Automated External Defibrillator (AED). Dry the victim and surrounding area well. Turn AED power on, apply pads and follow prompts. Make sure no one is standing in water or near the victim when using the AED.

NOTE: IF A LIFEGUARD IS ON DUTY, THE LIFEGUARD WILL IMPLEMENT THE REMOVAL METHODS FOR WHICH HE/SHE HAS BEEN TRAINED.

Sudden Illness

Sudden illness can occur to anyone, anywhere. You may not know what the illness is, but you can still provide care. If you think something is wrong or the person looks or feels ill, check the victim and look for a medical alert tag. Don't be afraid to ask questions to gain insight as to what is wrong; the condition can very quickly deteriorate.

There are many types of sudden illness, such as:
• Diabetic emergency

• Seizure
• Stroke
• Allergic reaction
• Poisoning

Signs and Symptoms of Sudden Illness
1. Feeling lightheaded, dizzy or confused.
2. Sweating or weakness.
3. Nausea, vomiting, or diarrhea.
4. Changes in skin color (pale, ashen, or flushed).
5. Severe headache, difficulty breathing, or pressure or pain in the chest that will not go away.
6. Seizures or changes in consciousness.
7. Paralysis, slurred speech, or blurred vision.
8. Abdominal pressure or pain that will not go away.

General Care Steps for Sudden Illness
When giving care for sudden illness, follow the general procedures for emergency situations. Keep in mind that you are not required to perform any skills beyond your level of training.
1. Use basic precautions for preventing disease transmission.
2. Care for life threatening conditions first.
3. Monitor airway, breathing, and circulation.
4. Watch for changes in consciousness.
5. Keep the victim comfortable and reassure the victim.
6. Keep the victim from getting chilled or overheated.
7. Do not give the victim anything to eat or drink unless he/she is fully conscious and is not in shock.
8. Care for any other problems that develop, such as vomiting.

The sudden illness information was taken from the American Red Cross Lifeguarding Training Manual.

Water Safety

Most state health codes classify a "public swimming pool" as any pool for which a direct fee is charged (i.e., class fees or instructor fees). Most of these same states require that a lifeguard be on duty at those pools at all times of use. There are situations where aquatic fitness is taught at facilities that do not have lifeguards on staff (hotels, spas, condominiums, apartment complexes, etc.). It would be prudent under these situations for the fitness professional to receive basic water rescue training at the minimum, and/or lifeguard certification.

Where possible, an instructor should adhere to the following guidelines:

1. Insure that a qualified lifeguard be on duty at all times during a class.

2. Insure that proper rescue equipment such as first aid kit, rescue tube, ring buoy, spine board and telephone is available at all times and that the lifeguard is trained and practiced in its use.

3. Know the Emergency Action Plan at each facility where he or she works and the responses expected of him/her.

4. Be able to recognize a water crisis.

5. Hold a current certificate in Cardio Pulmonary Resuscitation (CPR). Certifications in Basic Water Rescue and First Aid are also highly recommended.

The following information is NOT intended to be used as a replacement for taking a course in water safety or for hiring a properly trained lifeguard. Every instructor needs to know what to do when he or she is the closest person to the scene of a distressed or drowning victim. The following information will help the instructor review the basics he/she needs to know as a water exercise instructor.

AEA Standards and Guidelines: Lifeguard

Country, state, and local codes relating to lifeguard regulations should always be followed.

For maximal safety of participants and limited liability for the instructor and facility, AEA recommends that a certified lifeguard, in addition to the instructor leading the class/session, should be on duty at the pool facility when aquatic fitness classes/ workouts are being held.

If an additional certified lifeguard is not present during the aquatic fitness class/session, AEA recommends:

1. The instructor to be certified in water safety and basic water rescue techniques.

2. The instructor to remain on deck while leading the class/session unless it is a one-on-one session that requires in-water assistance or guidance.

3. The instructor be fully aware of the facility's emergency action plan and his/her role in this plan.

Recognition of a Water Crisis

1. A victim in distress is one who can swim or float but can no longer make forward progress. He or she may have a cramp, be fatigued, or have swallowed water. These victims have some water skills and may be able to wave or call out for help. This condition can quickly deteriorate if fear takes hold.

2. A drowning victim is typically a person with little or no swimming skills who suddenly finds himself in deep water and panics. A distress victim can become a drowning victim when he or she panics. Due to the **Instinctive Drowning Response** the victim can neither wave nor call out for help. He or she must be reached within 20 to 60 seconds, the average time a victim struggles before going to the bottom.

The Instinctive Drowning Response is characterized by the following:

- The victim's arms are uncontrollably extended to the side and alternately being raised and pressed down in an attempt to raise the head above water.

- The victim will inhale as the head sinks below the surface.

- Since speech is a secondary function of the respiratory system, speech is not possible unless the victim is getting enough air to first satisfy the need to breathe. The victim is actually being suffocated by the water and, therefore, not able to call out for help.

- The fact that the arms are raised and the head appears to be bobbing up and down will give the illusion of play. Nearby bathers are often unaware that a drowning is taking place just 10 to 15 feet away from them.

- A small child will struggle up to 20 seconds, and an adult may struggle as long as 60 seconds. When intoxicated, an adult will not struggle at all but slip quietly below the surface.

Assisting a Victim in Distress or a Drowning Victim

Once you have identified a distressed or drowning individual, you must make an attempt to get that person to safety. A reaching or throwing assist is the safest way to help that person. *If you are not trained, attempting a swimming rescue is NOT recommended and may create a double drowning situation.*

How to make a proper **reaching assist:**

1. Be sure you are not in danger of being pulled into the water yourself.
2. Keep your center of gravity low to the ground when you extend your arm, leg, towel, shirt, etc.
3. When extending a pole, place it on the edge of the pool and slide it out and under the victim's outstretched arms. DO NOT AIM FOR THE FACE OR CHEST AREA.
4. If you extend a shepherd's crook, have the crook turned away from the victim as it is extended. Once alongside the victim, turn the pole and rotate the crook and hook it around the victim's waist. Slide it up to the armpits and pull the victim in slowly.
5. If you are doing a wading assist, be sure you lean your body toward shore or safety prior to contacting your victim. Take an object with you to extend to the victim if possible. A flotation device is the best object to use for an extension.

How to make a proper **throwing assist**:

1. When throwing a ring buoy or heaving a jug with a rope attached, attempt to throw it just past the victim and pull it under his/her thrashing arms. Be sure you don't throw the buoy or jug with the entire rope. Either stand on the end of rope or have it attached to your wrist. Be careful not to hit someone!
2. When throwing a ring buoy without a line, you attempt to have it land and drift under the victim's arms. If you are unsuccessful and you can safely swim to the victim, you may swim out and push the buoy to the victim being sure the victim cannot grasp you. At that point you can tow the buoy and victim to safety, tell the victim to hold on to the buoy and kick his way back to safety, or wait for further help to arrive.
3. Any item that floats and is tossable can be used in a throwing assist including kickboards, boat cushions, personal flotation device (PFDs), and Thermos jugs. These are tossed with the hopes that they will land and drift under the victim's flailing arms.
4. A rope can also be placed inside an empty plastic gallon jug and tied around the handle to make a throw jug. Simply place the rope around the wrist and toss the entire bottle, rope, and all. If the victim is very far away, a little water may need to be added to give sufficient weight to carry the bottle.

If no equipment is available for your use but there are several people in the area, you can form a **human chain**. Form a line of bystanders placing the heaviest person in the shallowest water and the lightest swimmer farthest out in the water. Every second person faces the opposite direction, and wrists are grabbed. Once the victim is contacted, the person on shore begins pulling in the entire chain.

Emergency Action Plans

An emergency action plan is a preconceived plan of action for emergency situations. Its purpose is to assure first aid will be given in the most expedient manner and the staff will deal with emergencies in a coordinated effort. Each facility should be prepared for emergencies and each staff member should be well trained in the proper procedures.

Emergency action plans should include the following information:

1. Course of action for all staff on duty at the time.
2. Identification of primary and support staff duties.
3. Chain of command.
4. Emergency phone numbers.
5. Facility address and phone number.
6. Follow-up procedures to evaluate the accident, including the correctness of response and prevention of similar accidents.

As a fitness professional, you should know your duties at the time of an emergency and how you fit into the emergency action plan under each situation that may arise while you are on duty at that facility.

This might include:

1. Pullout rescues – simply getting a conscious person to safety.
2. Unconscious rescues – covers drowning and cases where the pullout rescue is not effective.
3. Chest pain – the basics of a heart attack.
4. Spinal injury management – a potential neck or back injury.
5. Evacuation due to fire, earthquake, lightning, or other natural events.
6. Chlorine gas leak – mandatory if the facility uses chlorine gas.
7. Sudden neurological event
8. Injuries from falls at the pool

Diabetes

Diabetes is a blood sugar disorder characterized by chronically elevated blood glucose levels in the body. This section briefly discusses diabetes with emphasis on how to recognize and treat diabetic conditions. (Chapter 12 gives more detail on diabetes as a disease.) Diabetes is treated with injectable insulin, and/or oral medications. Insulin helps the body maintain normal sugar levels. Diabetes can cause any number of disorders including blindness, heart disease, kidney disease, stroke, and peripheral vascular disease. Amputation of toes, the foot, or leg is common in diabetics due to both a poor blood supply to the extremities as well as diabetic neuropathy, which is lack of normal sensation. Thus, injuries can occur to the diabetics' feet without them being aware. Diabetic students need to wear shoes in aquatic fitness classes to protect the delicate skin on their feet and avoid any skin trauma and possible resulting infection. Rough pool surfaces and pool chemicals can sometimes make it impossible for the diabetic to exercise in the water. Finally, make sure the diabetics visually inspect their feet both before and after each class

Exercise increases the rate at which glucose leaves the blood and can be very beneficial for diabetics. Some diabetics actually require less insulin when exercising regularly. A balance of carbohydrate intake, exercise expenditure, and insulin/medication is required to maintain proper glucose levels. When this balance is not met, either the glucose can markedly fall (hypoglycemia) or rise (hyperglycemia). In general, one hour of exercise requires an additional 15 grams of carbohydrates. It is important to watch diabetic participants for symptoms. Diabetic coma, an extreme form of hyperglycemia, requires treatment with insulin. Emergency medical care should be called, and the person should be treated for shock. Conversely, severe hypoglycemia may present with bizarre behavior or even stroke-like symptoms. Treatment is glucose. As in any condition, if the person becomes unconscious, call for emergency medical assistance.

It is advisable for the fitness instructor to become familiar with the signs and symptoms of hypoglycemia and hyperglycemia and to know proper emergency procedures for both. If you are unsure whether hyperglycemia or hypoglycemia is occurring, administer sugar or fruit juice (if the person is still conscious) and call emergency medical care.

Some people suffer from hypoglycemia during or after exercise even though they do not have a diabetic condition. Low levels of blood sugar can cause lethargy, weakness, dizziness and in severe cases, fainting. Some

Hypoglycemia (Low blood sugar)	Hyperglycemia (High blood sugar)

Signs and symptoms:
    Sweaty, clammy skin
    Hunger
    Feeling confused
    Dizziness
    Rapid heart rate
    Feeling nervous and shaky
    Mood changes
	Signs and symptoms:
	    Fatigue
	    Extreme thirst (polydipsia)
	    Frequent urination (polyuria)
	    Hunger (polyphagia)
	(These 3 make up the 3 "polys" of DM)
	    Blurred vision
	    Sudden weight loss
	Other signs and symptoms are: wounds that will not heal, vaginal infections for women, sexual problems, and numbness or tingling in the hands or feet.

Treatment: 3 - 4 glucose tablets, 1/2 can of regular (not diet) soft drink, 4 ounce glass of regular fruit juice, or 3 - 5 hard candies you can chew quickly like peppermints. If in doubt always treat for low sugar since it can progress quickly and lead to seizures or unconsciousness.	Treatment: Treatment in the field is limited to establishing that the sugar is indeed elevated, by using a finger-stick glucometer. Further treatment would be carried out in a hospitalized setting, and includes insulin and intravenous fluids.

clients who have not eaten for several hours and come to exercise may suffer low-level hypoglycemia symptoms. You may want to encourage these participants to eat breakfast before class in the morning or consume a healthy snack before afternoon or evening classes. If a client shows signs or symptoms of low blood sugar, treat as indicated for hypoglycemia above.

Myocardial Infarction (Heart Attack)

Some heart attacks are obvious- sudden and intense. Most heart attacks start with mild discomfort and pain, leaving the affected person confused about what is wrong and waiting too long to get help. Recognition of the symptoms of heart attack is important and immediate action is critical.

Signs That a Heart Attack May be Happening: (American Heart Association)
Chest discomfort. Most heart attacks involve discomfort in the center of the chest that lasts more than a few minutes, or that goes away and comes back. It can feel like uncomfortable pressure, squeezing, fullness, or pain.
Discomfort in other areas of the upper body. Symptoms can include pain or discomfort in one or both arms, the back, neck, jaw, or stomach.
Shortness of breath. May occur with or without chest discomfort.
Other signs. These may include breaking out in a cold sweat, nausea, or lightheadedness.

If you suspect someone is having a heart attack, call emergency medical service immediately. Have the person lie down and monitor them closely. Encourage the victim to take their own nitroglycerin. Have the facility's AED available if their condition deteriorates. Start CPR if necessary.

Stroke

Prompt response and care for stroke victims is as imperative as prompt response for a heart attack. In either case, damage from lack of blood flow is minimized with prompt medical care. In the case of a stroke, the fight is to save brain tissue and permanent loss of function. If stroke is suspected, call emergency medical care immediately, lie the person down and monitor them carefully.

Stroke Warning Signs: (The American Stroke Association)
Sudden numbness or weakness of the face, arm and/or leg, especially on one side of the body.
Sudden confusion, trouble speaking or understanding.
Sudden trouble seeing on one or both eyes.
Sudden trouble walking, dizziness, loss of balance or coordination.
Sudden, severe headache with no history of similar headaches.

Cardiac Arrest

Cardiac arrest is abrupt cessation of the heart beat- the heart stops beating. If this occurs, call emergency medical care immediately and begin CPR. When the AED becomes available, power it on, attach the chest pads and follow the prompts. Signs of cardiac arrest include:
- Sudden loss of responsiveness. No response to gentle shaking.
- No normal breathing. The victim does not take a normal breath when you check for several seconds.
- No signs of circulation. No pulse.

Epileptic Seizures

In the event a seizure (epileptic or other) takes place in the water, the following steps should be followed. These vary slightly from those followed on land and are worthy of mention.
1. Your primary concern is to keep the victim's head above the water and the airway open. Do NOT attempt to remove the victim from the pool during a seizure.
2. As soon as the seizure is over, you need to check for breathing and pulse. Usually, all that is necessary is to maintain a patent airway via a chin lift or jaw thrust. The patient's own tongue is the source of airway obstruction most of the time. If rescue breathing is necessary, start it in the water. Do this for the duration of one minute while the spine board and assistants are gathered. Then you can stop rescue breathing for up to one minute to remove the victim and place blankets on him/her to maintain body temperature.

3. You ALWAYS call EMS in the event of a seizure that takes place in the water. This is because you have no idea how much water has been swallowed or inhaled. The aspiration of pool water in large quantities can be deleterious to proper gas exchange in the lung and lead to a severe lung infection.

Heat-Related Illness

Overexposure to heat, combined with inadequate hydration, can cause heat cramps, heat exhaustion, and heat stroke. Any one is susceptible to heat-related illness, although the very young and very old are at greater risk. Heat-related illnesses can become serious or even deadly if unattended. The key to avoiding these conditions is prevention. Prevention of hyperthermia in exercise includes acclimatization, identifying susceptible individuals, unrestricted fluid replacement, and a well-balanced diet.

Acclimatization simply means getting used to a new environment. Travel to a warmer climate during winter months will take time for acclimatization and would present a higher risk for heat-related illness. Proper exercise and heat exposure progression is important to preventing heat illnesses. Keep in mind that the time it takes for a person to acclimate to exercising in a new environment will depend on a number of individual factors including body weight, age, and fitness level.

The three stages of heat-related illness are:

- **Heat Cramps:** Heat cramps are muscle pains and spasms. It is generally thought that loss of body fluids from heavy sweating and exertion causes heat cramps.
- **Heat Exhaustion:** Usually caused when people lose body fluids through heavy sweating. The fluid loss causes a decrease in blood flow to vital organs resulting in a form of shock.
- **Heat Stroke:** The victim loses the ability to sweat and cool the body because the temperature control

Stages, Symptoms, and Treatment of Heat-Related Illness: (American Red Cross)		
Stage I- Heat Cramps	**Stage II- Heat Exhaustion**	**Stage III- Heat Stroke**
Symptoms: Muscle cramping, commonly in the abdomen and legs. Sometimes very painful.	Symptoms: Cool, moist, pale skin (might be red after physical exertion). Dizziness and weakness or exhaustion. Nausea. Headache. The skin may or may not feel hot. Normal mentation.	Symptoms: Vomiting. Decreased alertness level or complete loss of consciousness. (A mental status change is the significant finding here.) High body temperature. Skin may still be moist or the victim may stop sweating and the skin may be red, hot, and dry. Rapid, weak pulse. Rapid, shallow breathing.
Treatment: Stop activity and rest. Drink frequent, small amounts of cool water or a sports drink. Gently stretch the cramped muscle, holding the stretch for about 20 seconds. Gently massage the muscle. If no other symptoms are present, activity can be resumed after the cramp stops.	Treatment: Get the person to a cooler place. Have them rest in a comfortable position. If awake and alert, have them sip a half glass of water every 15 minutes. No liquids with alcohol or caffeine. Remove or loosen tight clothing, and apply cool wet cloths. Call emergency medical care if the person refuses water, vomits, or loses consciousness.	Treatment: This late stage of heat related illness is life threatening. Call emergency care immediately. While waiting for their arrival, apply cool cloths; only give them oral fluids if they are awake and have an intact gag reflex.

system stops working. The body temperature can elevate dangerously resulting in brain damage and death if the body is not cooled quickly. Heat stroke is a life threatening condition.

General care for heat emergencies includes cooling the body, giving fluids, and minimizing shock. Additional symptoms and treatment are listed in the table on page 182.

To prevent heat related illness, the American Red Cross suggests:
1. Dress for the heat. Wear light weight, light colored clothing and wear a hat.
2. Drink water. Carry water or juice with you and drink continuously even if you do not feel thirsty. Avoid alcohol and caffeine, which dehydrate the body.
3. Eat small meals more often. Avoid foods that are high in protein which increase metabolic heat.
4. Avoid using salt tablets unless directed to do so by a physician.
5. Slow down if you start to feel overheated.

The aquatic instructor teaching from deck in extreme environmental conditions is susceptible to heat illness. The instructor should drink plenty of fluids and submerge often to cool body temperature.

Hypothermia could be a risk in some environmental situations such as outdoor pools or in pools with cooler water. Hypothermia occurs when heat loss exceeds heat production. Water cools the body rapidly, and some participants may become chilled to the point of discomfort and shivering. Hypothermia can be a health hazard just as hyperthermia. If water and air temperatures combined create conditions that would facilitate hyperthermia or hypothermia, appropriate measures should be taken to ensure participant safety. The instructor should not conduct the workout if participant safety cannot be ensured.

Swimmer's Ear

Swimmer's ear is caused by a bacterial infection resulting from failure to dry the ear adequately following swimming or water submersion. (11) Symptoms of this condition include itching, a greenish colored discharged, pain with chewing, and a blocked feeling of the ear. (11) (1) Prevention of this condition includes drying ears thoroughly with a soft towel and using an alcohol solution following each swim. (1). Once this condition progresses to the point of pain with discharge from the ear, a physician should be seen for treatment. Topical and/or oral antibiotics may need to be prescribed, and ear plugs may be recommended to prevent future infections.

Lightning Strikes

Each day the earth is struck by lightning approximately 8 million times. Each charge carries with it 10-20 million volts of direct electrical current, along with 20,000 amps. Yearly, lightning accounts for 150-250 deaths in the US alone, with over 1000 people seriously injured.

Five mechanisms of injury are well known:
1. direct lightning strike-carries a high rate of injury and death;
2. contact strike-when the victim is touching an object that is struck;
3. side splash-when a victim is close to the object that is initially hit, and the bolt jumps from the first object to the next-i.e. from a tree to a victim underneath it;
4. ground current-victims standing near a strike may be injured from current flowing through the ground;
5. blast effect-the air near a strike becomes superheated and creates explosive forces, which can cause massive blunt injuries.

Although the amount of voltage and amperage is huge, the duration of exposure is very short, and accounts for the injury patterns typically seen. Massive burns are very unusual in lightning. Usually, the electrically sensitive tissues are most affected: the cardiac conduction system and the central nervous system. These areas are responsible for heart beating and lung breathing, which may both be stunned following a lightning strike.

Common injuries include:
• Neurologic—loss of consciousness, amnesia, brain hemorrhage
• Cardiac—cardiac arrest, abnormal heart rhythms
• Respiratory—respiratory arrest
• Eye—cataracts, retinal detachments, bleeding inside the eye
• Ear—ear drum rupture, ear bones disruption
• Extremities—vascular spasm, temporary paralysis, bone fractures
• Obstetrics—miscarriages

Less common injuries include heart attack, burns, blunt abdominal injuries, kidney malfunctioning, and crush injuries of extremities.

Obviously, to achieve the best outcomes from a lightning strike is to avoid it in the first place. Therefore, recognition of an impending storm is paramount. Keep in tune to the constantly changing weather and be responsible for the safety of your participants. When you hear thunder, you've been trained to realize that lightning is not far away. Rapid evacuation of your entire class from the pool and the surrounding wet deck to the safer environment of an indoor shelter is your most important next move. If lightning does strike and participants are injured, have someone contact 911 to get emergency help. Although the victims pose no danger to touch, be aware that lightning can strike in the same spot twice, so be careful, and be quick.

The usual mass-trauma triage protocols call for caring for those alive and leaving those dead alone. Lightning is the exception to that rule: immediate care for those apparent dead victims may be lifesaving since rescue breathing and chest compressions should be very helpful. When lightning strikes, the cardiac muscle is shocked into asystole (flatline) and the respiratory centers in the brainstem are also stunned. However, the heart muscle cells possess automaticity. This means they will restart on their own in a couple of minutes or less. However, the brain's recovery time is longer, so the body will suffer from hypoxia (lack of oxygen) unless rescue breathing is initiated and chest compressions started and continued until a pulse is palpated. This is an appropriate time to use your CPR training. If nothing is done for lightning victims, the cardiac activity, once spontaneously returned, will disintegrate into ventricular fibrillation (heart quivering, not beating), and lack of oxygen to the heart and brain will cause eventual death.

The eventual hospital treatment for lightning victims depends entirely on their injuries. Anyone who is struck or shocked in any way should be seen at the local ER—many injuries may be subtle and in the excitement of the event, may not even be realized initially. Allow the doctors to thoroughly examine lightning victims, run tests, and arrange for specialist consultations, when necessary.

Adapted from AKWA, Gary Glassman, MD

AEA Standards and Guidelines: Thunder/Lightning

AEA recommends that all patrons and facility staff be cleared from the pool and deck area (indoor and outdoor facilities alike) at the first sounding of thunder or first sighting of lightning. Patrons and staff should not re-enter the pool area until 15-30 minutes after the last sounding of thunder or last sighting of lightning; furthermore, re-entry should not be allowed unless there are evident signs of clearing and the sky is no longer dark and threatening.

Based upon the Lifesaving Resources, Inc. Standard Operation Procedure #006 Emergency Procedures During Thunder and Lightning Storms, 7/21/82.

Chronic Injuries

An **acute** injury is defined as one with sudden onset and short duration. An example of an acute injury is the student who slips on the deck while walking from the locker room to her water fitness class and sprains her ankle. The onset is sudden and the length of time to full recovery can be one to six weeks depending on the severity of the sprain.

A **chronic** injury is defined as an injury with a long onset and long duration. A student that suffers from tendonitis in his or her shoulder as the result of ten years of swimming with poor stroke mechanics is an example of a chronic condition.

As a fitness professional, you are bound to have a client twist an ankle, knee, or back, get a cut, or even possibly fall during a work out. These injuries are usually minor, and the instructor needs to simply use the RICE method for treatment, as described above. Less often, the instructor may experience a situation where the injury is serious enough to require an x-ray, or some type of medical follow-up. At this point the instructor may need to assist the client until additional help arrives, provide for calling a family member to help, or in extreme cases stay with the client until an ambulance arrives. In the event of an acute injury during class, the instructor should follow facility protocol for treating and reporting injuries. Know proper procedures in advance so you are prepared for an injury in class and can handle the situation properly and professionally (i.e. emergency action plans).

People who exercise on a regular basis, both students and instructors, often experience overuse injuries. Many overuse injuries are experienced in the lower extremity due to the design of the foot to absorb shock for the entire body when making contact with non-resilient surfaces. (11) It is important to understand that the body is a system, and the forces that impact the foot and ankle also affect the knee, hip, pelvis, and spine. Overuse injuries can be caused by repetition of the same movement(s) over time and are generally considered chronic injuries. These injuries can be prevented by proper training methods including cross training with various activities. Water exercise can provide an excellent medium for cross training as well as recovery from overuse injuries. The following section will provide the fitness professional with basic descriptions, symptoms, and treatment of common injuries and conditions associated with exercise in general and with aquatic exercise specifically.

Shin Splints

There are two basic types of **shin splints**: anterior shin splints and posterior shin splints. Anterior shin splints are characterized by pain in the front of the shin along the tibia bone and are the result of tiny tears or abnormal rubbing of the tibialis anterior muscle. Posterior shin splints are characterized by pain on the inside of the lower leg/ tibia and are the result of tiny tears or pulling of the tibialis posterior and soleus muscles.

The exact cause of shin splints is not known, but several possibilities have been presented in literature including: poor postural alignment, falling arches of the foot, muscle fatigue, overuse, body chemical imbalance, or lack of proper anterior and posterior muscle balance in the lower leg. (5) Other sources site pronation of the ankle as the primary cause of shin splints. Some exercisers will experience shin splints after a change in running shoes or surfaces, or from increasing intensity and/or duration of exercise too quickly. Some experts believe it is caused by posterior compartment syndrome (increased pressure in the deep muscles of the leg) where others believe it is cause by periostitis or inflammation of the bone covering of the tibia where the muscles attach. Shin pain can be misinterpreted as shin splints, where in fact the pain is due to a stress fracture.

In the aquatic environment shin splints can be aggravated by exercising in water that is too shallow (increased impact) or water that is too deep (exercising on the toes). Management of this condition is varied depending on the individual. (1) Typically, ice massage, stretching the anterior and posterior muscles of the lower leg, and rest are effective. Strengthening the anterior muscles in the lower leg with toe taps or the "penguin walk" will help to reduce the onset and recurrence of this condition. If the condition persists, it would be wise for the student to seek advice from a medical practitioner. Often custom made orthotics are prescribed to reduce ankle misalignment and to prevent reoccurrence. Changing exercise surface, shoes, or altering intensity and duration can also relieve this condition.

Plantar Fasciitis

The plantar fascia is a sheet of connective tissue covering the muscles on the sole of the foot. **Plantar fasciitis** is a condition that most commonly affects the sole of the foot. Many factors, such as leg length discrepancies, foot mechanics, lack of gastrocnemius and soleus flexibility, training shoes (fit, type, or lack of), stride length and running surfaces, have been studied in relation to the cause of plantar fasciitis. (1) Researchers have been unable to link any one factor with this condition.

Most of the time, a person with plantar fasciitis will complain of localized anterior heel pain. Pain is often worse in the morning when first getting out of bed and putting weight on the foot; however, pain usually decreases after the first few steps. Ice and rest generally help to alleviate symptoms. Stretching and properly fitted shoes that are not too stiff and provide good support help prevent this condition. (11) Orthotic supports that prevent ankle pronation and supination are often prescribed, as well as ultrasound therapy, alternative therapies, and anti-inflammatory medication. Once this condition becomes chronic, it can be very difficult to manage.

Tendonitis

Tendonitis is a chronic condition that involves inflammation of the tendon. Tendons in the body connect muscles to the bones. The most common cause of tendonitis cited is overuse. Swimmer's shoulder is a condition that involves tendonitis of the rotator cuff muscles caused by repetition of the arm stroke. Imagine the competitive swimmer's experience of 10,000 yards a day at roughly 18 arm strokes per length of the pool for a total of 7,200 arm strokes per day or 1,872,000 per year.

Causes of tendonitis can also include poor exercise form and technique, previous direct injury to the tendon from a fall or blow, improper foot wear, joint overuse, improper exercise progression, anatomical causes, and age-related changes to the tendons. Tendonitis that occurs as result of exercise usually affects the knee, elbow, and shoulder.

Arnheim (1) describes three stages of pain associated with tendonitis: pain following sports activity, pain during and after sports activity that still allows for normal performance, and pain during and after activity that inhibits performance.

Treatment of this condition includes ice, rest, ultrasound therapy, alternative treatments, anti-inflammatory medications, physical therapy, and sometimes surgery. To avoid tendonitis, strengthen and stretch affected areas, use progressive overload, vary the exercise program, and try not to cycle between periods of activity and inactivity. When symptoms appear, back off the aggravating activity and switch to an activity you can perform pain free.

Bursitis

Bursitis is caused by inflammation of the bursa, which is a synovial-lined sac of fluid that helps reduce friction between tendon and bone or tendon and ligament. Bursitis exhibits many of the same symptoms as tendonitis. Typical locations include the anterior knee, the posterior elbow and the lateral hip.

Bursitis usually results from a repetitive movement or is due to prolonged and excessive pressure (resting on the elbows, kneeling on the knees, or walking barefoot). Other causes include traumatic injuries and systemic inflammatory conditions such as rheumatoid arthritis.

Treatment usually involves rest of the affected joint and keeping pressure off the affected area. Movement or pressure only makes the condition worse. Ice controls the inflammation and reduces swelling. Often anti-inflammatory medications are prescribed and cortisone injections are given.

To prevent bursitis, learn proper form and technique, take breaks from repetitive movements, and cushion your joints (for example during prolonged kneeling.)

Conditions of the Patella (Knee Cap)

The knee cap is an important part of the knee joint because it functionally increases leverage. (see figure 11-2) It can allow for a 30% increase in strength when extending the knee such as when kicking a ball. The most common symptom of patellar irritation is pain when sitting for long periods of time and when descending stairs. People with this condition may experience swelling of the knee as well as a grating noise during flexion and extension of the knee.

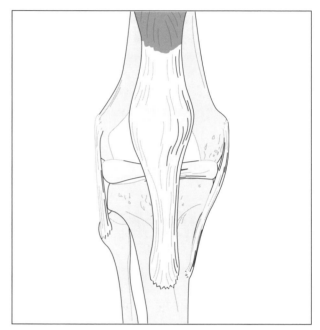

Figure 11-2 Anterior Knee Joint

The three most common patella conditions are:
Chondromalacia patellae (runner's knee), the most common of the three, occurs due to irritation and softening of the articular cartilage on the undersurface of the kneecap.

Patellar bursitis (housemaid's knee) is a condition of swelling and inflammation over the front of the knee. It is commonly seen in people who kneel for extended periods of time such as carpet layers or gardeners.

Patellar subluxation/dislocation, also called an unstable knee cap, is a condition where the knee cap does not track evenly with its groove on the femur.

Treatment of these conditions includes rest, ice, cross training, gradual progression back into activity, physical therapy, and anti-inflammatory medications. In some cases, surgery may be required.

Back Pain

Eight out of ten people suffer from **low back pain** in their lifetime (9). It is one of the most common symptoms of orthopedic patients. Although many symptoms of back pain generally resolve in a few weeks, it is a very disabling condition. Back pain is a very broad term for a large number of back conditions. This section gives general information on back pain and its treatment.

Diagnosis for back pain may include muscle strain (thought to be the most common cause of back pain), intervertebral herniated (see figure 11-3) or ruptured disk, spinal stenosis (narrowing of the spinal canal leading to compression of nerves), osteoarthritis, osteoporosis, and spondylolyis/ spondylolisthesis (an acquired malformation of the spinal column.)

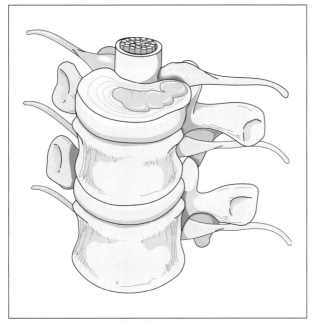

Figure 11-3 Herniated Disk

Treatments for the relief of acute pain may include pain medications, epidural steroid injections, rehabilitation and physical therapy, and if all else fails, surgery. Once acute symptoms dissipate, the most common treatment prescribed for low back pain is exercise. Maintaining proper strength and flexibility in the core musculature is paramount to back health. A strong core allows weight to be better distributed and less force placed on the spine.

Carpal Tunnel Syndrome

Carpal tunnel syndrome is an overuse condition that occurs in the wrist. The median nerve is compressed by the inflamed flexor tendons which all pass together through a tight fitting carpal tunnel. This results in pain, tingling, or decreased sensation from the thumb to the ring finger of the hand (10). Pain may extend up the arm and is often worse at night. (see figure 11-4)

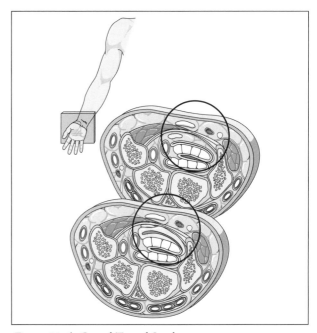

Figure 11-4 Carpal Tunnel Syndrome

Causes of carpal tunnel syndrome include diabetes, hypothyroidism, arthritis, pregnancy, and repetitive movement/use of the wrist. Eighty percent of patients with carpal tunnel syndrome are over the age of 40.

Conservative therapy for carpal tunnel syndrome includes simple exercises that can be performed at home. Padded wrist rests should be used while typing on the computer and sports related carpal tunnel syndrome can be prevented with proper technique and the use of wrist braces. This condition can occur during water fitness classes as a result of improper hand positioning while using equipment. Education and cueing of students on neutral hand position can prevent this condition from occurring. Treatment usually begins conservatively and becomes more aggressive if needed. It includes anti-inflammatory medications, wearing a brace, injection with a combined anesthetic/ steroid, and surgical release of the carpal tunnel.

Stress Fractures

A bone is typically broken due to exposure to a very high force strong enough to break the bone. Mechanisms may include a fall, a direct blow or a vehicular crash. Contrast this to a **stress fracture**, which occurs when lower level forces happen repetitively for a long period of time and is also known as a "fatigue fracture." Stress fractures are commonly seen in athletes who run and jump repetitively on hard surfaces; naturally they are most commonly seen in foot and shin bones. Symptoms include progressive pain and tenderness when pressure is applied to the bone. Swelling may or may not be present. Stress fractures may not appear on x-rays and may need to be diagnosed with an MRI.

A stress fracture can result from repeated stress due to hard surfaces, an acceleration in training, inadequate footwear, an existing condition, or dietary abnormalities and menstrual irregularities. The best treatment is rest. If the activity causes pain, it should be avoided. If walking causes pain, then crutches or immobilization may be necessary. Ice the affected area, use proper equipment including proper footwear, use progressive overload, and seek medical advice if pain persists or intensifies.

Fitness Professional Wellness

Lifeguard Lung Disease

A growing concern in the aquatic environment worthy of mention is Lifeguard Lung Disease. This risk is increasing with the growing number of indoor facilities that have water spray features. The bacteria that cause this condition appear to be suspended in water droplets and are breathed in. Prevention, through adequate and properly maintained filtration and ventilation systems, combined with early detection and treatment are important to avoid health risk.

Report:

Lifeguards and aquatic fitness professionals need to be aware of this illness. It is a risk from indoor pools. Once you have the disease there is nothing you can do to prevent if from worsening except permanently leave the contaminated pool area. It is an asthma-like condition. It can be treated if detected early, but permanent lung scarring can also occur if diagnosis and treatment aren't timely. Symptoms include: persistent coughs, chest tightness, eye irritation, headaches, shortness of breath, fever, tiredness, night sweats, weight loss, fatigue, achy flu-like symptoms, wheezing, and labored difficult breathing.

Diagnosis may be complicated by the fact that its symptoms are the same as asthma, influenza, or bronchitis. This is only occurring in people associated with <u>indoor pools and hot tubs</u>. Many of the people affected blamed their symptoms on cold or overwork. The bacteria are suspended in water droplets or vapor droplets. Turning a faucet is the easiest way to be exposed. Once affected it is very hard to completely get rid of the infection.

When bacteria suspended in water droplets are breathed in, the lungs get inflamed. It mainly affects those who spend dozens of hours at an indoor facility that is not properly filtered and ventilated. Concentrations of airborne bacteria by-products were highest near the lifeguard crow's nest, about 8 feet from the surface of the pool than at pool level. The bacteria may have been dead but were still capable of causing an immune reaction in the lung.

Source: National Jewish Medical and Research Center

<u>www.nationaljewish.org</u> / 1 800 222-Lung / <u>lungline@njc.org</u>

Overtraining

In the case of exercise, more is not always better. Inappropriate levels of training can lead to a potentially serious condition called **overtraining**. Overtraining is a condition where an individual trains too hard, too often, and/or too long. This ends in a state of staleness and general fatigue. The body can react negatively to excessive exercise and overtraining leads to decreased performance. Many overtraining syndromes are a function of the rate of progression- in other words, doing too much too quickly. This typically results in extreme soreness and fatigue.

Usually overtraining occurs in one of two ways: overload of a specific group of muscles or overload of the entire body. In either case, prevention of overtraining includes varying program components, practicing periodization, and incorporating appropriate rest into the workout. The mechanism for overtraining in resistance training is slightly different than the mechanism for overtraining in cardiorespiratory or endurance training due to the difference in metabolic systems used. There is no

100% accurate measurement for the onset of overtraining. Once symptoms occur, the most effective treatment is rest.

The causes of overtraining are multi-faceted and include physiological as well as psychological factors. It is important to keep site of the fact that exercise is one important component of overall health or wellness. Webster (1993) defines health as "a state of fitness of the body or of the mind." Realize that "health" takes on as many meanings as there are people on the planet earth. Consider that Webster's definition isn't very specific and doesn't include body measurements, weights, or body systems. In short, encourage your clients to exercise and provide them with accurate lifestyle information to help them improve and maintain overall health and total wellness. This is true for the fitness professional as well, who often gets trapped in overtraining syndrome by teaching too many classes and/or training sessions.

Treatment for overtraining would include cutting back on frequency, duration, or intensity of exercise sessions. If training for an athletic event, an exerciser can often benefit by changing the type or mode of exercise. Many athletes cross train in the water to get relief from impact and heat while maintaining functional capacity.

If an instructor or student exhibits any of the above symptoms, a re-evaluation of current exercise behavior may be considered. There is a fine line between abusive exercise/ exercise addiction and healthy exercise. Healthy exercise leaves an individual feeling refreshed, rejuvenated, mentally alert, and productive.

Vocal Use and Abuse

Vocal injury is recognized as any alteration in your normal manner of speaking.

Exercise leaders tend to take their voices for granted. Vocal abuse afflicts singers, actors, ministers, classroom teachers-anyone that has an occupation that requires an enormous amount of talking. Fitness professionals should become "vocal athletes" by learning the warning signs and symptoms of vocal abuse and taking proper care of their voice to prevent injury and the deterioration of the voice.

According to Dr. Ceila Hooper, Clinical Associate Professor of Speech and Hearing at the University of North Carolina at Chapel Hill, "The voice is a sound produced by the vocal folds which are bands of tissue located in the larynx, or voice box, in the neck. The speech functions of the larynx include the production of pitch, loudness, and voice quality. Voice problems

Symptoms of Over Training From Resistance Exercise:	Common Markers of Aerobic Endurance Overtraining:
Plateau followed by decrease of strength gains	Decreased performance
Sleep disturbances	Decreased percentage of body fat
Decrease in lean body mass (when not dieting)	Decreased maximal oxygen uptake
Decreased appetite	Altered blood pressure
Persistent cold	Increased muscle soreness
Persistent flu-like symptoms	Decreased muscle glycogen
Loss of interest in the training program	Altered resting heart rate
Mood changes	Increased submaximal exercise heart rate
Excessive muscle soreness	Altered cortisol concentration
	Decreased total testosterone concentration
	Decreased sympathetic tone (decreased nocturnal and resting catecholamines)
	Increased sympathetic stress response

Adapted from NSCA, 2004

in fitness professionals are usually caused by the strain of speaking over music, yelling, or speaking while positioning the body in neck-straining postures. These abusive habits may result in swellings or growths on the vocal folds which may develop into granulated tissue called **vocal nodules**. Any change in the sound of one's voice which persists for more than two weeks needs to be checked by a physician to rule out any serious medical condition." (see figure 11-5)

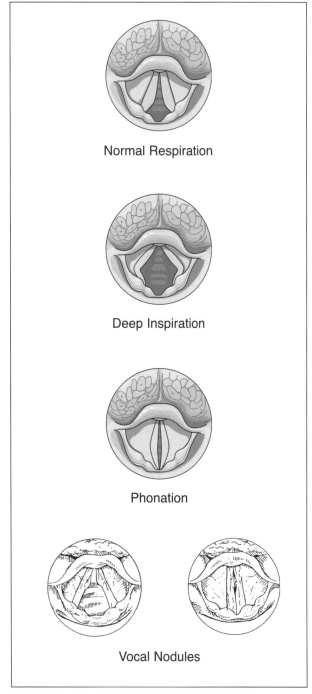

Normal Respiration

Deep Inspiration

Phonation

Vocal Nodules

Figure 11-5 Vocal Cord Positions

There are a variety of early symptoms which may indicate vocal misuse, abuse, or injury. The progression of symptoms is very gradual. Symptoms or warning signs of vocal abuse include:
- Harsh, gravelly, rough voice
- Habitual use of lower pitch
- Pain when swallowing
- Feeling of something in your throat
- Difficulty swallowing
- Dry mouth
- Clearing throat frequently (more than two times an hour)
- Frequent hoarseness, voice loss
- Pitch breaks, voice cracking
- Reduced range for the singing voice
- Voice not heard clearly (muffled)
- Frequently asked if you have a cold or to repeat a sentence
- Comments on how sexy your voice sounds
- Vocal fatigue (worse at night)
- Voice tired after talking a lot

If you determine you might be experiencing a voice injury, seek a professional opinion from an otolaryngologist. An otolaryngologist is an ear, nose, and throat specialist (ENT). He/she will examine your larynx. The larynx which is made of cartilage, muscle, and connective tissue houses the **vocal cords**. The vocal cords open and close in regular cycles. The otolaryngologist will most likely take a voice history and look at your vocal folds with a laryngoscope.

Tips to Reduce Vocal Abuse

Prevention of voice injury is your first line of defense. To reduce your risk of vocal abuse, you can/should:
- Keep your throat moist and your vocal cords lubricated. Drink plenty of water throughout the day.
- Avoid overuse. Limit the number of classes you teach and limit enthusiastic shouts and screams. Use body language and nonverbal cues.
- Renew your breath frequently.
- Use a microphone.
- If using music, keep it at a moderate level. Consider speaker placement and the location from which you project your voice.
- Check ventilation and chemical fume levels in the pool area.
- Project your voice with proper posture and body alignment. Maintain the neck in neutral alignment.

- Minimize background noise as much as possible.
- Limit talking when you have an upper respiratory infection. The vocal folds are already swollen and inflamed.
- Substitute a swallow for excessive throat clearing. Try to cough quietly to bring the vocal folds together gently.

The earlier vocal abuse is detected, the easier it is to treat this overuse injury. Many exercise leaders experience denial of voice-related problems. They may fear it will end their career as fitness professionals. Vocal therapy may help the instructor develop correct vocal technique and minimize vocal abuse.

What an Instructor May Learn From a Speech/Language Therapist

A speech/language therapist will help you determine if you are speaking at too high or too low a pitch, speaking with inadequate breath support, speaking with a relaxed throat and mouth position, and determine if you speak with too many hard glottal attacks. In addition, you may learn easy onset of voicing and other vocal warm ups, tips for those who suffer from allergies and gastroesophageal reflux, and help to determine if you talk from your throat instead of your diaphragm and abdominals. You would receive help with how to warm up your voice with vowel rich words and phrases. The therapist will explain why whispering and gargling strains the voice.

Summary

1. Acute injuries have sudden onset and a reasonably short duration. A chronic injury has a long onset and a long duration.

2. Common chronic injuries in exercise include shin splints, plantar fasciitis, tendonitis, bursitis, patellar problems, back pain, carpal tunnel syndrome, and stress fractures.

3. RICE is the common treatment for basic first aid.

4. CPR can be adapted to be administered in the shallow water.

5. An aquatic fitness professional should be aware of basic water safety and how to recognize a drowning victim.

6. Additional concerns and conditions in the aquatic environment include recognizing signs and symptoms, prevention, and basic treatment for heart attack, stroke, cardiac arrest, epileptic seizures, hyper and hypoglycemia, heat-related illness, and lightening strikes,

7. Recognize some features of instructor wellness including lifeguard lung disease, over training, and proper vocal care.

Review Questions

1. Which chronic condition is due to excessive, prolonged pressure or from repetitive movement?
2. What do the letters in RICE represent for basic first aid treatment?
3. You should remove a victim who is having an epileptic seizure from the water immediately. True or False.
4. You should always remove a victim from the water before administering CPR. True or False.
5. List three common markers indicating cardiorespiratory overtraining.
6. List 3 tips to avoid vocal abuse and injury.
7. Before using the AED machine, it is not necessary to dry the victim. True or False
8. Obtain a copy of your facility's emergency action plan and see if it adequately addresses all of the emergencies discussed here.

See Appendix E for answers to review questions.

References

1. Arnheim, D. (1989). *Modern Principles of Athletic Training*. 7th Edition. St. Louis, MO. Times Mirror/Mosby College Publishing.

2. Beachle, T. and R. Earle. (2004). *NSCA's Essentials of Personal Training*. Champaign, IL. Human Kinetics Publishers.

3. Cailliet, R. (1983). *Knee Pain and Disability*. 2nd Edition. Philadelphia, PA. F.A. Davis Publishers.

4. Durstine, J. and G. Moore. (2002). *ACSM's Exercise Management for Persons with Chronic Disease and Disabilities*. 2nd Edition. Champaign, IL. Human Kinetics Publishers.

5. Ekstrom, M. (1987). Lower Leg Pain Can Stop Athletes in Their Tracks. *The First Aider*. 56:5, 1.

6. Howley, T and D. Franks. (2003). *Health Fitness Instructor's Handbook*. 4th Edition. Champaign, IL. Human Kinetics Publishers.

7. Kasdan, P. (2004). *Disorders and Ailments-Plantar Fasciitis*. www.ourfootdoctor.com/yourfeet_plantar fasciitis.shtml. Ourfootdoctor.com.

8. Laird, C. (2002). *Webster's New World Dictionary and Thesaurus*. 2nd Edition. Indianapolis, IN. John Wiley & Sons Publishers.

9. Nachemasson, A. (1985). Advances in Low Back Pain. *Clinical Orthopedics and Related Research*. Volume 200. Baltimore, MD. Lippincott, Williams and Wilkins.

10. Prentice, W. (2001). *Rehabilitation Techniques in Sport Medicine with PowerWeb: Health and Human Performance*. 3rd Edition. New York, NY. McGraw-Hill Publishers.

11. Vinger, P. and E. Hoerner. (1986). *Sports Injuries: The Unthwarted Epidemic*. 2nd Edition. Chicago, IL. Year Book Medical Publishers.

Select Images provided by:
Kumm, R. (2005). *LifeART Super Anatomy 3*. Baltimore, MD. Lippincott, Williams & Wilkins. Website: www.lifeart.com

Resources

American Diabetes Association
www.diabetes.org

American Heart Association
www.americanheart.org

American Institute of Cancer Research
www.aicr.org

American Red Cross
www.redcross.org

American Stroke Association
www.strokeassociation.com

Hughston Sports Medicine Foundation
www.hughston.com

About, Inc./Orthopedics
www.orthopedics.about.com

Chapter 12: Special Populations

INTRODUCTION

Chapter 12 gives an overview of the unique needs of special population groups. Working with special populations can be very challenging, but can also be very rewarding. This basic overview serves to aid the fitness professional who may see special populations mainstreamed into regular programs.

Some fitness professionals will pursue specialized education and training in order to make a career out of servicing a specific population such as older adults, children, or clients with cardiovascular disease. This chapter touches on various conditions and age groups, but is far from a complete reference or specialized training for working with special populations. Fitness professionals should continue to pursue resources, education, and references to aid in developing safe and effective programming for individuals with various abilities and disabilities.

Unit Objectives

After completing Chapter 12, you should be able to:
1. Identify recommended water temperature, shallow water depth, tempo, and program formats for special populations.
2. Recognize characteristics, the benefits of exercise, and program considerations for the following special populations: Older Adults, Larger Adults, Children, Adolescents, Pre and Post Natal, Cardiovascular Disease, Pulmonary Disease, Musculoskeletal Disease, Metabolic Disease, Neurological Disease, and Immunological/Hematological Disorders.

Key Questions:
1. What is the difference between chronological and functional age?
2. Which is more relevant to the development of chronic disease: overweight or obesity?
3. Name three primary program considerations for children's exercise programming.
4. Are all adolescents at the same level of maturity physically and psychologically?
5. Why is exercise important for obese clients?
6. What are the benefits of water exercise for the pregnant client?

If every client had the same needs and requirements, developing exercise programs would be easy, requiring little expertise or thought. In reality, people come in various sizes, shapes, ages, and with various lifestyles. Since every client is unique, so are their goals, abilities, health problems, and disabilities. As a fitness professional, it is important to understand how exercise can help or hinder these variances. This will enable you to guide all individuals who cross your path to safe and effective exercise choices. It is important to recognize your limitations as a fitness professional and to refer clients to a more qualified trainer or instructor if necessary.

This chapter presents an overview of the common age groups and conditions you may encounter beyond the "typical" healthy adult including:
- Older Adults
- Larger Adults
- Children
- Adolescents
- Pre and Post Natal Clients
- Clients with Cardiovascular Disease, Pulmonary Disease, Musculoskeletal Disease, Metabolic Disease, Neuromuscular Disease, and Immunological/Hematological Disorders.

Older Adults

Recommended Water Temperature: A temperature range of 83-86 degrees F (28-30 degrees C) is recommended for moderate to high intensity exercise. A temperature range of 86-88 degrees F (30-31 degrees C) is recommended for lower intensity exercise.

Recommended Tempo: 120 to 145 beats per minute utilized at one half tempo.

Recommended Shallow Water Depth: Chest to armpit depth to allow for reduced impact and controlled movement.

Recommended Program Formats: Most program formats can be adapted for an older adult population. Continuous aerobic training can be performed at an intensity level well within a comfortable pace for participants. Interval training can be performed above and below the aerobic threshold. Circuit training can be performed at a moderate to low intensity. Many older adults enjoy participating in modified aquatic kickboxing, water striding, and muscular conditioning formats. Modified deep water exercise is also recommended.

Monitor intensity and incorporate rest periods in deep water if necessary.

Characteristics

The term "older adult" or "senior" can include adults ranging from age 55 to over 90, creating a large variation in age and ability. **Functional age** is measured by the ability of the individual to maintain daily activities related to independent living. **Chronological age** refers to the person's physical age as measured in years. Many older adults may have an advanced chronological age but a young functional age. The reverse is possible as well.

The American Medical Association's Committee on Aging found that it was almost impossible to distinguish between the effects of aging and the effects of physical inactivity. Many ailments attributed to aging (low energy, weakness, poor muscular strength, stress and tension, high cholesterol, diabetes, stiffness, constipation, hypertension, obesity, insomnia, back problems, and decreased range of motion) are often reported by middle-age adults who are physically inactive. Research has shown that exercise initiated at any age will provide physiological and psychological benefits. Many of these conditions can be improved or alleviated through regular physical activity.

As the body matures, changes occur as part of the aging process. The degree to which these changes occur varies with the age and from individual to individual. Some of these changes include:

Sensory Changes: Sensory perception changes with age. Visual changes may include decreased acuity or sharpness of perception, a decrease in the size or extent of visual field, and/or a decrease in judgment of the speed of moving objects. Hearing impairment affects a large percentage of older adults with decreases in acuity or sharpness and sound discrimination. A decrease in number and sensitivity of nerve cells leads to slower data transmission causing changes in mobility, response time, spatial awareness, and balance. There is an overall decrease in functional coordination between nerves and muscles.

Physical Changes: Older adults experience decreases in height and increased midsection measurements due to spinal compression. Body composition changes occur typically with an increase in body fat and a decrease in muscle tissue. Hair can thin and lose color and the skin loses elasticity. Bone density decreases bringing an increased risk of bone breaks. Muscular strength, endurance, and flexibility can decline.

Heart Changes: The heart grows larger with age due to heart muscle being replaced with fat and connective tissue. This results in a loss of contractibility and a decline in pumping capacity. Maximal attainable heart rate declines with age, and blood pressure increases due to loss of elasticity and a narrowing of the blood vessel walls. The immune and respiratory system becomes less effective.

Psychological Changes: Although psychological changes are hard to document, many older adults experience depression, anxiety, insomnia, as well as other psychological conditions.

Benefits of Regular Exercise

Physical activity slows the aging process. Properly designed aquatic fitness programs can help the older adult retain physical and psychological functioning. The initiation of resistance training programs for older adults has led to significant documented strength gains for persons well into their nineties. Becoming more active at any age is beneficial. Physical activity helps the older adult retain sensory, physical, and psychological functioning.

Water exercise classes are appealing to seniors for several reasons. Water is a forgiving medium; reducing joint compression and the downward pull of gravity. Many participants who are unable to exercise on land can be comfortably active in the water. The water's pressure helps reduce swelling of inflamed joints. The water provides tactile feedback and improves sensory functioning. A class environment helps alleviate loneliness, depression, and anxiety, and allows socialization with peers. Aquatic fitness can be fun and motivating while providing several physical benefits. Aquatic fitness can help the older adult improve self-esteem, quality of life, and foster a better outlook on life.

Program Considerations

Because of decreased balance, vision, and hearing, make sure your older adult participants are familiar with pool safety before starting class. Instructions should be given in a way that is easy for them to hear, see, and understand. Five minutes spent prior to class acclimating new students to their surroundings may prevent accidents and alleviate the need for rescue or emergency assistance. Making participants aware of emergency procedures will make them feel more secure and enable them to help you, and each other, should a crisis arise. You will want to make them aware of the following:

- Pool layout including pool depth and slope.
- The location of the lifeguard.
- Procedures for emergencies.
- Deck layout and deck hazards including slippery areas.
- The location of pool lifts, ramps, and accessible ladders for the shallow and deep ends.

Several changes in class formatting are recommended for the older adult. Programming can be made more specific by incorporating exercises that offset the effects of aging. Class formatting and music selection should be dictated by the need and desire of class participants. Recommendations include:

- The warm up should be longer. Additional time is needed to progressively warm up all joints in the body.
- In the cardiorespiratory segment of class, offer low impact options for participants who cannot safely or comfortably do high impact activities.
- Include movements that change direction to improve balance and coordination.
- Use holding patterns to allow enough time for transitions and readjustment of body alignment.
- Incorporate muscular balance into the routine for strength and flexibility.
- Incorporate strengthening and stretching exercises to improve posture and prevent rounded shoulders.
- Encourage all participants to work at a comfortable intensity level.
- Utilize all three planes for movement to encourage increased range of motion.
- Avoid exercises that will aggravate arthritis, back, hip, and knee problems.
- Adapt exercises as many older adults have hip and knee replacements.
- Encourage socialization and interaction between participants.
- Watch for chilling during cool down and post-stretch exercises.
- When teaching from the deck, watch participants for prolonged neck hyperextension.

Older adults benefit from eye contact and instructor interaction. Choose music that is the proper tempo and appealing to your participants. Remember that older adults often have additional health-related issues that must be considered as well in programming.

Larger Adults

Recommended Water Temperature: A temperature range of 80-86 degrees F (26.5-30 degrees C) is recommended for obese participants. Overheating can be an issue for obese participants, even in the water, due to increased thermal insulation. Water temperatures over 86 degrees may be more appropriate for toning, stretching, and less vigorous types of class formats. Program design should be carefully considered if water temperature exceeds 90 degrees. The intensity of the class should be inversely proportional to the water temperature. As water temperatures increase, intensity should decrease.

Recommended Tempo: The lower and middle range of typical recommended tempo ranges (125-150 bpm shallow and 100-130 bpm deep) are recommended for obese participants due to larger body mass and more surface area. Approaching 150 bpm for shallow and 130 bpm for deep water may be inappropriate for most larger adult participants.

Recommended Shallow Water Depth: Waist to armpit depth. Optimal depth will be influenced by a client's total buoyancy as well as height.

Recommended Program Formats: Interval programming works well for a multi-fitness level class for obese participants. Working above and below aerobic threshold, above and at aerobic threshold, and within the target heart rate range will accommodate most levels of fitness. Circuit training also allows for multi-fitness levels to be successful within a class. Deep water training is a non-impact, challenging option for larger adults. Although many larger adults feel very buoyant, the use of buoyant equipment may still be necessary to maintain proper alignment and form. Be sure to have belts that are large enough or can be adjusted or combined to accommodate all participants.

Characteristics

Overweight is a condition where an individual's weight exceeds the population norm or average, which is determined by height/weight tables based on gender, height, and frame size. Although a standard approach, the definitions lack the ability to account for significant muscle mass. A better measure might be percentage body fat, but this approach has not replaced the simple approach.

Obesity is a condition where there is "an excess of body fat frequently resulting in a significant impairment of health," a level of 20% or more above ideal body weight. Obesity is generally defined and accepted as above 20% body fat for males, and above 30% body fat for females. There is some variance in obesity thresholds as determined by different organizations or criteria. The prevalence of obesity is approaching an epidemic level in the US, with obesity on the rise in many other developed countries.

Obesity is typically measured through Body Mass Index (BMI) or percentage of fat as compared to lean tissue mass. Overweight is determined with a BMI of 25- 29.9, and obese with a BMI of 30 or higher.

Although not all larger adults are unhealthy, there are various health risks that have been associated with obesity. These risks include:

- Premature death
- Type 2 Diabetes
- Heart disease
- Stroke
- Hypertension
- Gall bladder disease
- Osteoarthritis
- Sleep apnea
- Asthma
- Breathing problems
- Cancer (endometrial, colon, kidney, gallbladder, and postmenopausal breast cancer)
- High blood cholesterol
- Complications of pregnancy
- Menstrual irregularities
- Stress incontinence
- Psychological burden including depression and social stigmatization

Adapted from www.nih.gov

Benefits of Exercise

There are many ways in which exercise is beneficial to the obese participant. Exercise helps to promote negative energy balance and aids in weight loss efforts. With exercise, there is a higher likelihood that weight lost is fat weight, and muscle weight is spared or improved. Additional benefits include:

- risk reduction for chronic disease
- improved circulation
- stronger heart and lungs
- increased stamina, strength, and endurance
- lower resting blood pressure and pulse
- improved body composition
- increased life span
- self-confidence and awareness

- positive changes in mood
- relief of depression and anxiety
- increased mental well-being
- positive coping strategies

The advantages to exercising in the water for the larger adult include:
- Reduced impact pressure and load due to the water's buoyancy.
- The benefits of hydrostatic pressure to increase circulation and reduce swelling.
- The cooling effect of the water- it is a more comfortable exercise medium for many larger adults.
- The fact that water "covers up" or hides the body making many larger adults feel less self-conscious when they exercise.

Program Considerations

Dress is an important issue with this population. It is important that fitness professionals appropriately convey a message that will make the overweight client feel at ease. Dress appropriately as the fitness professional, keeping your larger participants in mind. Exposing their body in the pool area may be the number one deterrent or excuse for not participating in an exercise program. Let participants know where they can find large lycra bike shorts, supportive exercise bras that can be used in the water, and how to cover up their swim suit or other clothing with a T-shirt. Having that information available will help keep many from making excuses not to attend.

Be aware that some larger adults may have special needs in exercise programming. Remind them to wear shoes on the pool deck to prevent slips and falls. Using Vaseline may help to prevent chaffing where areas of the body may rub together during repetitive movements. Help them with positioning in the pool so they are not too buoyant to keep up with the class.

General program considerations include:
1. Obese individuals need safe and comfortable access to enter and exit the pool. Steps, ramps, and ladders in the shallow area of the pool serve this purpose. Some participants may require assistance to raise their body weight out of the water.
2. Some participants may need alternatives for impacting. Body mass can affect range of motion, and modifications may need to be given for some stretching and toning exercises.
3. Avoid exercises that would cause discomfort or discourage participants with larger bodies. Do include movements for coordination, balance, range of motion, and improved body alignment.
4. Stress proper body alignment and form. Cue proper knee and foot position as many participants have lower leg and ankle misalignments.
5. Use appropriate music and movement tempo. Some larger participants may be more comfortable at a slightly slower tempo due to a larger body mass and additional frontal surface area which will increase intensity.

Adapted from Aquatic Exercise Association's Larger Adult Instructor Training Course

There are fewer restrictions for overweight exercisers in water as compared to land. Repeated high impact movements, excessive side to side movements, and calisthenics that require extended periods of single limb support should be avoided on land. The buoyancy of the water allows for the use of high impact in moderation for most students, reduces the risk of side to side movements, and supports weight for single limb activities. Participants can usually assume a supine position for longer periods of time in water and not experience as much weight pressing on the internal organs as on land. Water provides many benefits, increased programming options, and additional movement possibilities for the overweight exerciser.

It is important not to assume that all overweight participants are unfit. Many, however, have never been encouraged to participate in any kind of exercise activity. The instructor should be well versed on exercise progressions in the aquatic environment, such as pelvic tilts progressing to curl ups; shorter levers and range of motion leading to longer levers and range of motion; and no impact leading to lower impact and then bounding moves. Participants should be guided to safely progress to better quality muscle contractions and more intense activity.

The obese participant should be given the opportunity to work at a moderate intensity for as long as is tolerable. Duration and intensity should be gradually increased as the participant becomes more fit. Longer duration, moderate intensity exercise is beneficial in fat loss efforts as well as tolerability and comfort. Let students know that they may feel very heavy as they leave the pool the first few times, and they should leave the water slowly. The student may start to feel tired and out of energy at about 20 minutes if they have not been active. The body will take about a month to be able to effectively utilize fats for energy.

While it may take some effort to develop strategies to motivate the obese participant, it is extremely rewarding to participate in the process that leads to success and a healthier life.

Children

Recommended Water Temperature: A water temperature range of 83-86 degrees F (28-30 degrees C) is recommended for children's aquatic fitness programs.

Recommended Tempo: The recommendation for a typical shallow and deep water tempo applies to children as well. However, most children's programs (especially with younger children) may not follow a regular tempo or beat for fitness activities.

Recommended Shallow Water Depth: Various depths of water can be used for children's programming.

Recommended Program Formats: The primary formats used for younger children's programming follow a start-stop or go fast-go slow type of activity pattern. This reflects the natural tendency of how children prefer to move and play. As children mature and their attention spans increase, various continuous training formats can be introduced.

Characteristics

In general there are a vast number of differences as well as similarities between adults and children participating in fitness programs:

- Children need to be careful of overheating because they have underdeveloped thermoregulatory systems. Children should drink water before, during, and after exercise.
- Children have smaller hearts and lungs that work extremely fast. They require more ventilation than adults to deliver a given amount of oxygen. Their heart rates are higher than adults and they have an increased ventilatory rate, which supports the notion that they have inferior ventilatory efficiency.
- Children tend to have 20-30% greater energy expenditure than adults during aerobic activities.
- It is a child's natural preference to participate in start/stop activities. They do not typically engage in sustained forms of exercise. Children should use RPE to convey how they feel.

- Children have impaired cardiac output and stroke volume and they have lower blood oxygen carrying capacity. Children's aerobic fitness components differ from adults.
- Girls and boys differ in levels of endurance fitness. In 1988, research done by Dr. Washington found that the average pre-pubertal boy has greater levels of endurance fitness than the average girl.
- Recent information indicates that both boys and girls demonstrate significant gains in strength after weight training. (Westcott, 1992). The basic principles of strength training, as recommended by ACSM, apply to adults as well as children. Submaximal loads should be used for children and form and technique should be the primary emphasis.

Adapted from Aquatic Exercise Association's Children's Aquatic Fitness Instructor Training Course

Benefits of Exercise

Obesity is becoming a significant health care concern for children as well as adults. The level of physical fitness in children has declined significantly and the prevalence of obesity is rising rapidly. A decrease in physical education programs, after-school activities, and outdoor play combined with the availability and convenience of unhealthy fast food and snacks increase the risk for children to become obese, unfit, and consequently unhealthy. Many physical educators and fitness leaders are concerned that children are not as active as they should be. Inactivity can lead to the same health problems for children as for adults with an even shorter expected life span, more dire consequences, and a higher, longer term expense burden on the health care system.

Exercise provides the same or similar benefits to children as it does for adults. The aquatic environment is ideal for enticing children to play and be active. Most children love the pool and water activities.

Program Considerations

Factors that affect children's programming content and format include attention span, physical capabilities, level of socialization, and socioeconomic background. Programming is primarily dependent on the age of the child. Programs should be developed to promote fitness, social skills, motor skills, and healthy habits for each age level. A preschooler's fitness needs are similar to a preteen's fitness needs, but the manner of programming used to meet these needs is very different. Emphasis should be placed on developing and maintaining healthy habits for children of all ages, that will carry into adulthood.

Following are programming characteristics and considerations for children according to age group needs.

Ages Birth-2

This is a great age to introduce water. Working with a parent, a child can develop many positive skills while receiving one on one instruction and direct parental attention. Water exposure for this age group fosters trust, reduces the fear of water, and helps to strengthen the bond between parent and child. Activities should include lots of toys and play. Attention span can be as short as 10 seconds; short activities that are mixed and repeated work best. Beginning motor skills for swimming are taught and interspersed with eye-hand and lower torso skills.

Ages 3-5

At this age, it is imperative to keep the class "moving" because of short attention spans. Pay close attention to how your students are reacting and if they start to lose interest, switch quickly to another activity. Have all equipment ready and in place so you can switch activities quickly. Thorough class planning is critical. Have a few extra activities ready to go in case you have extra time, as some activities may not take as long as you expect. You may want to avoid having the children help with equipment- it will use up a lot of class instructional time trying to get them organized. Plan activities that include all students and avoid situations where they have to wait for turns. Children this age don't like to wait for anything and will become disruptive. Additional characteristics include:

- Children from ages 3-5 have rather unrefined gross motor and manipulative skills. For example, they will tend to catch a ball with their body and arms rather than their hands.
- Programs should include activities that incorporate gross motor skills and the use of large muscles to offer the opportunity to begin to refine skills. Running, chasing, hopping, and directional changes are examples of these activities. Balls, bean bags, hoops, and other medium sized objects offer the chance to practice manipulative skills.
- Since children in this age group have high levels of imagination and curiosity while being imitative,

opportunities such as acting like animals or pretending to be superheroes support expression of ideas while using the body.

- These children are also very active and have high levels of energy. Using continuous activities to hold their attention, alternating between high and low intensities is important.
- Structured rest should be included by adding "quiet" activities or games interspersed through out the program.
- A short attention span is characteristic of the child from 3-5. Activities should change every 60-90 seconds and should include simple games, songs, and movements.
- Children this age are also individualistic or egocentric and need experiences to learn to share. Parallel play alongside rather than with other children begins to teach awareness of others.
- The key is to keep things simple, but fast moving and ever changing.

Suggestions for components of programming to incorporate for ages 3–5 years old:
1. Introduction to class, review rules, quickly talk about what you will do today. Designate an area to which they will return to sit and receive quick instructions between each activity, such as against a wall or in a circle. Communicate set areas or boundaries you want the children to stay within.
2. Gross motor skills including locomotor activities with music.
3. Gross motor activities including eye-hand and eye-foot coordination with equipment.
4. Obstacle courses or other agility/coordination activities.
5. Movement exploration with music, stories, and/or equipment.
6. Fine motor skills with equipment or music. (Wee Sing finger plays or manipulation of fine motor equipment.)

Ages 6-9

At this age you will be able to start introducing more advanced concepts such as games and fitness activities. You will want to include some structured fitness activities such as a block of resistance exercises with paddles, but should intersperse structured activities with play activities. Children this age are becoming more social and like group problem solving activities. They do well working in a circuit format and are usually motivated to go from station to station, especially if the stations are fun. They like relay activities and races. Additional characteristics include:

- Children are becoming more concerned with self-confidence at this age, but still want to have fun.
- Gross motor skills are becoming more refined and graceful so activities can introduce sport skills and drills.
- Combinations of basic movements can be put together.
- Eye-hand coordination is improving so manipulation of smaller objects is possible as well as using activities to improve accuracy. Tossing balls through a hoop or at a target are great skills to include.
- This age group has better balance and body control so activities such as "statue maker" or "red light-green light" could be incorporated.
- Many children this age will have a tendency towards poor posture so activities should focus on body mechanics and the development of endurance and strength.
- The child age 6-9 is becoming more socially mature and begins to consider the interest of a group.
- They have an increased attention span so games can become longer and the rules can be more complex. Circuit activities work well.
- You can include team activity, but division into teams needs to consider a greater gender-related difference in skills and competitive spirit. Boys may compete to fatigue. Ability grouping and balancing teams needs to be considered. "Choosing" teams should be avoided and more random ways of dividing students should be used.
- The spirit of adventure is high so new activities and games requiring some courage and creativity work well.
- These children are intellectually curious and can begin to do problem-solving activities and create their own games and goals.

Suggestions for components of programming to incorporate for ages 6–9 years old:

1. Introduction to class, go over well defined rules and consequences, talk about what you are going to do today.
2. Informal thermal warm up activity and a pre-stretch including a few static stretching exercises if water temperature allows.

3. Children this age will still want to do interval type activities by nature. Avoid long periods of continuous intensity activity. Incorporate activities where they alternate working really fast, fast, slow, and really slow. Tell a story where they are an active character and have them "act out" the part incorporating different intensities of activities. Use fast and slow music or whistles to keep them motivated and giggling.
4. Introduce a block of muscular fitness exercises with "toys" or equipment, starting to emphasize form and technique, and moving relatively quickly from exercise to exercise. Do fewer repetitions alternating between exercises and sets to hold their attention.
5. Age appropriate games, relays, circuits, or races.
6. Cool down with static held stretches if water temperature allows.

Ages 9-12

Ages 9-12 years will have longer attention spans and can work on more structured activities. Rules to games can be more complex and they can handle form and technique training for muscular fitness, cardiorespiratory fitness, and flexibility exercises. Form and technique should be emphasized over high intensity for muscular fitness activities. You can alternate individual activities with group activities. Relays, circuits, and intervals still work well with this age group, although you can start to introduce some continuous training as well. Having fun is still a primary issue. Children in this age group will be at varying degrees of physical and emotional maturity. Additional characteristics include:

- This is an age group of diversity. Many children will be undergoing bodily changes in the form of puberty while others will look and think like younger children.
- Division of this group may be dependent upon the method used in a particular area in school. Some schools combine 6th–8th grades in Junior High while others are strictly 7th and 8th.
- There is a tremendous amount of social pressure in this age group such as wanting to fit in with others while at the same time expressing individualism.
- Older children like basically the same kinds of activities as the younger ages with rules of the games changed to become more competitive.
- Music should reflect the interests of the group and children can be encouraged to bring in music to be screened for content and then shared.

- Circuit and interval training work well with this age group. These formats can be designed in ways similar to adults, but taught in a group format first and then later as an individual effort.
- Children this age like the idea that they can socialize with friends while exercising.
- Coordination is more highly developed and there is a keen interest in proficiency in skills. These children have a desire to learn more difficult skills and need more coaching on refinement of those skills.
- There are greater sex differences in skills and interests. Separation of the sexes within classes might be beneficial for competitive contact activities since boys may play more vigorously than girls.
- Games that lead up to sports are typically well-received. Girls typically enjoy advanced dance patterns.
- Good skills, as well as physique, are important to social acceptance, particularly for boys.
- Some instruction concerning the understanding of the fitness components, changes in growth, and varied abilities can be included. Flexibility is naturally decreasing so there is a need to maintain a level of flexibility within structural limitations. Muscular growth is occurring, particularly in boys. Focusing on proper form and technique with strength and endurance activities is important for both genders.
- Group spirit is high and allegiance to the group is strong. There is a need to belong to a stable group, make rules and decisions, and abide by them. Allowing the children to participate in setting rules allows for greater buy in of the process. Letting children help select activities will improve their self worth and insure greater participation.
- As children enter 7th and 8th grade, the sexes differ in both skill and interest. Interest in the opposite sex is increasing.
- Girls may show lack of interest in some activities due to cultural influences. There are greater feelings of insecurity by both genders and a desire to be a part of a group.
- There is also a need to be accepted by the teacher. This can be shown in different ways, both positive and negative, through trying to gain attention.

Suggestions for components of programming to incorporate for ages 9-12 years old:
- Introduction to class, go over well defined rules and consequences, talk about what you are going to do today.

- Informal, <u>social</u> thermal warm up activity and a pre-stretch including a few static stretching exercises, if water temperature allows. Work on proper stretching techniques.
- For cardiorespiratory training, you can include a series of intervals or stations as well as a block of interesting continuous training. Jumping jacks, knee lifts, kicks and other typical aerobic movements can be introduced. Keep it moving and fun.
- Games always make exercise fun. Incorporate games in which all students can easily participate and succeed. You may want to consider games that are active as well as social and require group problem solving.
- Muscular fitness training should focus on form and technique. Intensity should remain moderate. Keep the exercises fun and challenging.
- Cool down including a static stretch emphasizing proper form and technique.

A fitness professional can serve as a positive, healthy role model for children of any age. Adapt popular land games for the water and use lots of inventive equipment. Variety and stimulation are important factors, but repetition builds motor skills. Be creative and find different ways to practice the same skill. Keep in mind peer interaction and individual needs, but most importantly, have fun!

Adolescents

Recommended Water Temperature: A temperature range of 83-86 degrees F (28-30 degrees C) is recommended for moderate to high intensity exercise. A temperature range of 86-88 degrees F (30-31 degrees C) is recommended for lower intensity exercise.

Recommended Tempo: 120 to 150 beats per minute utilized at one half tempo for shallow water programs. 100 to 130 beats per minute utilized at one half tempo for deep water programs. Tempos may vary with program format.

Recommended Shallow Water Depth: Chest to armpit depth to allow for reduced impact and controlled movement. A minimum depth or 6.5 (1.98 meters) is recommended for deep water programming. Water depth may vary with program format.

Recommended Program Formats: Younger teens typically do not like to do one type of exercise or program for an extended period of time. As maturity is approached, the teen is more open to a regular conditioning program as developed for adults.

Characteristics

Adolescence, or the teen years, is a time of rapid bodily growth and development in which the body matures both physically and sexually. Generally, adolescence is defined as occurring somewhere between the ages of 8 and 19 for females, and 10 and 22 years for males. There is a great deal of variation in regards to the age at which children enter into adolescence with the onset of puberty. Adolescence is typically considered over when adulthood is reached. Although teens follow the same general growth pattern, each individual's timing in this process is unique. Often it is important to consider physical, emotional, sexual, social, and mental maturity as opposed to chronological age alone.

Some characteristics for adolescents or teens include: (Adapted from Darst and Pangrazi)
- Large differences in social development can be seen among teens.
- Early-maturing students are usually heavier and taller. They also have larger amounts of muscle and bone tissue. Often, early maturers will carry a greater percentage of body weight as fat tissue.
- Generally, early maturing males have mesomorphic (muscular) physiques.
- Early-maturing females are often characterized by endomorphy (shorter and heavier).
- Differences in body size and composition probably account for male-female performance differences that require strength and power.
- Obese teens are usually more mature for their age than normal-weight teens.
- Activity has little or no impact on the stature of maturing adolescents, but does positively affect fitness levels.
- Motor performance of males increases with skeletal maturity. Motor performance for females seems not to be related to physiological maturity. It appears that late maturing females have higher motor performance.
- Due to physiological differences, teens are at a disadvantage when exercising in hot environments as compared to adults.
- Competitiveness is common, as is fighting with parents and peers.

- Younger teens (Junior High) have rapid and uneven growth leading to decreased effectiveness for learning motor skills. High growth velocity allows shorter time to adjustment to bodily changes. Many teens are self conscious about their bodies, and posture can be a problem for teens who are self-conscious about their height.
- Because of hormonal fluctuations, early teens can become easily angry, fearful, and upset.
- There is a lot of peer pressure and influence during adolescence. Grooming, clothes, and appearance become more important. Independence from adults is desired.
- Older teens (High School) have finished their growth spurt and are reaching physical maturity. They have passed the period of physical awkwardness and feel more comfortable with their abilities.
- Older teens have fewer mood swings and seem to be a little more emotionally stable. Most have completed puberty and are more comfortable with their body and the direction of their life.

Benefits of Exercise

There is a growing prevalence of obesity among adolescents in developed countries. The rise in obesity is accompanied by a rise in health risk for this age group as well. There is concern that unhealthy teens will become unhealthy adults. One of the best things an exercise professional can give to an adolescent is a positive attitude about their body and exercise. Exercise can help with weight management and the development of healthy levels of lean tissue mass. It is very important for adolescents to develop healthy eating and exercise habits to carry into adulthood to aid in the reduction of chronic lifestyle diseases.

Additional benefits of exercise for adolescents include:
- Strength training causes muscle hypertrophy gains similar to that in adults, with similar detraining effects as well.
- Aerobic power in teens can be increased by 10-20% through a regular training program, however responses to training will be very individual. It is possible to train two teens with the same program and end up with different results.
- Bone tissue in teens increases in diameter and density in response to physical activity, and can help guard against osteoporosis in adult life. Exercise assures optimum growth of bones during the maturation process.

- Exercise can build self-awareness, self-confidence, and a healthy body image. Physical activity has many physical and psychological benefits for the adolescent exerciser.

Program Considerations

Consider different programming options for younger adolescents as compared to older adolescents. Most younger teens tend to dislike doing one type of exercise program for an extended period of time. The concept of games and making exercise fun still applies to a great extent for this age group. Most older adolescents have developed adequate physical and mental stamina to be more open to participating in a typical conditioning program. Adolescents tend to like sports conditioning formats, like kick boxing and sports games, as opposed to typical aerobic choreographed routines. In order to keep adolescents interested, a program should be conducted in a games/fun format. Teens do well with circuit, strength, interval, and deep water activity based class formats.

Pre and Post Natal

Recommended Water Temperature: A temperature range of 78-84 degrees F (25.5-29 degrees C) is recommended for moderate to high intensity exercise. For moderate to high intensity exercise, avoid pool temperatures above 85 degrees F.

Recommended Tempo: The lower and middle range of typical recommended tempo ranges (125-150 bpm shallow and 100-130 bpm deep) are appropriate. Approaching 150 bpm for shallow and 130 bpm for deep water may be inappropriate for pregnant participants.

Recommended Shallow Water Depth: Chest to armpit depth to allow for reduced impact and controlled movement.

Recommended Program Formats: High intensity formats or programs that elevate and lower the heart rate should be minimized for pregnant participants. Comfortable, continuous, moderate intensity aerobic exercise is recommended with emphasis on postural muscles, slower transitions, and relaxation exercises.

Characteristics

A woman's body goes through many changes during the three trimesters of pregnancy. There are physiological changes in many organs and systems in the mother's body to allow for supplying the fetus with proper nutrients and waste removal. There are many structural changes that occur to accommodate housing the fetus. For most pregnant women, exercise is a healthy choice that better enables the body to adapt to the necessary bodily changes. Exercise can also foster a positive self-image and mental outlook to ease the psychological burden of pregnancy.

Characteristic changes include:
- Heart rate increases both at rest (10-15% increase) and during exercise.
- Lung capacity decreases due to an increase in size of the abdomen.
- Mechanical changes include weight gain, enlarged uterus and breasts, skin thinning, and postural changes.
- Postural changes include kyphosis and forward head from increased size and weight of the breasts, and lordosis as the size and weight of the abdomen increases. A shift in center of gravity and/or center of buoyancy may accompany these changes.
- Blood volume and cardiac output increases. Adequate oxygenation is important. Increased blood volume is a partial cause for the swelling, cramping, and supine hypotension (abnormally low blood pressure) that occurs during pregnancy. Increased blood volume can also cause dizziness with sudden changes in movement, increased water dissipation, and increased saliva and vaginal discharge.
- Blood vessels soften and enlarge to accommodate increased blood volume resulting in varicose veins, hemorrhoids, swelling, and decreased venous return.
- After the first trimester the supine position may result in a significant decrease in cardiac output. Motionless standing is associated with an even greater decrease in cardiac output than the supine position.
- Blood pressure increases are possible. Pregnancy induced hypertension is a risk.
- The prostaglandin hormone "relaxin" is released during the first trimester, relaxing the musculo-skeletal system by softening ligaments and loosening joints, preparing the body for childbirth. This makes the musculoskeletal system vulnerable to injury. Abrupt moves and power moves should be avoided.
- The mother has an increased basal metabolic rate requiring more calories to sustain herself and the

fetus, an increase in heat production, and a higher risk of hypoglycemia (low blood sugar).

- Adequate consumption of water is very important.
- Supportive clothing, including shoes, is imperative.
- Many physiological and morphological changes persist for 4-6 weeks postpartum. Softening of the connective tissue continues 6-12 months postpartum.

Adapted from Aquatic Exercise Association's Programming for Pre and Post Natal Instructor Training Workshop.

Benefits of Exercise

It was once thought that exercise during pregnancy was not good for the mother or the baby. Due to medical and scientific research, most doctors have reversed this opinion. Many are encouraging women with normal, low-risk pregnancies to exercise consistently through pregnancy and to resume exercise soon after giving birth. The aquatic environment provides additional benefits to the pregnant client. The benefits of regular exercise during pregnancy include:

- Regular exercise increases circulation capacity allowing for an increased ability to deal with physiological stress, such as in delivery.
- Exercise reduces swelling and problems associated with varicose veins and hemorrhoids. Exercise in the water has been shown to be even more effective because water pressure further aids in the reduction of swelling.
- Exercise increases metabolism for better weight regulation.
- Exercise eases gastrointestinal problems and constipation.
- Exercise aids with coordination and facilitates reflex pathways. The water facilitates these benefits by removing the fear of falling. The viscosity of the water allows for slower, more deliberate and controlled movements that enhance stabilization, balance, and coordination during exercise.
- Exercise strengthens muscles, tendons, and ligaments to reduce backaches and muscle and joint pain. Water provides a multidirectional resistance to aid in the development of muscle balance. Shallow and deep water provide resistance for the abdomen and core muscles, strengthening them to support the weight of the uterus and maintain proper posture.
- Research indicates that pregnant women who exercise perceive labor as less painful, have shorter, easier labors with less medical intervention, have

babies with higher neonatal Apgar scores, and have quicker recoveries.

- Aquatic exercise additionally provides a low impact environment, the cooling effect of the water to reduce fetal heat stress, a reduced heart rate response with similar oxygen consumption, and hydrostatic pressure to reduce swelling in the extremities.

Program Considerations

If you mainstream pregnant and postpartum participants into your general fitness classes, consider meeting with them before they join the class, or providing them with a hand out, to explain their special needs. Most facilities will require physician's consent. You can provide written information, such as the American College of Obstetricians and Gynecologists (ACOG) guidelines, and ask them to collaborate with their care giver to decide how the guidelines best apply to their individual situation. The ideal situation is to have a separate class for pre and postpartum clients, if possible, to build a social and support system through their pregnancy and after the baby is born.

Programming for pre and post natal clients is dictated by the ACOG Guidelines. It is recommended that all fitness professionals follow these exercise guidelines which were created in 1985 and most recently revised in 2002.

Recommendations for Exercise in Pregnancy and Postpartum
Source: American College of Obstetricians and Gynecologists, Home Exercise Programs, Washington, DC, 2002

1. During pregnancy, women can continue to exercise and derive health benefits even from mild to moderate exercise routines. Regular exercise (at least three times per week) is preferable to intermittent activity.
2. Women should avoid exercise in the supine position after the first trimester. Such a position is associated with decreased cardiac output in most pregnant women; because the remaining cardiac output will be preferentially distributed away from splanchnic beds (including the uterus) during vigorous exercise, such regimens are best avoided during pregnancy. Prolonged periods of motionless standing should also be avoided.
3. Women should be aware of decreased oxygen available for aerobic exercise during pregnancy. They should be encouraged to modify the intensity of their exercise according to maternal

symptoms. Pregnant women should stop exercising when fatigued and not exercise to exhaustion. Weight-bearing exercises may under some circumstances be continued at intensities similar to those prior to pregnancy throughout pregnancy. Non weight-bearing exercises such as cycling or swimming will minimize the risk of injury and facilitate the continuation of exercise during pregnancy.

4. Morphologic changes in pregnancy should serve as a relative contraindication to types of exercise in which loss of balance could be detrimental to maternal or fetal well being, especially in the third trimester. Further, any type of exercise involving the potential for even mild abdominal trauma should be avoided.

5. Pregnancy requires an additional 300 kcal/day in order to maintain metabolic homeostasis. Thus, women who exercise during pregnancy should be particularly careful to ensure an adequate diet.

6. Pregnant women who exercise in the first trimester should augment heat dissipation by ensuring adequate hydration, appropriate clothing, and optimal environmental surroundings during exercise.

7. Many of the physiologic and morphologic changes of pregnancy persist 4-6 weeks postpartum. Thus, prepregnancy exercise routines should be resumed gradually based on a women's physical capability.

Contraindications to Exercise
The following conditions should be considered contraindications to exercise during pregnancy:
• Pregnancy-induced hypertension.
• Pre-term rupture of membranes.
• Pre-term labor during the prior or current pregnancy or both.
• Incompetent cervix/cerclage.
• Persistent second or third trimester bleeding.
• Intrauterine growth retardation.

In addition, women with certain other medical or obstetric conditions, including chronic hypertension or active thyroid, cardiac, vascular, or pulmonary disease, should be evaluated carefully by their physician in order to determine whether an exercise program is appropriate.

Summary
In the absence of either obstetric or medial complications, pregnant women can continue to exercise and derive related benefits. Women who have achieved cardiovascular fitness prior to pregnancy should be able to safely maintain that level of fitness throughout pregnancy and the postpartum period. Depending on the individual's needs and the physiologic changes associated with pregnancy, women may have to modify their specific exercise regimens. Despite findings that suggest lower birth weights among offspring of women who continue to exercise vigorously throughout pregnancy, there currently is no data to confirm that, with the specific exceptions mentioned here, exercising during pregnancy has any deleterious affects on the fetus. While maternal fitness and sense of well-being may be enhanced by exercise, no level of exercise during pregnancy has been conclusively demonstrated to be beneficial in improving perinatal outcome.

ACOG Guidelines Update 2002
Exercise During Pregnancy and the Postpartum Period
The current Centers for Disease Control and Prevention and American College of Sports Medicine recommendation for exercise, aimed at improving the health and well-being of non-pregnant individuals, suggests that an accumulation of 30 minutes or more of moderate exercise a day should occur on most, if not all days of the week. In the absence of either medical or obstetric complications, pregnant women also can adopt this recommendation.

Given the potential risks, albeit rare, thorough clinical evaluation of each given pregnant woman should be conducted before recommending an exercise program. In the absence of contraindications, pregnant women should be encouraged to engage in regular, moderate intensity physical activity to continue to derive the same associated health benefits during their pregnancies as they did prior to pregnancy.

In general, participation in a wide range of recreational activities appears to be safe. The safety of each sport is determined largely by the specific movements required by that sport. Participation in recreational sports with a high potential for contact, such as ice hockey, soccer and basketball, could result in trauma to both the woman and fetus. Similarly, recreational activities with an increased risk of falling, such as gymnastics, horseback riding, downhill skiing, and vigorous racquet sports have an inherently high risk for trauma in pregnant and non-pregnant women. Those activities with a high risk of falling or for abdominal trauma should be avoided during pregnancy. Scuba diving should be avoided throughout pregnancy because during this activity the fetus is at increased risk for decompression sickness secondary to the inability of the fetal pulmonary circulation to filter bubble formation.

Exertion at altitudes of up to 6,000 feet appears to be safe; however, engaging in physical activities at higher altitudes carries various risks. All women who are recreationally active should be made aware of signs of altitude sickness for which they should stop the exercise, descend from the altitude, and seek medical attention.

Moderate weight reduction while nursing is safe and does not compromise neonatal weight gain. Finally, a return to physical activity after pregnancy has been associated with decreased incidence of postpartum depression, but only if the exercise is stress relieving and not stress provoking.

Conclusions and Recommendations

Recreational and competitive athletes with uncomplicated pregnancies can remain active during pregnancy and should modify their usual exercise routines as medically indicated. The information on strenuous exercise is scarce; however, women who engage in such activities require close medical supervision.

Previously inactive women and those with medical or obstetric complications should be evaluated before recommendations for physical activity during pregnancy are made. Exercise during pregnancy may provide additional health benefits to women with gestational diabetes.

A physically active woman with the history of or a risk of preterm labor or fetal growth restriction should be advised to reduce her activity in the second and third trimesters.

In addition to the ACOG Guidelines for Exercise, consider the following when planning exercise programs for pregnant and post partum clients:
- Include exercises such as pelvic tilts, kegels, scapular retraction, and abdominal strengthening to offset postural changes and weight redistribution.
- Be aware of options for abdominal exercise in the water, discussed later in chapter.
- Focus on assuring muscle balance, proper alignment, and controlled movements.
- Be cautious of weight bearing exercises, and caution against over-stretching.

- Be aware that synovial fluid decreases, so longer warm ups are needed to lubricate the joints.
- Evaluate and consider the pros and cons for the use of additional resistance equipment such as rubber bands around the ankles as well as drag and buoyant equipment.
- Try to have the pregnant clients maintain their exercise levels prior to pregnancy. Clients may increase intensity only if done gradually and with care, and should be monitored carefully.
- Avoid over-heating and encourage proper hydration.

The abdominal muscles are important to condition because they play an important role in maintaining correct pelvic tilt and spinal alignment and help prevent low back pain. Supple abdominal muscles that have maintained optimum contractibility and blood circulation will lengthen easily during pregnancy and shorten more readily afterward. ACOG recommends that after the first trimester, supine training should not be performed (on land) because the weight of fetus and anatomical structure of the pregnant woman can depress the vena cava which may inhibit blood supply to both mother and fetus. Fortunately, due to the buoyant environment of water and actual position of the body, the fetus does not depress as extensively on the vena cava. Therefore it is generally considered safe for a pregnant woman to continue to perform "supine" abdominal exercises in the pool as long as she remains comfortable, can breath easily, and does not hold her breath. Communicate to the class that if an individual experiences any dizziness, nausea, or lightheadedness during this type of training, the woman should immediately shift positions. As an added precaution, this supine aquatic position should only be maintained for a maximum of two minutes before changing positions. If supine abdominal training is not allowable, feasible, or comfortable, provide options such as standing crunches using bouyant devices for resistance. Some caregivers recommended that pregnant women who have diastasis recti (vertical separation of the rectus abdominis muscle) continue to perform abdominal exercises, but they should "proximate" during the movement. "Proximate" refers to physically holding the separated abdominal together with the hands or a support belt. Individuals should consult with their primary caregiver as some medical doctors still recommend avoiding abdominal exercises in this situation. Always check with the participant's physician prior to recommending this type of exercise. Should the caregiver recommend that a participant not utilize this exercise position, the instructor should provide other alternatives for the individual.

Pre-pregnancy training should be gradually resumed based upon the individual's capabilities and the care giver's recommendations. Resumption of water exercise will be influenced by healing of the episiotomy and the level of vaginal discharge (lochia). Exercise tends to improve sleep patterns, reduces stress and tension, and can help relieve postpartum depression. Getting together with other new moms can provide support, encouragement, and advice on many aspects of motherhood.

Cardiovascular Disease

Recommended Water Temperature: A temperature range of 83-86 degrees F (28-30 degrees C) is recommended for moderate to high intensity exercise. A temperature range of 86-88 degrees F (30-31 degrees C) is recommended for lower intensity exercise.

Recommended Tempo: 125 to 150 beats per minute utilized at one half tempo for shallow water exercise.

Recommended Shallow Water Depth: Chest to armpit depth to allow for reduced impact and controlled movement.

Recommended Program Formats: Continuous moderate level aerobic conditioning is generally prescribed for clients with cardiovascular disease. For unfit individuals, rest periods may need to be incorporated, or interval training above and below the lower target heart rate threshold may provide tolerable programming.

Characteristics

Cardiovascular disease (CVD) is a general term for diseases of the heart and blood vessels. ("Cardio" means heart and "vascular" means vessel.) Cardiovascular disease includes high blood pressure, atherosclerosis, heart attack, stroke, congestive heart failure, rheumatic heart disease, and congenital defects. Some of these diseases affect the blood vessels while others affect the heart itself.

CVD has been the major cause of death in the U.S. for decades. Coronary artery disease (CAD) ("hardening" of the arteries in the heart), also known

as coronary heart disease (CHD), affects more than six million Americans. In 2003, about 950,000 Americans died of CVD, accounting for over 40 percent of all deaths. The main causes of CVD are atherosclerosis and hypertension. (see definitions below) Atherosclerosis contributes to high blood pressure, and high blood pressure contributes to atherosclerosis.

Cardiovascular diseases are a result of both genetic and environmental factors. Lifestyle habits (low fat, high fiber diet, and exercise), along with medications, can play a major role in terms of prevention. In addition, lifestyle changes can help maintain optimal cardiovascular function following cardiac rehabilitation. The risk factors associated with cardiovascular disease were discussed in Chapter 10.

Terms Associated with Cardiovascular Disease

1. **Angina**: Medically known as angina pectoris, it is a feeling of pressure or tightness in the chest. This cardiac pain can radiate to the arm, shoulder, upper back, or jaw.
2. **Arteriosclerosis**: An arterial disease in which the blood vessel walls become thickened and hardened.
3. **Atherosclerosis**: A form of arteriosclerosis in which fatty deposits of cholesterol and calcium develop on the blood vessel walls.
4. **Coronary Artery Thrombosis**: An obstruction from a blood clot in the coronary artery.
5. **Coronary Heart Disease (CHD)**: Also known as coronary artery disease (CAD) in which atherosclerosis develops in the arteries of the heart.
6. **Embolism**: A sudden obstruction of a blood vessel, usually caused by a clot carried in the blood stream.
7. **Heart Attack**: Medically known as myocardial infarction in which a section of the heart dies due to lack of blood supply.
8. **Hypertension**: Higher than normal blood pressure.
9. **Stroke**: An obstruction of an artery in the brain.
10. **Thrombosis**: A clot in a blood vessel.

Stroke

A **Stroke** or Cerebrovascular Accident (CVA) is due to a disruption of blood supply to the brain. When blood does not supply oxygen and other nutrients to cells, nerve cells in the affected area cannot function properly and may be permanently damaged. It is imperative that individuals who suffer a stroke receive immediate transport to a medical facility to receive medical care. The longer the event continues untreated, the higher the risk of brain tissue damage and permanent disability. In the event of immediate medical care, for some a complete recovery is possible.

Recognition of a stroke is imperative to immediate medical care. Although subtle changes during stroke may be missed, there are some obvious changes that can be noticed. These changes include:
- A lack of alertness and ability to follow commands.
- Eye movements that are not symmetrical or double vision noted.

- Weakness in one arm or leg, or both.
- Sudden loss of balance or vague dizziness.
- Numbness in an extremity or neglect of one side of the body.
- Loss of speaking skills and/or loss of comprehension.
- Facial asymmetry may be seen in the smile or tongue.

Stroke is the major cause of long-term disability in developed countries. A stroke usually affects the motor power (muscular control) on one side of the body. Muscles on the affected side may have no tension or strength or they may become tense and rigid. Balance may also be affected and speech communication may be impaired.

A Closer Look at Atherosclerosis

Atherosclerosis is a condition that affects all of us. Unfortunately, some people suffer such high levels that they die from it. Atherosclerosis begins with the buildup of soft fatty streaks along the inner walls of the arteries. The sites at which the arteries branch contain the highest concentration of these streaks. With time, the streaks enlarge and become hardened plaques. Plaques are mounds of lipid material, mostly cholesterol and fat, which mix with smooth muscle cells and calcium to become hard and nonpliable. Although arteries normally expand with each heartbeat in order to accommodate the pulses of blood that flow through them, the plaque filled, hardened arteries cannot. This drives up blood pressure. This increased pressure further damages the arterial walls, which encourages more plaque formation at that point. And so the process escalates. The critical point of coronary artery disease begins when plaques have covered over 60% of the coronary artery walls. The increased pressure buildup in the artery can cause part of the arterial wall to become weakened and balloon out, forming an aneurism which can eventually burst. A burst aneurism in the aorta, femoral arteries, or brain can lead to massive bleeding and quick death.

Atherosclerosis also brings about abnormal clotting processes. Normally, there is a balance between the process of clots forming and dissolving. Atherosclerosis disturbs this balance as platelets, the

cell-like bodies which cause clots to form, are wrongly triggered when they encounter plaques in the bloodstream. Also, substances released by the platelets may contribute to plaque growth.

One of these clots may attach to a plaque in an artery and gradually grow until the artery is completely blocked. This would not allow blood flow to the affected tissue. The tissue will slowly die and be replaced by scar tissue. A stationary clot is called a thrombus, and when it closes off an artery, it is called a thrombosis.

A clot can break off and travel through the bloodstream until it reaches an artery that is too small to allow passage. This traveling clot is called an embolus. Once again, the affected tissues will lose their blood supply and die. An embolus in this condition is called an embolism. If the thrombosis or embolism occurs in the heart, we say the person had a heart attack. If it occurs in the brain, we call it a stroke. When significant amounts of heart or brain tissue are affected, the victim dies.

Hypertension accelerates the atherosclerosis process. The increased pressure in the arteries causes arterial lesions to develop which cause plaques to grow faster. Additional pressure can also cause aneurysms to burst. Sometimes, heart attacks and strokes occur with no apparent blockage. Instead, an artery, for a yet unknown reason, goes into a spasm and restricts or cuts off blood supply to the brain or heart.

Blood Cholesterol Levels

Cholesterol occurs in various forms in the bloodstream. Both total cholesterol levels and the levels of certain types of cholesterol molecules increase or decrease the rate of atherosclerosis. Cholesterol is a lipid and is insoluble in water. Therefore, in order for cholesterol and other fats to be transported in the blood, they must combine with proteins and phospholipids to form a molecule that will dissolve in water. These molecules are called **lipoproteins**.

There are three major classes of lipoprotein. These include **chylomicrons**, **low density lipoproteins** (LDL), and **high density lipoproteins** (HDL). Chylomicrons carry food fats from the intestines into the bloodstream and to the liver and other tissues. Although LDL and HDL carry lipids in the blood, they have different make-ups and different effects on atherosclerosis. LDL are lighter and more lipid filled. LDL carry cholesterol and triglycerides from the liver to the tissues. It is the cholesterol in LDL that finds its way into the plaques of atherosclerosis. Hence, LDL cholesterol has been named the "bad cholesterol."

HDL are smaller, denser, and packaged with more protein. HDL act as scavengers and pick up excess cholesterol and phospholipids from the tissues and return them to the liver for disposal. HDL have earned themselves the label of being "good cholesterol." High blood cholesterol levels, particularly a high ratio of LDL to HDL, are associated with CVD.

Cholesterol Levels
Cholesterol levels are measured in milligrams (mg) of cholesterol per deciliter (dL) of blood.

Total Cholesterol Level	Total Cholesterol Category
Less than 200 mg/dL	Desirable
200-239 mg/dL	Borderline high
240 mg/dL and above	High

LDL Cholesterol Level	LDL Cholesterol Category
Less than 100 mg/dL	Optimal
100-129 mg/dL	Near optimal/above optimal
130-159 mg/dL	Borderline high
160-189 mg/dL	High
190 mg/dL and above	Very high

HDL Cholesterol Level	HDL Cholesterol Category
Less than 40 mg/dL	A major risk factor for heart disease.
40 - 59 mg/dL	The higher, the better.
60 mg/dL and above	Considered protective against heart disease.

Adapted from National Cholesterol Education Program, 2004.

Women and Cardiovascular Disease

In the past, most heart disease research had focused on men. More recently, many new eye-opening facts are emerging about women and heart disease. These facts include:
- CHD ranks first among all disease categories in hospital discharges for women.
- CHD is higher in minority women, substantially higher in black women.
- In 2000, CHD claimed the lives of 505,661 females; all forms of cancer claimed 267,009.
- 38% of women will die within one year after a heart attack, compared to 25% of men.
- Most women are older and sicker than men by the time of diagnosis (approximately 10 years older).
- Women are twice as likely to die of a first heart attack than men.
- Women frequently have different symptoms, often more vague.
- Women respond differently to treatment.
- Quite often, women have different outcomes and recoveries.
- The medical profession still battles a history of "gender prejudice."
- Women have a tendency to wait longer to seek medical attention.
- Women are likely to have a second heart attack within the first year.

(Aqua Hearts®, 2001)

Benefits of Exercise

Lack of physical activity is a risk factor for coronary heart disease. The benefits of regular exercise in the treatment and prevention of cardiovascular disease are well documented in research. Guidelines for physical activity and exercise to reduce the risk of chronic disease are discussed in Chapter 4. Additional exercise related benefits that reduce risk or aid in treatment of CVD include:
- Regular aerobic exercise can reduce blood pressure if hypertensive.
- Regular aerobic exercise can help raise HDL and lower LDL and is especially important for those with high triglyceride and/or low HDL levels who are overweight with a large waist measurement (central obesity).
- Warm water exercise can reduce muscle tension and increase flexibility for stroke victims.
- The psychosocial and psychological benefits of exercise are important to combat depression and

confusion accompanying the necessary lifestyle changes that lie ahead for clients that have been diagnosed with cardiovascular disease.

- Enhanced circulation due to hydrostatic pressure massaging the venous system.
- Hydrostatic pressure promotes deeper breathing as it exerts force on respiratory walls and resists respirations.
- Improved balance.
- Weight loss.
- Improved flexibility and upper body strength in patients post open heart surgery post sternotomy.
- Reduced sternal discomfort post open heart surgery.

Cardiovascular Disease and Obesity

Central obesity refers to the condition of fat being stored on the abdomen and is sometimes referred to as the "apple" profile. This apple shape is in contrast to those individuals who store their fat on their hips and buttocks which is referred to as the "pear" profile. Central obesity has been highly associated with CVD.

Program Considerations

Cardiovascular diseases cause the majority of deaths in our society with coronary heart disease (CHD) as the leading cause of premature death in the United States. Individuals with cardiovascular disorders may be medically compromised by participating in an exercise program. For this reason, any individual with a history of cardiovascular problems should see his/her physician before participating in an exercise program. Cardiac disease advances, unless people are very proactive in making lifestyle changes. The fitness professional can be instrumental in risk factor education to promote healthy lifestyle changes. Additional considerations include:

- It is best to have a physician determine the upper limit for exercise heart rate. If a physician has recommended exercise, it is appropriate to make contact with that doctor regarding concerns you might have for the participant. Upper limits of exercise are often individually determined by symptoms.
- For many programs, initially, a target heart rate 30 beats above resting is used. Use 20+ HRrest for clients taking atenolol or beta blockers.

- Fitness professionals may want to acquaint themselves with medications prescribed for control of heart rate and blood pressure. Often these medications affect resting and exercise heart rates making RPE a better indicator of intensity than heart rate methods alone.
- Cardiac patients should participate in a medically supervised program for at least Phase I and II Cardiac Rehabilitation. These patients participate at a facility with medical supplies and care readily available, and are monitored by a medical professional during exercise.
- In Phase III-VI Cardiac Rehab, an exercise participant should be able to exercise at a 5 MET level (measure of exercise intensity) as a standard of care set by American Association of Cardiovascular and Pulmonary Rehabilitation (AACVPR). The average cardiac patient typically graduates from a Phase II program at a 4-5 MET level. It is considered safe to put that participant in the water and assume they will be able to handle the additional resistance and workload. Research indicates that performing calisthenics in chest deep water is 4.6-6.8 MET level. Every cardiac rehabilitation program can be configured differently. Some Phase II programs are only six sessions and may involve exercise at a lower or higher MET level than 4-5 at completion of the program. If a person can comfortably handle walking for 1/2 hour at 2-3mph, a 20-30 minute mile, then they can typically handle water aerobics. This is a generic guideline to follow.
- Research indicates that deep water running elicits an 11-13.1 MET level with 76-83% HRmax. A more fit cardiac participant that is well healed from a heart attack, more athletic, and able to exercise at a higher MET level can exercise in deep water.
- Increased water depth, cool water temperatures, and stress in an unfamiliar environment may affect angina threshold.
- It is recommended that a person waits six weeks after a heart attack for water exercise because it takes six weeks for the myocardium to heal after an MI (Myocardial Infarction or Heart Attack.)
- Three months is recommended after open heart surgery to start a water program mostly because of the healing of the sternotomy. There may be danger of slipping in a wet environment, the stress of a patient pulling themselves up on a ladder, or falling on the vulnerable sternum. It typically takes three months to heal the sternum.

- Participants that have had stents and angioplasties without heart attacks, may want to avoid getting into the water for two weeks following the procedure. This allows time for the puncture site to fully heal. These puncture sites can break open up to two weeks and can have serious complications with bleeding. If they have had heart attacks and had a stent or angioplasty to interrupt the MI, then the rule of waiting six weeks, as for heart attacks, is applicable.
- It is not recommended that cardiac patients engage in cardiorespiratory exercise or resistance training at maximal levels. Submaximal levels, well within the individual's capability should be prescribed and practiced.
- Additional information for program considerations for the cardiac patient can be found in the ACSM Guidelines for Exercise Testing and Prescription in the chapter "Exercise Prescription for Cardiac Patients."

Pulmonary Diseases

Recommended Water Temperature: A temperature range of 83-86 degrees F (28-30 degrees C) is recommended for moderate to high intensity exercise. A temperature range of 86-88 degrees F (30-31 degrees C) is recommended for lower intensity exercise. Water temperature should increase as intensity of exercise decreases.

Recommended Tempo: Tempo will need to be self paced.

Recommended Shallow Water Depth: Armpit depth can be used for clients that can tolerate the additional work for the breathing muscles. A lower depth may be needed initially until the client adapts.

Recommended Program Formats: Program formats will vary depending on limitations and abilities. Some clients will be able to tolerate a cardiorespiratory format, while others may only be capable of performing basic toning and stretching exercises.

Characteristics

Pulmonary diseases limit the body's ability to provide oxygen to the body's tissues. Although you will see different classifications of pulmonary diseases, they generally fall into two categories. These categories include chronic obstructive pulmonary disease (COPD), including emphysema, and chronic bronchitis and asthma. (National Heart, Lung, and Blood Institute) There are various other lung diseases and disorders including cystic fibrosis, lung and heart transplant, lung cancer, mesothelioma, tuberculosis, and many others that will not be discussed in this manual.

According to the American Lung Association, lung disease is the number 3 killer in the United States, responsible for 1 in 7 deaths. The ACSM recommends that all clients with pulmonary disease receive physician's clearance prior to participating in an exercise program. The body's need for oxygen intake and carbon dioxide removal is increased during exercise, so clients with pulmonary disease must learn how to cope with diminished lung capacity and increased oxygen demands. Gas exchange impairments also create problems for the cardiovascular and muscular systems. Many people with pulmonary disease can safely exercise and benefit from a regular exercise program.

Chronic Obstructive Pulmonary Disease (COPD)

Chronic obstructive pulmonary disease is a lung disease in which the lung is damaged, making it hard to breath. In the emphysema type of COPD, the walls between many of the air sacs or alveoli in the lungs are damaged. The normal small air sacs are replaced with fewer larger air sacs with less surface area. The ability to exchange oxygen and carbon dioxide is impaired causing shortness of breath.

In chronic bronchitis, the airways have become inflamed and thickened and there is an increase in mucus production. This contributes to excessive coughing and difficulty getting air in and out of the lungs.

Cigarette smoking is the most common cause of COPD. Breathing in irritants to the lungs over a long period of time causes the airways to become inflamed and narrowed, and destroys the elastic fibers that allow the lungs to stretch and then return to resting shape. Other exposure that may contribute to COPD includes:

- Working around certain kinds of chemicals and breathing in the fumes for many years.
- Working in a dusty area over many years.
- Heavy exposure to air pollution over time.
- Exposure to second hand smoke.

People with an inherited tendency toward COPD (presence of a gene-related disorder) are at higher risk for developing COPD and will develop the disease more rapidly. Symptoms of COPD include cough, sputum (mucus) production, shortness of breath (especially with exercise), wheezing, and chest tightness.

Asthma

Bronchial asthma is a syndrome characterized by reversible obstruction to airflow and increased bronchial responsiveness to a variety of allergy and environmental stimuli. (10) Asthma is a lung disease that can be life threatening. It causes breathing problems which need to be dealt with on a daily basis. These breathing problems are called attacks or episodes of asthma.

Asthma symptoms include coughing a lot during or after exercise, shortness of breath, wheezing, and tightness in the chest. Asthma symptom triggers include viruses, colds, allergies, or gases and particles in the air. Triggers may include other causes and can often be difficult to figure out. Discovering what triggers attacks helps the asthma sufferer control and prevent asthma episodes.

Clients can be placed in one of three categories when considering exercise: (10)
- Exercise-induced asthma (EIA) without any other symptoms.
- Mild asthma (ventilatory limitation does not restrain submaximal exercise).
- Moderate to severe asthma (ventilatory limitation restrains submaximal exercise.)

These categories help to dictate intensity and duration for asthmatic clients. The causes of exercise-induced asthma are not known. EIA typically occurs 5- 15 minutes following exercise.

Benefits of Exercise

Most clients with pulmonary diseases benefit from regular exercise programs. Inactivity can lead to a vicious cycle for these clients. Shortness of breath and fatigue during exercise leads to cessation of exercise, resulting in diminished lung capacity, making it more difficult to exercise. Pacing, in daily activities and exercise, is an important skill for clients with diminished lung capacity to learn. Ability will fluctuate day to day and even hour to hour. Benefits of exercise for clients with pulmonary disease include:
- Cardiovascular reconditioning.
- Desensitization to dyspnea (shortness of breath).
- Improved ventilatory efficiency.
- Increased muscular strength and endurance.
- Improved flexibility.

- Improved body composition.
- Better balance.
- Enhanced body image.
- Increased feelings of well-being.

Clients with controlled exercise induced asthma should see relatively normal conditioning gains. "When EIA is controlled, asthma has no effect on the adaptations to exercise training." (10) Clients with COPD may see impairments in exercise response due to hypoxemia (inadequate oxygen in the blood), therefore a very conservative exercise progression is key to adaptation. Adaptation capability is determined by the severity of the disease and individual characteristics.

Program Considerations

Intensity, duration, and frequency of programming for clients with pulmonary diseases are directly dictated by individual client factors. Medications, the exercise environment, exercise tolerance at any given time, the need for breathing treatments or oxygen, fatigue level, and many other factors make exercise programming for this population a dynamic effort. Often a respiratory therapist (provides optimum oxygenation), an occupational therapist (helps the client pace through activities of daily living), and an exercise professional will work together to progress a client with pulmonary disease. Following are a few additional considerations for clients with pulmonary disease.
- Clients with COPD may feel better exercising at certain times of the day or shortly after they have taken their medication. Maximal limits of exercise are set as tolerated by symptoms.
- It is typically recommended that asthmatic exercisers take medication 10 minutes prior to exercise and carry an inhaler at all times. The client should consult his/her physician.
- Asthma may develop during prolonged exercise. The threshold for producing asthma symptoms is typically around 75% of predicted max heart rate.
- The hydrostatic pressure of the water may make it more difficult for clients with lung disease to breathe when submerged. Ventilatory muscular fatigue is common due to the increased work of breathing. Time may be needed to condition the breathing muscles, with ventilatory muscle training to work against the water's resistance, before starting a conditioning program. Clients may need to start in waist deep water and work up to chest deep water.

- The warmth and humidity in the aquatic environment may make it easier for some clients with lung disease to breathe.
- Clients may be sensitive to chemical fumes in the aquatic environment. Be aware of ventilation issues and help asthmatic exercisers recognize and control their triggers.
- Clients with pulmonary disease can exercise more comfortably and successfully when they are desensitized to dyspnea, fear, and other limiting symptoms. The exercise professional can play an important role in helping the client build confidence and tolerance.
- Clients should be instructed in "pursed-lips" breathing. (Breathe in through the nose keeping the lips together except at the very center, exhaling by blowing the air out with a firm steady effort.) This type of breathing slows the breathing rate and helps with a sense of control.
- Improved coordination, balance, form, and technique will help to conserve energy and provide more oxygen to working muscles.
- Choose activities that are perceived as enjoyable, have reasonable RPE values, and will improve the ability to perform usual activities of daily living. Walking is strongly recommended. (2)

Musculoskeletal Disease

Recommended Water Temperature: A temperature range of 83-86 degrees F (28-30 degrees C) is recommended for moderate to high intensity exercise. A temperature range of 86-88 degrees F (30-31 degrees C) is recommended for lower intensity exercise. Water temperature will increase as intensity of exercise decreases.

Specific Recommendations: Minimum arthritis guidelines are 83-88 degrees F (28-31 degrees C) as set by the Arthritis Foundation. The Aquatic Therapy and Rehabilitation Institute recommends 86-90 degrees F (29-32 degrees C) for a low level, low intensity class.

Recommended Tempo: Tempo will vary with client's abilities. A tempo well within the capability of the individual is recommended. In group settings, allowances for self-pacing are prudent.

Recommended Shallow Water Depth: Armpit depth for shallow water exercise. Lower depths may put additional strain on the musculoskeletal system. A minimum depth of 6.5 feet (1.98 meters) is recommended for deep water exercise.

Recommended Program Formats: Program formats will vary depending on limitations and abilities.

Characteristics

Musculoskeletal diseases include an array of conditions affecting muscles, tendons, ligaments, bones, and/or joints. Several acute and chronic musculoskeletal conditions and injuries were discussed in Chapter 11. Three primary conditions will be discussed in this chapter; arthritis, low back pain, and osteoporosis. These three diseases will be considered from a chronic perspective. Because these diseases are different in recommendations for exercise and programming considerations, each one will be considered independently.

Arthritis

Arthritis is a disease resulting in inflammation in the joints and surrounding connective tissue. This definition is applied to over one hundred different conditions which cause aching and pain to joints and connective tissues. Symptoms include persistent pain and stiffness; tenderness and/or swelling in one or more joints (especially neck, lower back, and knees); tingling sensations in fingertips, hands and feet; unexplained weight loss; fever; and weakness. Arthritis is often called the country's number one crippling disease.

The two most common forms of arthritis are **osteoarthritis** and **rheumatoid arthritis**. Osteoarthritis is also known as degenerative joint disease. It tends to be localized to an affected joint or joints, and originates with deterioration of the cartilaginous material around the joint. If osteoarthritis progresses, it often results in surgery or joint replacement.

Rheumatoid arthritis tends to be a multijoint, multisystem inflammatory disease. It arises from pathological activity of the immune system against joint tissue and sometimes organ systems. (10)

Clients with arthritis can benefit from regular exercise. Increases in strength and endurance will increase quality of life and will enable the exerciser to more easily perform activities of daily living. Vigorous activity is not recommended during acute joint inflammation or arthritis "flare ups."

Pain and stiffness can lead to biomechanical inefficiency which can lead to an increase in the metabolic cost of physical activity. Exercise mode should be chosen dependant upon the site and severity of the disease. Many persons with arthritis tend to avoid exercise due to chronic pain and impairment. Often joint range of motion is impaired by swelling, inflammation, and stiffness. Exercise professionals should take care as clients with arthritis may be more susceptible to injury, especially in affected joints.

The benefits of exercise include improved health, cardiorespiratory endurance, muscular strength and endurance, flexibility, decreased joint pain and swelling, and improved quality of life. Although exercise may be tedious when managing arthritis, physical inactivity promotes poor health and may make the disease even harder to tolerate. A carefully planned and progressed exercise program can be very beneficial for arthritics.

The Arthritis Foundation recommends warm water exercise as the exercise choice for people who have arthritis and want to maintain optimal flexibility, strength, and endurance. This organization has designed a training program to certify water exercise instructors to lead exercise classes appropriate for this population. Warm water exercise is commonly prescribed and tolerated by participants with arthritis.

Low Back Pain Syndrome

It is estimated that 80 percent of adults will suffer from at least one episode of low back pain that will be severe enough to cause absence from work. Low back pain is one of the primary causes of disability in the United States and is one of the most widely experienced health-related problems in the world. Low back pain can be acute or chronic in nature. It is often viewed as a multifaceted condition including physical, psychological, behavioral, and social aspects and causes. It is commonly treated with medications and/or therapeutic modalities, or through addressing various psychological and behavioral factors.

Many low back problems are caused by poor muscular tone and flexibility in the primary core muscles. Because of this, exercise is often prescribed as a treatment and prevention. Programming typically includes toning exercises for the abdominals, gluteus maximus, hamstrings, and back extensor muscles with flexibility exercises for the hip flexors, quadriceps, and lower hamstrings. Clients with low back pain may need to alter exercise positions or substitute exercises that support the low back to avoid pain. Activities that increase low back pain should be avoided or eliminated. Educational information for proper posture, lifting techniques, and low back health are helpful.

During low back pain flare-ups, exercise may need to be modified or stopped until the symptoms are under control. It has been found that tolerance for exercise is dictated by individual beliefs and attitudes. Severe pain will affect form, technique, and exercise ability. Most clients with low back pain syndrome can effectively progress to higher levels of fitness and well being. For many low back pain sufferers, exercise needs to become a way of life for prevention and management of the condition.

Recent research indicates that deep water training may be a beneficial modality for clients with low back pain. It was found that deep water substantially decreases the compressive load on the spine, making deep water exercise a valuable tool in training progressions. Deep water training is also very effective for training the core musculature which is important to good posture and back health. For additional information, see Chapter 16.

Osteoporosis

Osteoporosis ("osteo" means bones and "porosis" means porous) is a systemic skeletal disease characterized by low bone mass and deterioration of bone strength, leading to bone fragility and an increased risk of fracture. (7) Some loss of bone mass is typical in aging adults due to the declining activity of the bone-forming cells after the age of 35. In America, it is predicted that over 18 million people have osteopenia and 10 million more have osteoporosis. There is a subtle difference, with osteopenia being defined as bone mineral density >1 standard deviation above young-normal and osteoporosis being defined as bone mineral density >2.5 standard deviation above young-normal as defined by the World Health Organization. In a sense, osteopenia is the early or beginning stages of osteoporosis.

Osteoporosis occurs when calcium is lost from the bones. There are actually two kinds of bone loss which occur at different sites in the bone. The calcium loss eventually weakens the structure until the bone becomes so porous that it breaks under the simple weight of the body. Hip bones can shatter and cause a person to fall to the floor. Vertebrates can suddenly disintegrate and crush down on nerves to result in debilitating pain and a decrease in height.

Risk factors for osteoporosis include:
• Genetics including northern European or Asian descent, fair complexion, family history of osteoporosis, or a small thin frame.

- Advancing age.
- Amenorrhea, estrogen deficiency, and early menopause.
- Lifestyle factors such as chronic smoking, lack of physical activity, and excessive alcohol consumption.
- Dietary factors including low dietary calcium intake.
- Chronic use of certain medications.

Gains in bone strength and density occur throughout the first 20 to 25 years of life. At this time calcium is deposited in the bones. Around the mid-30's bones stop growing, and as time goes on, bone tissue is lost causing a decrease in strength and density. Women are most affected by this process as menopause brings about a decrease in estrogen levels. This decreased estrogen level speeds the rate of calcium loss from the bones. A decrease in estrogen levels is also experienced by anorectics, women who over exercise and restrict their body weight so unreasonably that they develop athletic amenorrhea, and by women who have had their ovaries surgically removed.

Unfortunately, the condition of bone loss is unavoidable. The key to the prevention or diminution of osteoporosis is to slow down the rate of bone loss and to deposit as much calcium in the bones as possible during childhood and early adulthood. Diets that are high in calcium during these critical times will assure dense bones. Research has also shown that extra calcium may be beneficial in the ten years following menopause.

Although calcium supplements are available, the calcium in dairy products is most easily absorbed. The RDA for males and females is 1200 mg up through age 25 and 800 mg afterwards. Pregnant and lactating women are advised to consume 1200 mg/day. A glass of milk, a cup of yogurt or keifer, and approximately an ounce and a half of cheese each provide 300 mg of calcium. Other food sources of calcium, although not as rich as milk, are corn tortillas made with lime, tofu, greens, and sardines and other fish with bones. Individuals who cannot tolerate milk should talk to their physician about a supplement.

The primary concern for exercise programming in this population is the degree of musculoskeletal limitation imposed from previous fractures if they have occurred, if the disease has impaired locomotor abilities, and the presence of kyphosis. Many elderly people with osteoporosis will avoid physical exercise because of the increased risk and fear of falling. This can lead to an increased risk in cardiovascular and other chronic diseases.

Exercise is beneficial in the management of osteoporosis for several reasons. One of the most beneficial aspects of exercise is that improved balance, muscular strength, coordination, posture, and performance accompanying regular training decreases the risk of falls and injury. This is important to decreasing fractures, surgery, loss of function, and death. It is unclear whether exercise alone actually increases bone density. It is reasonably clear that exercise at least slows bone loss. Osteoporosis itself is not known to have any effects on the useful benefits of cardiovascular exercise and muscular conditioning. Favorable training effects should still be attainable. Kyphosis, however, may cause mechanical limitations for the respiratory system.

Most clients will need to start with a low intensity program and safely progress to higher levels of function or fitness. A balanced program for cardiorespiratory endurance, muscular fitness, and flexibility is recommended. The client's physician and physical therapist should provide input as to the safety and viability of the proposed program. Typically, 4 sessions of aerobic training and 2-3 sessions of resistance training are prescribed weekly. The mode is dependant upon the client's abilities. Activities requiring forward flexion and twisting of the spine should be avoided. Adaptations and the sparing of bone mass are specific to the part of the body being used in the exercise. Keep the exercise area free from hazards to reduce the risk and anxiety of falling. Support and spotting should be offered for exercises with a high risk of losing balance or falling.

The water has presented a double edged sword for use as a modality for training clients with osteoporosis. On one hand, the water provides a relatively safe environment minimizing fear and injury in falls, providing kinesthetic feedback, providing buoyancy for reduced joint stress, and providing resistance for muscular conditioning. On the other hand, it is questioned as to whether the bone loading potential in the water is sufficient enough to build or preserve bone mass. Research has indicated favorable and unfavorable results, depending on study design. At present, it appears that water exercise does provide sufficient stimulus to maintain and possibly build bone mass based on the results of limited research. As the mechanisms that cause osteoporosis continue to become clearer, so will the recommendations for exercise and the benefits of water exercise.

Metabolic Disease

Recommended Water Temperature: A temperature range of 83-86 degrees F (28-30 degrees C) is recommended for moderate to high intensity exercise. A temperature range of 86-88 degrees F (30-31 degrees C) is recommended for lower intensity exercise. Watch for heat stress.

Recommended Tempo: Tempo will vary with client's abilities. A tempo well within the capability of the individual is recommended. In group settings, allowances for self-pacing are prudent.

Recommended Shallow Water Depth: Armpit depth for shallow water exercise. A minimum depth of 6.5 feet (1.98 meters) is recommended for deep water exercise.

Recommended Program Formats: Continuous cardiorespiratory exercise, resistance training, and flexibility exercises through a variety of program formats are recommended.

Characteristics

Metabolic diseases include diabetes mellitus, obesity, blood lipid disorders, thyroid disorders, and end-stage metabolic disease (renal failure and liver failure). Obesity and blood lipid disorders were discussed previously, so this section will focus on diabetes mellitus.

Diabetes Mellitus is characterized by abnormalities in insulin production by the pancreas, insulin action, or both. This causes a problem with metabolism and results in glucose intolerance. Chronic hyperglycemia is associated with long-term damage, dysfunction, and failure of various organs including the eyes, kidneys, nerves, heart, and blood vessels. The classic symptoms of diabetes include intense thirst, high urine output, and unexplained weight loss. Diabetes is diagnosed through fasting and other types of blood glucose measurements.

The complete lack of insulin production in the case of Type I Diabetes (Insulin Dependant Diabetes Mellitus – IDDM) requires the person having the disease to take insulin injections or use an insulin pump in order to sustain life. It is primarily thought to be genetically determined. Although it can occur at any age, it usually occurs before the age of 30. IDDM affects 5-10% of the 16 million people with diabetes in the United States.

The more common type of diabetes is often called "late onset" diabetes. The low production of insulin and decreased cellular receptivity to insulin in Type II Diabetes (Non-insulin Dependent Diabetes Mellitus – NIDDM) sometimes requires insulin through injection. There are also oral medications available to enhance production and utilization of insulin, helping the diabetic avoid or delay the need for insulin injections. The cause of NIDDM is unclear. The development of insulin sensitivity is believed to be caused by several factors including obesity and genetics. In most cases, Type II Diabetes develops after the age of 40. It is often undetected until it has been present for some time causing organ damage before it is diagnosed.

Gestational diabetes occurs during pregnancy. The risk factors include family history, obesity, and previous large birth weight babies. Gestational diabetes differs from Type I and II in that it resolves after pregnancy.

Benefits of Exercise

Diabetes, like hypertension, responds very well to exercise therapy. Exercise is considered to be a cornerstone to diabetic care. Exercise provides many benefits including:

- Possible improvement in blood sugar control for Type II Diabetes.
- Improved glucose sensitivity and often a reduced need for insulin.
- Improvements in body composition with decreases in body fat leading to better insulin sensitivity.
- Reduction in the risk of cardiovascular disease.
- Stress reduction and consequent better control of diabetes.
- Prevention of Type II Diabetes.

Program Considerations

Exercise has an insulin like effect, increasing the risk of hypoglycemia (low blood sugar). One of the primary concerns for diabetics when exercising is to prevent hypoglycemic events. Hypoglycemic events may be minimized by:

- Measuring blood glucose before, during, and after exercise. A client with Type I Diabetes needs to have blood glucose reasonably controlled in order to exercise safely.
- Avoiding exercise during periods of peak insulin activity.
- Unplanned exercise may have to be preceded by extra carbohydrates and post exercise insulin may need to be decreased.

- If exercise is planned, insulin doses should be reduced before exercise according to the intensity and duration of exercise as well as personal experience.
- Easily accessible carbohydrates may need to be consumed during exercise.
- After exercise, a carbohydrate rich snack may be needed.
- Exercise with a partner and carry medical identification and a fast acting carbohydrate.

Additional concerns include:

- Wear proper footwear and practice proper foot hygiene. This is especially true in the aquatic environment. Recommend clients wear shoes at all times in the locker room, the pool, and on deck to avoid stepping on small objects such as pierced earrings. Since peripheral circulation is affected, especially in the feet, any type of injury or infection may be difficult to heal and may lead to amputations.
- Be aware that medications like beta blockers may interfere with the ability to discern hypoglycemic symptoms.
- Diabetics are typically at higher risk for heat related disorders and should avoid exercising in excessive heat.
- Exercise programs for diabetics should be individualized based on medication schedule, diabetic complications, and individual characteristics.

Neuromuscular Diseases

Neuromuscular diseases affect the transmission of nerve impulses from the central nervous system to muscle fibers, causing muscle impairment, spasticity, loss of function, and paralysis. Accommodating clients with neuromuscular disease may require some extra thought and consideration in terms of safety and movement adaptation. Participant safety needs to be considered at all times in the aquatic environment. Approved lifesaving devices may need to be worn by some clients to insure safety and reduce the risk of a water emergency.

Physician's consent should be obtained prior to participation in an exercise program. Water is a wonderful modality for many of these clients allowing them to regain function through water exercise that is not possible through land exercise. Often water enhances quality of life and gives the client with a potentially debilitating disease a huge psychological and emotional boost.

Several neuromuscular diseases are briefly described below. If you choose to work with a client with one of these conditions, it is highly recommended you work hand in hand with the client's therapist and/or physician. There are many associations available to call or consult on line for additional information and recommendations.

Muscular Dystrophy (MD) is an inherited disorder that affects skeletal muscle structure. Muscle cells are progressively destroyed and replaced with fat tissue, and may appear larger than normal. It is characterized by progressive weakness and degeneration of the skeletal or voluntary muscles. Impairment of muscle function usually occurs when about 33% of the muscle mass has been lost. In some forms of MD, the muscles of the heart and other involuntary muscles can be affected. It can affect people of all ages.

There is no cure for MD and treatment includes drug therapy to slow the progression, physical therapy, occupational therapy, and cardiac and respiratory care if necessary. Research indicates that moderate resistance training and stretching can be beneficial for clients with MD. There is no evidence that exercise accelerates the rate of decline and many participants experience mild improvements in strength and activities of daily living.

It is recommended that exercise programs for clients with MD provide manageable short-term goals, stretching to prevent contractures, and slow progression to moderate levels of resistance training. If the client is too weak to use conventional weights, then program focus should shift to movement through full range of motion against the resistance of gravity or the water to prevent contractures. Strenuous exercise should be avoided in conditions of high heat and humidity.

Multiple Sclerosis (MS) is a chronic, potentially debilitating disease that affects the central nervous system (brain and spinal cord). The body directs antibodies and white blood cells to break down proteins in the myelin sheaths surrounding the nerves in the brain and spinal cord. Inflammation and injury to the sheath causes scarring (sclerosis), and the damage slows or blocks muscle coordination, visual sensation, and other nerve signals. The disease can range in severity from mild illness to permanent disability. The disease usually first occurs in adults between the ages of 20 and 50.

Initial symptoms of MS include:
• Numbness, weakness, or paralysis in one or more limbs.
• Brief pain, tingling, or electric shock sensations.
• Quick, involuntary muscle jerks.
• Impaired vision with pain during eye movement.
• Disordered eye movements, causing double vision or moving field vision.
• Fatigue and dizziness.

If the disease progresses, muscle spasms, slurred speech, vision loss, problems with bladder, bowel, or sexual function, and paralysis may occur.

Risk factors for MS include heredity and environmental factors such as viruses and bacteria that may trigger the disease if you are susceptible. Exercise has no effect on the prognosis or progression of MS. A three part process including medical management, education, and exercise is typically prescribed for managing MS. Exercise is believed to be beneficial for improving physical fitness and functional performance. When developing programming for a client with MS, remember that fatigue, sensory loss, spasticity, and impaired balance can affect exercise tolerance and performance. Safe access for entering and exiting the pool must be available. Choose class lengths and times of day keeping in mind that the MS client will fatigue easily. Program focus should be on maintaining or developing cardiorespiratory endurance, muscular strength and endurance, and joint flexibility to increase energy and efficiency. Heat intolerance is also a factor, and most MS clients will be more comfortable exercising in water temperatures at or below 84 degrees F. Cool water is key in keeping core body temperature from rising, minimizing the risk of increasing the symptoms of MS while exercising.

Epilepsy is a neurological condition that makes people susceptible to seizures. It is one of the most common disorders of the nervous system affecting people of all ages and ethnic backgrounds. Seizures are caused by a brief electrical disturbance in the brain and can vary from a momentary disruption of the senses, to short periods of unconsciousness or staring spells, to convulsions. People with epilepsy can have just one type of seizure or more than one type.

Epilepsy can be inherited, caused by tumors or strokes, or have no known cause. It is not a mental disorder, but a sudden change in how the brain cells send electrical signals to each other. It is primarily treated with seizure-preventing drugs, but can also be treated with surgery, diet, or electrical stimulation to the vagus nerve.

As long as seizures are kept under control, it is widely believed that a client with epilepsy can participate in almost all exercise and sports programs. Concern is that the person would be harmed or injured if they have a seizure while exercising. Refer to Chapter 11 for procedures in the event of seizures while in the water. Swimming under water, boxing, and heading the ball in soccer are not recommended. Activities involving heights such as rock climbing, diving, some gymnastic activities, horse back riding, as well as water activities require special monitoring. It is more common for a seizure to occur during rest following exercise than it is for it to occur during exercise. Regular exercise is beneficial for inhibiting seizure activity and tends to suppress the electrical activity. Factors that increase the risk of seizure include:
• Strobe lights
• Hyperventilation prior to breath holding
• Hypoglycemia
• Hypoxia
• Frustration
• Anger or fear
• Hyperthermia
• Extreme fatigue
• Breath holding during resistance training
• Changes in women's menstrual cycle
• Excessive alcohol intake
• High blood pH

Physical activity is important because poor cardiorespiratory fitness appears to be related to the frequency of seizures. Typical gains in fitness and conditioning are expected from training. Although the American Medical Association has approved of epileptics participating in contact sports, the safest activities tend to be individual sports.

Cerebral Palsy (CP) is a general term referring to abnormalities of motor control caused by damage to a child's brain early in the course of development. The damage may occur during fetal development, during the birth process, or during the first few months after birth. (Mayo Clinic) It may take one or a combination of three major forms. Spastic individuals suffer from hypertonia (excessive muscle tensions). Athetoid individuals have involuntary, uncontrolled movements of hands or feet and often have slurred speech and defective hearing. Ataxic individuals have a disturbed sense of balance and faulty depth perception and walk with a staggered gait.

CP is difficult to diagnose in the first 6 months after birth and is usually found when the child is one or two. Symptoms may include delays in motor skill development, weakness in one or more limbs, standing and walking on tiptoe, one leg dragging while walking, excessive drooling or difficulties swallowing, and poor control over hand and arm movement. CP can develop after meningitis, but for most children a specific cause is unknown.

Exercise response for clients with CP is lower than able bodied participants. The client with CP may have difficulty with performing skilled movements, may have muscle imbalances, and poor functional strength. Some clients may report an increase in spasticity after exercise, especially strenuous exercise. Clients will benefit from programs designed to develop cardiorespiratory endurance, muscular fitness, and flexibility. There is strong evidence of psychological benefits and physiological improvements in literature supporting exercise programs for clients with CP. Long-term programs have been shown to reduce muscle spasms and the need for antispasmodic medication. Program progression should be slow and emphasis should be placed on exercises for improving daily function and independence.

Parkinson Disease is a disorder that affects nerve cells in the part of the brain controlling muscle movement. (Mayo Clinic) The four cardinal signs of Parkinson Disease include resting tremor (usually of the hands and head), muscle rigidity (hardness or stiffness of the muscles), slowness of movement, and postural instability. It is often identified by tremors of hands and sometimes head and legs. The disease is progressive, with tremors followed by muscular rigidity, slowness of movement, and loss of facial expression. Posture and gait become problematic, but general health is not greatly affected. Many people have years of productive living with good quality of life after being diagnosed.

Parkinson Disease is generally associated with a reduction in the neurotransmitter dopamine. Symptoms may fluctuate from day to day, week to week, or even hour to hour. Treatment currently consists of medications and implantation of a brain stimulator (similar to a heart pacemaker) to provide deep brain stimulation to control symptoms. At this time, researchers believe that Parkinson Disease may result from a combination of genetic and environmental factors, or from a number of drugs

taken over a long period of time or in excessive doses. Unlike genetic and environmental factors, drug causes usually reverse when the drug is no longer taken. (Mayo Clinic)

Effects of cardiorespiratory conditioning vary at this time in literature. It is not clearly known how exercise benefits the client with Parkinson Disease. It is recommended that exercise programming for this population include flexibility, aerobic training, functional training, strengthening, and neuromuscular training. Water provides a great medium for training clients with Parkinson Disease, and it is important to remember that clients may be at various stages of disease progression. Breathing and relaxation exercises help with muscle rigidity, and exercises should be included for posture and gait. Exercises to develop and maintain range of motion are essential for individuals with Parkinson Disease. Creating a positive social environment may help with the depression and social isolation often experienced with this disease.

Amyotrophic Lateral Sclerosis (ALS), sometimes called Lou Gehrig's disease, is a rapidly progressive, invariably fatal neurological disease that attacks the nerve cells responsible for controlling voluntary muscles. It is characterized by the gradual degeneration and death of motor neurons. (National Institute of Neurological Disorders and Stroke-NINDS) Eventually all voluntary muscles are affected leaving the person bed ridden. Eventually muscles in the diaphragm and chest wall fail, requiring the patient to breathe with the aid of a respirator. Most people with ALS die within five years of the onset of symptoms. People of all ages and ethnic backgrounds can be affected. Men are affected more often than women. In 90-95% of all ALS cases, the disease occurs at random with no clearly associated risk factors or known cause. (NINDS)

Exercise will be limited by the client's level of muscular strength, muscular fatigue, spasticity, and decreased coordination and balance. There is no evidence that exercise slows or reverses the disease. Exercise can minimize muscle atrophy by maximizing the function of the still innervated muscle fibers, and may possibly help the client retain function for a longer period of time. Program considerations should include maintaining aerobic endurance and strength and function of the ventilatory muscles. Maintaining range of motion in joints, even if function is lost, will aid in the caretaker's ability to dress and care for the patient.

Poliomyelitis (Polio) is a highly infectious disease caused by a virus. It invades the nervous system and can cause total paralysis in a matter of hours. It can strike at any age, but primarily affects children under the age of 3. (12) Many people who have the virus are unaware they are affected. Approximately one in two hundred with the virus will experience symptoms and may become permanently paralyzed, especially in the legs. There is no cure for polio, but it can be prevented through immunization.

For those affected with paralysis, moist heat and physical therapy are used to stimulate the muscles. Antispasmodic drugs are administered to promote muscle relaxation. These treatments improve mobility, but do not reverse polio paralysis.

Adults who suffered polio as a child are at increased risk for **Post-Polio Syndrome** (PPS). Symptoms are similar to symptoms of the disease including fatigue, muscle and joint pain, weakness, intolerance to cold, and sleeping disorders. PPS is characterized by the onset of additional muscle pain and weakness beyond symptoms that may occur from the original disease.

Clients with symptomatic PPS usually have reduced leg strength and aerobic capacity. Although research is minimal, it is believed that clients with PPO can significantly increase leg strength and function and aerobic capacity. Programming should be designed to promote overall health and fitness and reduce the risk of diseases associated with physical inactivity. Programming for PPO clients includes a narrower range of exercise intensities which should not typically exceed moderate intensity. If exercise intensities are too high, there is risk of premature acceleration of motor unit loss.

Non weight bearing and aquatic exercise are recommended. If there is no new weakness or pain, an exercise intensity of 60-70% of peak oxygen consumption can be prescribed. If symptoms are present, an intensity of less that 50% is recommended. Continuous training may need to be broken down into intervals of 2-5 minutes. Programming will be largely dictated by symptoms and the amount of muscle recruitment possible. Exercise every other day is recommended with a frequency of 3 times/week. Increased pain or fatigue should alert the client to decrease intensity and duration. If symptoms persist for more than two weeks and are exacerbated by exercise, then exercise should be terminated and the client should be referred to his/her physician. (10)

Head Injury (HI) can result from a blow to the head, producing a concussion, skull fracture, or contusion. Areas of functioning that may be affected include: consciousness, motor ability, sensation, intelligence, and emotion. Usually muscle tone is exaggerated as well as reflex action, which produces involuntary movement. Joints may stay in flexion or extension positions. Impairment of movement is marked by lack of coordination. Individuals with head injury usually respond best in familiar surroundings, doing repetitive tasks with few distractions (especially noise).

Spinal Cord Injury (SCI) can be caused from disease or trauma and usually results in paraplegia or quadriplegia. SCI affects many systems of the body and may require tremendous effort to survive. The psychological stress on a person with an SCI is immense. If the problems involved, such as bowel and bladder control and pressure sores, can be sufficiently solved to enable the individual with SCI to enter water for exercise, it can become the best "normalizing" environment in which to restore movement. Proper flotation equipment should be worn at all times. The benefits of exercise play a major role in health and quality of life. Weight gain for individuals with SCI is a major inhibiting factor that is easily addressed through exercise in water. Exercise for the spinal cord-injured person steps up metabolism and burns calories in the same way it does for the non-injured individual.

Immunological/ Hematological Disorders

Cancer

Cancer is a group of diseases characterized by uncontrolled growth and spread of abnormal cells. If the spread is not controlled, it can result in death. (American Cancer Society) There are hundreds of different types of cancers and cancer affects people of all ages and ethnic backgrounds. The occurrence of cancer increases as an individual ages, with most cases occurring in adults beginning middle age. Approximately 76% of cancers are diagnosed at age 55 and older. (American Cancer Society) The risk for developing cancer is classified in two ways.

Lifetime risk refers to the probability that you will develop or die from cancer over the course of your lifetime. Lifetime risk for men in the United States is a little less than 1 in 2. Lifetime risk for women is a little more than 1 in 3.

Relative risk compares the risk of developing a specific cancer in persons with a certain exposure or trait to the risk in persons who do not have this exposure or trait. Relative risk statistics are published by the American Cancer Society.

Risk factors for cancer include smoking, heavy alcohol consumption, diet, sun exposure, physical inactivity, obesity, and environmental and occupational risks. All cancers caused by cigarette smoking and heavy alcohol consumption are believed to be completely preventable. Scientific evidence suggests that about 1/3 of all cancer deaths in the US are related to nutrition, physical inactivity, overweight, and other lifestyle factors. Skin cancer can be prevented by limiting exposure to the sun's rays or wearing sun screen. Cancers attributed to infectious exposures can be prevented through behavioral changes, vaccines, and antibiotics. Your risk for cancer depends on a number of factors, including your family medical history, your environment, and the lifestyle choices you make. (American Cancer Society)

Research indicates that almost all individuals with cancer can benefit from exercise. Benefits of exercise for clients with cancer include:

- Increased functional capacity- improved work capacity and lower heart rates at a given exercise intensity.
- Decreased body fat.
- Increased lean muscle tissue.
- Decreased nausea and fatigue.
- Improved natural defense mechanisms.
- Improved sense of control.
- Improved mood.
- Improved self-esteem.
- Self-reported improved quality of sleep.

A comprehensive review of literature in 2000 by Courneya et al "reveals that exercise has a positive effect on a broad range of quality-of-life parameters after patients are diagnosed as having cancer." Physicians who prescribe exercise for their cancer patients see improvements in motivation and adherence. General exercise prescription is moderate intensity exercise 3 to 5 days/week for 20 to 30 minutes per session. The effects of cancer on exercise response are dependant upon the type of cancer, location of the cancer, and individual characteristics of the client. Exercise programs will need to be individualized for each client. A concern with cancer survivors is that they may have impairments in cardiovascular and pulmonary function as the result of treatment.

Additional general program considerations include:
- Exercise may need to be modified according to fatigue during periods of treatment.
- Adjustments may need to be made for surgical impairments or the presence and location of an implanted catheter for chemotherapy treatment.
- Exercise response will be affected by whether the person has local or metastatic disease.
- Goals of exercise may be altered depending on whether the client is receiving initial treatment, is in remission, or is receiving treatment for a recurrence.
- Program objectives should include returning the client to former levels of physical and psychological function, and to preserve or enhance function.

There are instances when exercise is contraindicated in cancer clients. Work hand-in-hand with the client's oncologist and physician to provide safe and effective care. Some contraindications with exercise program adjustments are listed below.

Contraindications to Physical Exercise Following Cancer Diagnosis
(Courneye, et al. Physician and Sports Medicine. Vol 28- No. 5- May 2000)

Contraindication	Comment
Complete blood counts:	
Hemoglobin level < 8.0 g/dL	Avoid activities that require significant oxygen transport (ie, high intensity)
Absolute neutrophil count < 0.5 x 109/ microliters	Avoid activities that may increase risk of bacterial infection (eg, swimming)
Platelet count < 50 x 109/microliters	Avoid activities that increase risk of bleeding (eg, contact sports or high-impact exercises)
Fever > 38°C (100.4°F)	May indicate systemic infection and should be investigated; avoid high-intensity exercise
Ataxia, dizziness, or peripheral sensory neuropathy	Avoid activities that require significant balance and coordination such as treadmill exercise
Severe cachexia (loss of > 35% of premorbid weight)	Loss of muscle mass usually limits exercise to mild intensity, depending on degree of cachexia

Continued on next page

Continued from previous page

Dyspnea	Investigate cause; exercise to tolerance
Bone pain	Avoid activities that increase risk of fracture such as contact sports and high-impact exercises
Severe nausea	Investigate cause; exercise to tolerance
Extreme fatigue and/or muscle weakness	Exercise to tolerance

Fibromyalgia Syndrome

Fibromyalgia Syndrome (FMS) is a chronic condition characterized by fatigue and widespread pain in muscles, ligaments, and tendons. To be classified with fibromyalgia, a patient must have 11 of 18 specific areas of the body with pain or pressure, and must have widespread pain lasting at least three months. (15)

Signs and symptoms of fibromyalgia include widespread pain, fatigue and sleep disturbances, irritable bowel syndrome (IBS), chronic headaches and facial pain, heightened sensitivity, depression, numbness or tingling in the hands and feet, difficulty concentrating and mood changes, chest or pelvic pain, irritable bladder, dry eyes, skin, and mouth, painful menstrual periods, dizziness, and a sensation of swollen hands and feet.

It is believed that a number of factors, as opposed to just one single cause, contribute to the development of fibromyalgia. These factors may include: (15)
• Chemical changes in the brain.
• Sleep disturbances.
• Injury.
• Infection.
• Abnormalities of the autonomic (sympathetic) nervous system.
• Changes in muscle metabolism.

Fibromyalgia occurs more in women than in men and tends to develop in people between the ages of 20 and 60. Cases have been reported in children. Disturbed sleep patterns are believed to increase risk for the development of fibromyalgia, but it is not clear whether it is a cause or the result of the disease. Family history is also considered a risk. Chronic pain syndromes such as fibromyalgia create challenging and frustrating therapeutic dilemmas. Because of the array of symptoms, many types of treatment are prescribed

including medication, relaxation techniques, and physical conditioning.

Benefits of exercise for this population include: (10)
• Reduced number of tender points and decreased pain at tender points.
• Decreased general pain.
• Improved sleep and less fatigue.
• Fewer feelings of helplessness and hopelessness.
• More frequent and meaningful social interactions.
• Lessened impact of the disease on daily activities.

Goals for exercise programming for clients with fibromyalgia are similar to the goals for most chronic diseases- restore and improve function and mental outlook. Like arthritis clients, fibromyalgia clients find it very comforting and supporting to exercise in warm water. Additional program considerations include:
• Non or low impact, low to moderate intensity exercise is typically prescribed including water exercise, walking, and cycling.
• Resistance training using low weight, elastic bands, or gravity emphasizing proper form and technique will help to build muscular endurance and increase pain tolerance. Flexibility exercises should also be included.
• Adherence is typically low in this population. Supervised exercise, or exercise in group sessions tends to increase adherence. Support groups and client education are also helpful.
• The initial level of exercise should be determined by client characteristics and pain tolerance. For most clients, progression should be very conservative beginning at a low intensity level.
• Avoid early morning exercise and repetitive overhead activities to reduce the level of attrition.
• Symptoms may worsen initially when first starting an exercise program. Clients with fibromyalgia should consider pacing their exercise sessions with daily activity obligations.

Chronic Fatigue Syndrome

Chronic Fatigue Syndrome (CFS) is a poorly understood condition characterized by severe and disabling fatigue that persists or recurs for six or more consecutive months, and is not relieved by rest. (6) CFS makes one feel too tired to do normal activities and become easily exhausted with no apparent reason. It can remain active for months and in some cases even years.

Symptoms for CFS come and go or remain constant for at least six months. These symptoms include headache, tender lymph nodes, fatigue and weakness, muscle and joint aches, and inability to concentrate. Once thought of as "yuppie flu" in the early 1980's, doctors now have seen the syndrome in people of all ages and social and economic classes. Similar illnesses, known by different names, date back to the early 1800s. (20)

Although the causes are unknown, there are hypotheses for what may cause the disease. Major hypotheses for what trigger and sustain CFS include:

- Persistent viral infection including human herpesvirus-6, an enterovirus, the Epstein-Barr virus, or a retrovirus.
- Chronic immune dysfunction with abnormal cytokine production and activity.
- Neuropsychiatric disorder where depression and psychiatric problems may precede or play a role in sustaining the illness.
- The "hybrid" model that suggests both physical and psychological factors play a role in triggering and sustaining the disease.

Chronic fatigue syndrome is difficult to diagnose because it has symptoms similar to many other diseases. It is typically treated with medications, cognitive behavioral therapy (a psychological counseling or therapy), and graduated exercise therapy. It is recommended that CFS clients eat a balanced diet, get plenty of rest, exercise regularly, and pace themselves physically, emotionally, and intellectually because too much stress can aggravate symptoms. (NIAID) Although improvements in physiological parameters and function may be modest for a client with CFS, most report dramatic improvements in perceived outcomes in quality of life from a regular exercise program.

Additional exercise program considerations for clients with CFS include:

- Studies indicate that cardiac, pulmonary, muscular, metabolic, immune, and endocrine responses to acute exercise are similar to those seen in normal individuals with profound deconditioning. (10)
- Exercise at an intensity and duration that will not cause additional fatigue. Mild to moderate exercise is typically prescribed with a slow, conservative progression. All parameters of fitness should be addressed.
- Chronic mild fever is not uncommon in CFS clients. Instruct clients to take their temperature before exercise. If the temperature is over 100.4 degrees F (38 degrees C), vigorous exercise should

be avoided and replaced with gentle stretching. (7)
- Primary exercise objectives should include maintenance of function and prevention of physical deterioration.
- Fatigue and discomfort may be more acute following exercise sessions in the initial stages of an exercise program. Warn your client about this in advance.
- CFS clients tend to overestimate their ability and set unrealistic expectations.
- Encourage exercise sessions during periods of the day when symptoms seem less severe.

Acquired Immune Deficiency Syndrome (AIDS)

Acquired Immune Deficiency Disease (AIDS) develops from HIV or Human Immuno-deficiency Virus. Although positive gains have been made in the prevention, diagnosis, and treatment of AIDS, a vaccine or cure is still unavailable. The mechanism of AIDS results in immunosuppression which leads to increased risk of opportunistic infections, decreased food consumption and lean body mass, further decreased immune system function and advanced body tissue wasting, with disease progression and eventual death.

There are three stages of HIV that should be considered in exercise programming. Stage I is asymptomatic HIV seropositive (positive in blood). The individual is infected with HIV and is contagious to others. HIV is transmitted through sexual or bloodbourne routes. Stage I can last for 10 years or longer. There are usually no effects on exercise performance or changes in exercise prescription for clients with Stage I HIV.

Stage II is early symptomatic HIV. In this stage intermittent or persistent signs and symptoms are experienced. Symptoms include fatigue, diarrhea, weight loss, fever, and lymphadenopothy (disease of the lymph nodes.) In Stage II, the disease progression can often be checked for several years. Clients in Stage II may have a reduced exercise capacity, reduced oxygen consumption, and reduced heart rate and breathing reserve.

Stage III is the development of AIDS. Symptoms become more severe and there is typically a dramatic reduction in exercise capacity. There are more severe limitations in oxygen consumption and altered neuroendocrine responses. The client will experience physical exhaustion and muscular fatigue.

Although the risks and benefits of exercise for clients with HIV are not fully understood, there is general consensus that training is beneficial. Benefits include an increase in cells mediating natural immunity, higher rates of natural killer cell activity, increased protection against upper respiratory tract infection, and reports of fewer colds and sick days. Regular cardiorespiratory exercise, resistance training, and flexibility exercises will help to augment lean body tissue, oxidation, and endurance capacity. Routine moderate exercise may possibly delay the onset and severity of symptoms.

Additional program considerations include:

- It is best to start exercise programming in Stage I as soon as the condition is diagnosed.
- The program needs to be individualized taking into consideration the client's stage, symptoms, blood profiles, and treatments.
- Intense exercise or prolonged activity over 90 minutes is not recommended. (10)
- Exercise is contraindicated if the client's temperature is elevated or the client is in the acute phase of a secondary infection such as cold or flu.
- Bear in mind that the client is more susceptible to colds and infections.
- Exercise programming should be re-evaluated and adjusted as the disease progresses.

HIV is a contagious disease. As a fitness professional, universal procedures and precautions should be followed at all times to prevent the spread of HIV. Following are the guidelines from the Centers for Disease Control (CDC) for preventing the spread of HIV.

1. There are certain body fluids to which the guidelines pertain. These body fluids include blood or other bodily fluids containing visible blood, semen and vaginal secretions, tissues and certain specific body fluids including synovial, cerebrospinal, pleural, pericardial, peritoneal, and amniotic.
2. There are body fluids to which precautions do not apply. These include feces, nasal secretions, sputum, sweat, tears, urine, vomit, and saliva (unless any of these contain visible blood.)
3. Use protective barriers to prevent exposure to the body fluids to which universal precautions apply. These may vary based on the situation.
4. Immediately and thoroughly wash hands or other skin surfaces which may have been exposed to any of the fluids to which universal cautions apply.
5. Use a 1:10 dilution of household bleach to decontaminate equipment and surfaces.

HIV and Public Facilities

1. HIV is not spread through casual contact.
2. The virus is easily killed by chlorine bleach, alcohol, and other common disinfectants. Washing carefully and using a disinfectant will kill the virus before it can enter your body.
3. HIV is transmitted only through exposure to infected blood, sexual intercourse, or breast milk. In addition, direct and indirect contact with an injured person's body fluids should be avoided. Every precaution should be taken.

2001 Lifeguard Training Manual, American National Red Cross (3)

Summary

1. Program considerations for older adults include: a proper acclimation to the pool environment, a longer warm up, low impact options, postural exercises, and functional exercises. Older adults benefit from the social aspect of exercise.

2. Program considerations for larger adults include: comfortable access to enter and exit the pool, modifications to account for larger bodies, cuing for proper form and alignment, and possibly a slightly slower music tempo due to lager frontal surface area.

3. When designing programming for children, age is a primary consideration. Attention span, physical capabilities, level of socialization, and socioeconomic background will affect the type of programming offered.

4. Younger adolescents will need exercise programming that still includes games and fun. Older adolescents may be ready to start participation in more standard fitness programs as prescribed for adults.

5. The American College of Obstetricians and Gynecologist (ACOG) guidelines and recommendations should be followed for pre and post natal clients.

6. Clients with cardiovascular and pulmonary disease can benefit from a well designed exercise program. It is best to have a physician determine the upper limit for exercise based on client symptoms.

7. Most clients with musculoskeletal disease can benefit from an exercise program that improves stamina, strengthens weak muscles, and stretches tight muscles to improve muscular balance and overall functional capacity.

8. Clients with diabetes mellitus require proper footwear for aquatic exercise to protect the delicate skin on their feet. Exercise should be coordinated with insulin intake and a high carbohydrate snack.

9. Water temperature and program considerations vary in neuromuscular diseases and immunological/ hematological disorders depending on the disease type.

Review Questions

1. Name the 4 primary categories for changes that occur as the body matures.
2. Cardiorespiratory exercise in water temperatures above 90 degrees F (32 degrees C) is safe and prudent for larger adults. (True or False)
3. Which cardiovascular disease is caused by blockage to arteries in the brain?
   a. Coronary artery disease
   b. High blood cholesterol
   c. Stroke
   d. Myocardial infarction
4. Which neurological disease is characterized by a loss in muscle function due to the deterioration of the myelin sheaths around the nerves?
   a. Muscular Dystrophy
   b. Multiple Sclerosis
   c. Cerebral palsy
   d. Epilepsy

See Appendix E for answers to review questions.

References

1. American Cancer Society. (2005). *Cancer Facts and Figures 2005*. Atlanta, GA. American Cancer Society.

2. American College of Sports Medicine. (2006). *Guidelines for Exercise Testing and Prescription*. 7th Edition. Baltimore, MD. Lippincott, Williams & Wilkins.

3. American Red Cross. (2001). *Lifeguard Training Manual*. Washington DC. American Red Cross.

4. Ashlie, D. (2004). *Aqua Hearts® Instructor Training Manual*. Instructor Training Workshop. Vancouver, WA.

5. Bellenir, K. (2004). *Fitness Information for Teens: Health Tips about Exercise, Physical Well Being and Health Maintenance*. Detroit, MI. Omnigraphics Publishers.

6. Cleveland Clinic Department of Patient Education and Health Information. (2004). *Muscular Dystrophy*. Cleveland Clinic Health Information. Cleveland, OH. www.clevelandclinic.org/health/health-info/docs/2100/2112.asp?index=877

7. Cotton, R. (1999). *Clinical Exercise Specialist Manual*. 1st Edition. San Diego, CA. American Council on Exercise.

8. Courneye, K., J. Mackey and L. Jones. (2000). Coping with Cancer: Can Exercise Help? *The Physician and Sportsmedicine Journal*. (28) 5.

9. Darst, P. and R. Pangrazi. (2001). *Dynamic Physical Education for Secondary Students*. 4th Edition. San Francisco, CA. Pearson-Benjamin Cummings Publishers.

10. Durstine, J. and G. Moore. (2002). *ACSM's Exercise Management for Persons with Chronic Disease and Disabilities*. 2nd Edition. Champaign, IL. Human Kinetics Publishers.

11. Epilepsy Foundation Staff. (2004). *Epilepsy: An Introduction*. Landover, MD. Epilepsy Foundation. www.epilepsyfoundation.org/answerplace/intro toepilepsy.cfm

12. Global Polio Eradication Initiative. (2005). *The Disease and the Virus*. Geneva, Switzerland. World Health Organization. www.polioeradication.org/disease.asp

13. Goldenson, R., J. Dunham and C. Dunham. (1978). *Disability and Rehabilitation Handbook*. New York, NY. McGraw-Hill Publishers.

14. Mayo Clinic Staff. (2005). *Cerebral Palsy*. Mayo Clinic. Mayo Foundation for Medical Education and Research. www.mayoclinic.com/invoke.cfm?id=DS00302

15. Mayo Clinic Staff. (2005). *Fibromyalgia*. Mayo Clinic. Mayo Foundation for Medical Education and Research. www.mayoclinic.com/invoke.cfm?id=DS00079

16. Mayo Clinic Staff. (2005). *Multiple Sclerosis*. Mayo Clinic. Mayo Foundation for Medical Education and Research. www.mayoclinic.com/invoke.cfm?id=DS00188

17. Mayo Clinic Staff. (2005). *Parkinson's Disease*. Mayo Clinic. Mayo Foundation for Medical Education and Research. www.mayoclinic.com/invoke.cfm?id=DS00295

18. National Heart, Blood and Lung Institute. (2005). *COPD*. Washington, DC. Department of Health and Human Services. www.nhlbi.nih.gov/health/dci/Diseases/Copd/Copd_WhatIs.html

19. National Heart, Blood and Lung Institute. (2005). *How is High Blood Cholesterol Diagnosed?* Washington, DC. Department of Health and Human Services. www.nhlbi.nih.gov/health/dci/Diseases/Hbc/HBC_Diagnosis.html

20. National Institute of Allergy and Infectious Diseases. (2004). *Chronic Fatigue Syndrome*. Office of Communications and Public Liaison. National Institute of Health. Bethesda, MD. www.niaid.nih.gov/factsheets/cfs.htm

21. National Institute of Neurological Disorders and Stroke. (2004). *Amyotrophic Lateral Sclerosis Fact Sheet*. Office of Communications and Public Liaison. National Institute of Health. Bethesda, MD. www.ninds.nih.gov/disorders/amyotrophiclateral sclerosis/detail_amyotrophiclateralsclerosis.htm

22. Quinn, E. (2004). *Exercise as Cancer Treatment*. About.com. www.sportsmedicine.about.com/cs/exercisephysiology/a/aa090501a.htm

Chapter 13: Basic Nutrition and Weight Management

INTRODUCTION

As an aquatic fitness professional, you want to have a firm understanding of basic nutrition and weight management. Sharing sound nutritional information with your clients may motivate them to make healthy food and health enhancing choices. Good nutrition is important to both physical and emotional health. Wise food choices assure that your body is adequately "fueled" in order to carry out daily functions and a healthy exercise session. Proper nutrition and weight management reduces risk for many lifestyle- and obesity-induced chronic diseases.

Americans spend billions of dollars annually on weight control. There are between 15,000 and 20,000 different weight loss methods when you consider all the books, plans, programs, and products that are available. Weight management resources represent a never-ending supply of opinions and angles. Researchers are constantly developing new theories and many have devoted their life's work to discovering the mystery of weight management. It is important for a fitness professional to be able to sort fact from fiction when helping a client with weight management tactics and strategies.

Unit Objectives

After completing Chapter 13, you should be able to:
1. List the 6 basic nutrients found in food.
2. Explain the Dietary Guidelines for Americans and how to use them to ensure nutrition adequacy in the human diet.
3. Explain the role of nutrition in reducing the risk of lifestyle-related disease.
4. Understand the importance of proper hydration and replacing fluids during exercise.
5. Define overweight and obesity and discuss the theories of obesity.
6. Be familiar with the benefits of exercise in weight management.
7. Identify unsafe dieting practices and list symptoms for common eating disorders.
8. Recognize and discuss guidelines for safe and effective weight management.

Key Questions
1. Name three foods rich in nutrients for each of the following: carbohydrate, fat, protein.
2. What are the Dietary Guidelines for Americans?
3. Name 3 chronic diseases for which proper nutrition can reduce your risk.
4. What are basic guidelines for fluid replacement during exercise?
5. What role does exercise play in weight management?

As an aquatic fitness professional, you are not in the business to make nutrition and weight management your career. However, because of the multitude of dieters you'll come across, this chapter condenses a mass of information and presents the key points for basic nutrition and weight management. Aquatic fitness professionals are encouraged to pursue continuing education in the field of nutrition and weight management and forge relationships with Registered Dietitians and other nutrition professionals to refer clients.

Nutrients in Food

Simply, **nutrition** is defined as the study of nutrients in foods and their functions in the body. A complete definition, at least for those professionals whose goals are to improve the health of their clients, would also include the study of human behaviors related to food. Usually people who eat well and exercise are more mentally alert and better able to deal with the every day stresses of life. Life itself can be emotionally taxing and hard on the immune system. Inadequate nutrition only exacerbates the situation. It is important to note that this chapter is only a very basic introduction to the subject of nutrition and that nutrition is a relatively young science. Although many facts on nutrition are known, there is still a lot to learn. Most nutrition research has been conducted in this century and the body of knowledge keeps growing and changing. This is the reason that you may sometimes get confused about the apparent contradictions in reports of different studies. Therefore, it is important to keep an open yet analytical mind about this subject. All in all, you will find that eating in accordance with the U.S. Dietary Guidelines (in relationship to one's specific stage in the lifecycle, i.e., child, teen, pregnant women, etc., and health status) will assure adequate balance and moderation in a diet for normal, healthy individuals.

The human body requires six classes of **nutrients** in order to assure normal growth and function. Nutrients are the components of food that help to nourish the body by performing any of the following functions: providing energy, serving as building material, helping maintain or repair body parts, promoting or sustaining growth, and regulating or assisting in body processes. The nutrient classes are carbohydrates, proteins, fats, vitamins, minerals and water. Carbohydrates, protein, fats and vitamins are considered organic compounds as they contain carbon. All organic compounds are made by living things.

A very important function of some of these nutrients is to provide energy. Green plants are able to capture the energy of the sun and store it in the chemical bonds that form carbohydrates, protein and fat. Animals, including humans, get their energy by eating plants or by eating animals that feed on plants.

During digestion and metabolism, foods undergo mechanical (i.e., chewing) and chemical processes to break them down and release the stored energy in their chemical bonds. This energy is used to form the high energy bonds in ATP. As mentioned in Chapter 2, it is the energy derived from the ATP molecule that is used to drive all the body's functions and processes, and we make that ATP by metabolizing energy sources from food (carbohydrates, protein, and fat).

Energy is measured in calories or units of heat. Strictly speaking, a calorie is the amount of heat energy required to raise the temperature of one gram of water 1 degree Celsius. A gram (g) is the weight of a cubic centimeter (cc) or milliliter (ml) of water under defined conditions of temperature and pressure. (For perspective, one raisin or small paper clip weighs about 1 gram). Food quantities are measured in grams.

Food energy is measured in kilocalories (kcalories, abbreviated kcal; kilo stands for 1000). Therefore a kilocalorie is the amount of heat required to raise the temperature of a kilogram (a liter) of water 1 degree Celsius. Kilocalories are simply referred to as calories (cal) in general speaking and writing and will be referred to as calories in this chapter as well.

The energy found in nutrients is a follows: one gram of carbohydrates yields 4 calories, one gram of protein yields 4 calories, and one gram of fat yields 9 calories. Vitamins, minerals, and water do not contain calories. Alcohol, although not a nutrient, is touted for potential drug benefits, and yields 7 calories per gram, unlike any other drug on the market.

Carbohydrates

Carbohydrates are compounds composed of simple sugars or multiples of sugars. Carbohydrates are made by green plants in a process called photosynthesis (photo means "light", synthesis means "making"). Chlorophyll, the green pigment found in plants, traps the sun's energy in order to make carbohydrates from carbon dioxide and water. The energy invested into the bonds to form the carbohydrates is the same energy that's released when the carbohydrate is metabolized.

Sugars

Simple carbohydrates are called monosaccharides, single sugar units, or disaccharides (pairs of single sugar units linked together). Mono means "one," di means "two" and saccharide means "sugar" unit. **Glucose**, fructose and galactose (the "ose" ending means sugar) are the monosaccharides. Glucose is the key body carbohydrate. All dietary sugars and starches are converted to glucose during digestion or shortly after absorption. It is mainly glucose that is formed by photosynthesis. Fructose is the sugar found in fruit and honey.

While fructose and glucose occur freely in nature, galactose is usually bound to glucose molecules to form the disaccharide lactose, or milk sugar. The remaining disaccharides are maltose and sucrose. (Note: most of the fructose we eat is in the form of sucrose). Maltose is composed of two glucose units and is found wherever starch is being broken down (as in digestion). Sucrose, or table sugar, is composed of a fructose and a glucose molecule bonded together.

Starch

Starch is simply composed of glucose units bound together in long strands. It is this grouping of glucose units which gives rise to the name complex carbohydrate. Another term that you may hear for starch is polysaccharide (poly means "many"). Starch is the plant storage form of glucose. It is found in grains, cereals, legumes and tubers (root vegetables such as potatoes, sweet potatoes, etc.).

Complex carbohydrates in food are broken down in the intestinal tract by various enzymes to form disaccharides and then monosaccharides in order to be absorbed through the intestinal wall into the bloodstream. Glucose is circulated around the body as is, while galactose and fructose are sent to the liver to be converted to glucose or fat (depending on the body's needs).

All cells are able to break down the circulating glucose molecules for energy. Liver and muscle cells are able to form and store glycogen from the circulating glucose. **Glycogen**, sometimes called animal starch, is the storage form of glucose found in animals. It is similar to the starch of plants, but its

chains are longer and more highly branched. The liver also converts excess glucose into fat so it can be stored in the fat cells for later energy use.

It is important to note that glucose is the body's preferred fuel source. The brain and central nervous system depend almost entirely on glucose as its energy source. Glucose can be derived from proteins if necessary, however it is an expensive source. Also, there are health risks associated with high protein intake. Fat, the body's other fuel source, raises the risk of various degenerative diseases when eaten in excess, so carbohydrates should provide the bulk of energy in the diet. Various national and international governmental and private health agencies recommend that at least 55% of the calories in a diet should come from carbohydrates with an emphasis on the carbohydrates found in fruits, vegetables, grains, and cereals, as these foods contain many more important nutrients besides carbohydrates. (4) If a client were on a 2000 calorie per day diet, approximately 1100 (2000 x .55) calories should come from carbohydrate. This would equate to approximately 275 (1100 ÷ 4 calories/gram) grams of carbohydrate per day.

Fiber

Fiber is another polysaccharide or strand of sugars. Fiber contributes to the support structures of the leaves, stems, seeds, and roots of plants, which typically cannot be broken down by the human digestive tract. The digestive enzymes in humans are not able to split apart the glucose units that make up the fiber, so most fiber passes through the human body without being broken down for absorption.

There are two forms of dietary fiber: soluble and insoluble. These terms refer to the ability of the fibers to dissolve in water. Each type of fiber has important health benefits.

The insoluble fibers, cellulose and hemicellulose, are found in brown rice, fruits, legumes, seeds, vegetables, wheat brans, and whole grains. These fibers provide roughage in the form of the string of the celery, the skins of corn kernels and legumes, and the outer layer of brown rice. Insoluble fibers soften stools; regulate bowel movements; speed transit of fecal matter through the colon; reduce the risk of diverticulosis, cancer, and appendicitis; and improve the body's handling of glucose which is helpful for people with diabetes.

Pectins, gums, and mucilages are water soluble fibers. They are found in barley, fruits, legumes, oats, oatmeal, rye, seeds, and vegetables. The water soluble fibers help to lower blood cholesterol levels, slow glucose absorption, and slow the transit of food through the upper digestive tract. The decreased transit time through the tract is beneficial as it offers the feeling of fullness for a longer period of time and can help an individual to eat less.

The USDA Food Guide recommends 31 grams of total dietary fiber per day for the average healthy adult. (4) Encourage your students to consume both types of fiber in order to receive the complete range of possible health benefits. Extreme amounts of fiber intake should not be encouraged in order to avoid the possible deficiencies of other nutrients displaced by putting too much emphasis on fiber-rich foods.

Lipids

Fats belong to a family of greasy compounds called lipids, which are soluble in fat-like solvents but not in water. The lipids include triglycerides (fats and oils), phospholipids (i.e., lecithin), and the sterols (i.e., cholesterol). Fats (including oils) and cholesterol are the primary dietary lipids.

In food, fat contributes to the taste and smell of food, stimulates the appetite, provides satiety (feeling of fullness), and helps to make food tender. In the body, fat is the primary form of stored energy for muscular work, serves as an emergency food supply in times of illness and diminished food intake, acts as a carrier for fat soluble vitamins, forms the major material of cell membranes, and is converted to the other compounds as needed. Also, fat pads inside the body protect the internal organs, while the fat layer under the skin insulates against cold temperature.

Gram for gram, fat contains more than twice the calories of either carbohydrate or protein. A fat molecule is tightly packed together and stores more energy in a smaller space. It is important to note that the body is much more efficient at burning dietary fat compared to dietary carbohydrate. In fact, there is recent research that alludes to the possibility that the body is able to use the whole 9 calories from a gram of fat, but may only be able to use 3 calories of energy from the 4 calories in a gram of carbohydrates.

The USDA Food Guide recommends total fat intake be 29% of total calories per day for the average healthy adult. It is also recommended that saturated fat not exceed 7.8% of the 29% of total fat. (4) If a client were on a 2000 calorie per day diet, approximately 580 (2000 x .29) calories should come

from fat. This would equate to approximately 64 (580 ÷ 9 calories/gram) grams of fat per day, with no more than 17 of those fat grams from saturated fat.

Triglycerides

Triglyceride is the chemical term for fat, either from your diet or in the body. Triglycerides, like glucose, contain carbon, hydrogen, and oxygen. Triglycerides are composed of three long carbon chains that are attached to a small, water soluble carbohydrate derivative called glycerol. (Glycerol is only three carbons long.) The three long carbon chains are called fatty acids and they end in a specific configuration of carbon, oxygen, and hydrogen that make them an acid. Also, there are hydrogen molecules attached to the carbons all along the chains.

The fatty acids in triglycerides are **unsaturated** or **saturated**, and we refer to them as saturated or unsaturated fats. Saturated fatty acids have a hydrogen attached to every available bond on the carbons. Unsaturated fats have fatty acid chains that possess one or more points of unsaturation. At this point, a double bond exists between two carbons which exclude two hydrogen molecules from the chain. If there is only one point of unsaturation in the chain, then it is a **monounsaturated** fatty acid. If there are two or more points of unsaturation, then it is a **polyunsaturated** (poly means "many") fatty acid. The chemical structure of a molecule determines its physical properties. The degree of saturation determines the temperature at which the fat melts. The less saturated the fat is, the more liquid it is at room temperature. Conversely, the more saturated a fat, the more solid it is at room temperature.

Let's look at some examples of these fats. Beef fat is more saturated and harder than chicken fat at room temperature. Vegetable oils are rich in monounsaturated and/or polyunsaturated fatty acids which make them liquid at room temperature. Food processing companies also saturate fats. For example, margarine is made by hydrogenating an oil (adding hydrogen, saturating the fatty acid). The more hydrogenated the oil, the harder the margarine. Liquid margarine which squeezes out of a bottle (less saturated) is softer than tub margarine (more saturated) which is softer than stick margarine (most saturated). This is why the squeeze bottle margarines are a better, heart-healthy choice, because less saturated fats are healthier.

In general, vegetable and fish oils are rich in

mono- and polyunsaturates while animal fats are mostly saturated (not just meat, but also butter, cheese, sour cream, mayonnaise, eggs, gravy, and any other animal fat). Olive oil and canola oils are rich in monounsaturated fats and have been shown to be effective in lowering cholesterol levels, but they also should be consumed in moderation because, like all fats, they are high in calories. Food labels should be checked in order to identify and avoid foods that contain the highly saturated palm and coconut oils. Labels should also be checked for unhealthy trans fats which are discussed in more detail below.

Phospholipids

Phospholipids are fat molecules that contain a fatty portion (non-water soluble) and a water soluble portion that contains phosphorus. Phospholipids are integral components of cell membranes, as this structure allows them to keep fats dispersed in water so they can be transported across cell membranes. You may be familiar with the phospholipid, lecithin.

Sterols

Sterols are lipids that come in large complicated molecules which consist of several interconnected rings of carbon with attached side chains of carbon, hydrogen, and oxygen. Vitamin D, cholesterol, and the sex hormones are sterols or composed of sterols. Cholesterol, a sterol, is a part of every cell structure and is especially important to nerve and brain cells. It is also the major component of the plaques that narrow the arteries in atherosclerosis (hardening of the arteries). As cholesterol is only made by animals, those interested in reducing their dietary cholesterol would reduce their intake of animal products.

Proteins

Proteins are compounds of carbons, hydrogen, oxygen, and nitrogen arranged into strands called **amino acids** (amino means nitrogen containing). There are 22 different amino acids that comprise the proteins of living tissue. Their basic structures are all the same and consist of an amino group (the nitrogen containing part) attached to an acid group. They differ in their distinctive side chains that are attached to the basic structure. The great variety in proteins is due to the infinite combinations of amino acids in their chains.

Proteins have many functions in the body. They serve as a structure for most body cells and tissue; i.e.,

tendons ligaments, muscles, the core of bones and teeth, hair filaments, organ tissues, etc. Proteins also work as enzymes, antibodies, transport vehicles (for lipids, minerals, and oxygen), regulators for fluid and electrolyte balance, and some hormones. Protein forms the netting on which blood clots form.

Protein can also be used as an energy source. This occurs when insufficient carbohydrate and fat are consumed to meet the body's energy needs. The nitrogen of a number of the amino acids is removed and the remainder of the molecule is converted to glucose which is then broken down for energy. As previously mentioned, protein is an expensive source of energy, both in terms of dollar costs, and in terms of what it costs the body to use it as a fuel (waste products must be excreted), although it is burned for fuel when calorie or carbohydrate intake is restricted. (Note: During high intensity or anaerobic exercise, protein cannot be used as a fuel since it requires oxygen to be broken down and metabolized.)

Of the 22 amino acids, the body is able to manufacture 13 from fragments derived from carbohydrates, fats, or even other amino acids. There are nine remaining amino acids which are considered essential or indispensable as they cannot be synthesized by the body. These essential amino acids must be eaten in adequate amounts. Animal proteins provide all the amino acids including the essential ones. Therefore, individuals who eat red meat, chicken, fish, milk, eggs, and any other animal products will meet the need for essential amino acids. This statement assumes that adequate amounts of carbohydrates and fats are also being consumed.

On the other hand, vegans (strict vegetarians who eat no animal products at all, including chicken and fish) should understand that they need to be more careful about choosing protein sources. Vegetable proteins lack one or more essential amino acids. But by combining two so-called complementary proteins (they complement each other), vegans can eat all 9 amino acids needed for human protein growth. As an example, corn lacks the amino acid lysine, while beans lack the amino acid methionine. But by eating beans with a corn tortilla, you've created a meal containing a complete (all 9 of the essential amino acids) protein. These complementary proteins do not necessarily need to be eaten at the same time but should be eaten in the same day. Some other complementary protein combinations include rice and beans, bread and peanut butter, lentils and rice, humus (a middle eastern paste made of pureed garbanzo beans, ground sesame seed, garlic, and lemon) served with pita bread, bean burrito (tortilla and refried beans). The USDA Food Guide recommends that protein comprise 18% of calories consumed per day by the healthy adult. (4) If a client were on a 2000 calorie per day diet, approximately 360 (2000 x .18) calories should come from protein. This would equate to approximately 90 (360 ÷ 4 calories/gram) grams of protein per day.

Vitamins

Vitamins are essential noncaloric organic nutrients needed in tiny amounts in the diet. Inadequate intakes of vitamins can result in deficiency diseases. Vitamins act as regulators in many of the body's processes that are necessary to maintain life. Tables 13-1 and 13-2 contain basic function and dietary reference intacts for vitamins, minerals and nutrients.

There are two classes of vitamins: water soluble and fat soluble. Water soluble vitamins are generally absorbed directly into the bloodstream. As they are not stored in the tissues to any great degree, excesses are excreted in the urine. Therefore, there is less chance of toxicity. Fat- soluble vitamins follow the same absorption pathway as fats. They are absorbed into the lymph and travel in the blood in conjunction with protein carriers. Fat-soluble vitamins are stored in the body's fatty tissues. Excess amounts can lead to toxic concentrations and accompanying detrimental effects.

Table 13-1

Nutrients for Health *		
Protein	meat, poultry, fish, eggs, milk, yogurt, cheese, dried beans, and dried peas	Provides energy at 4 calories per gram. Important for growth and maintaining every cell in your body. Is the building block for enzymes – substances that help produce energy and build tissues.
Carbohydrate	breads, pasta, cereals, potatoes, corn, squash, fruits and dried fruits.	Provides energy at 4 calories per gram. Is a major source of energy for the body.
Fat	shortening, oil, margarine, butter, and salad dressing	Provides energy at 9 calories per gram. Is part of every cell. Transports fat-soluble vitamins. Provides efficient storage of energy and insulates the body. Calories from carbohydrates and protein not needed for energy are stored as fat.
Water	beverages, fruits, and vegetables	Water is part of every cell and tissue in the body. Water carries nutrients to cells and removes waste products. It is essential for maintaining body temperature.
Calcium	milk, yogurt, cheese, salmon and sardines with bones, spinach, collard greens, and almonds	Builds and maintains strong bones and teeth. May help prevent high blood pressure and certain types of cancer.
Iron	liver, beef, pork, oysters, dried beans and peas, spinach, molasses, and enriched cereals.	Is the part of the blood cell that carries oxygen to the cells. Increases resistance to infection. Helps the body turn food into energy.
Potassium	vegetables, milk, yogurt, meat, poultry, fish, and fruits	Helps the body maintain normal blood pressure.

Vitamin A	liver, carrots, sweet potatoes, bok-choy, spinach, milk, tomatoes, broccoli, cantaloupe, nectarines, and water melon.	Is a key part of the eye's ability to see at night. Helps keep skin healthy and helps the body resist infections. May help prevent some types of cancer.
Thiamin (Vitamin B$_1$)	pork, sunflower seeds, green peas, black-eyed peas, breads, pastas, and cereals.	Is a key part of the enzymes that are needed to turn carbohydrates into energy. Helps the nervous system function normally.
Riboflavin (Vitamin B$_2$)	beef, pork, milk, yogurt, and cottage cheese	Is a key part of enzymes that cells use to produce energy. Plays a roll in healthy skin and eyes.
Vitamin C	oranges, grapefruit, papaya, mangos, strawberries, broccoli, brussel sprouts, and green peppers.	Helps wounds heal. Helps the nervous system function normally. May help prevent cancer.
Vitamin D	milk, fatty fish, eggs, liver, and butter	Is a key nutrient in helping the body absorb and use calcium to make bones grow and stay strong.
Niacin	poultry, fish, beef, pork, and nuts	Helps the body produce energy from carbohydrate and fat. Plays a role in maintaining healthy skin, nerves, and digestive system.
Fiber	breads, fruits, and vegetables	Is the non-digestible portion of food that helps maintain regularity and keeps the digestive tract healthy. Some types of fiber may help prevent cancer and lower blood cholesterol.

* Guide to Good Eating, Daily Food Guide Pyramid Leader Guide, Courtesy of National Dairy Council.

Vitamins C, E, selenium, and beta carotene (not a vitamin) serve as **antioxidants** in addition to their other roles. Antioxidants are compounds that protect other compounds from oxygen so that they are not broken down (oxidized).

Unstable **free radicals**, highly reactive molecules often containing oxygen, are produced by normal body processes. Physical stresses including injury, infection, radiation exposure, and even excessive exercise can speed the formation of the free radicals in affected tissues. These free radicals can set off destructive chain reactions which do damage to the cell membranes and disable the cell, if adequate antioxidants aren't present. Antioxidants protect the cell membrane lipids and proteins, DNA, or cholesterol molecules by "soaking up" and recycling the excess oxygen or other by-products. In other words, these vitamins are oxidized or broken down instead of the cells. In addition to the destruction of cell membranes, there are many other ways free radicals can harm the body, including precancerous changes in DNA and inflammation in blood vessel plaque triggering atherosclerosis.

Table 13-2

Dietary Reference Intakes for Vitamins and Elements (Minerals) For Healthy Adults		
Nutrient	RDA/AI	Upper Limits**
Biotin	30 (mg/d)	Not Determinable due to lack of data of adverse effects.*
Choline	550 (mg/d) males 425 (mg/d) females	3500 (mg/d)
Folate	400 (mg/d)	1000 (mg/d)
Niacin	16 (mg/d) males 14 (mg/d) females	35 (mg/d)
Pantothenic Acid	5 (mg/d)	Not Determinable due to lack of data of adverse effects.*
Riboflavin (B$_2$)	1.3 (mg/d) males 1.1 (mg/d) females	Not Determinable due to lack of data of adverse effects.*
Thiamin (B$_1$)	1.2 (mg/d) males 1.1 (mg/d) females	Not Determinable due to lack of data of adverse effects.*
Vitamin A	900 (mg/d) males 700 (mg/d) females	3000 (mg/d)
Vitamin B$_6$	1.3-1.7 (mg/d) males 1.3-1.5 (mg/d) females	100 (mg/d)
Vitamin B$_{12}$	2.4 (mg/d)	Not Determinable due to lack of data of adverse effects.*
Vitamin C	90 (mg/d) males 75 (mg/d) females	2000 (mg/d)
Vitamin D	5-15 (mg/d)	50 (mg/d)
Vitamin E	15 (mg/d)	1000 (mg/d)
Vitamin K	120 (mg/d) males 90 (mg/d) females	Not Determinable due to lack of data of adverse effects.*
Boron	Not Determinable due to lack of data of adverse effects.*	20 (mg/d)
Calcium	1000-1200 (mg/d)	2500 (mg/d)
Chromium	35-30 (mg/d) males 25-20 (mg/d) females	Not Determinable due to lack of data of adverse effects.*
Copper	900 (mg/d)	10,000 (mg/d)
Fluoride	4 (mg/d) males 3 (mg/d) females	10 (mg/d)
Iodine	150 (mg/d)	1100 (mg/d)
Iron	8 (mg/d) males 18 (mg/d) females (to age 50) 8 (mg/d) females (over age 50)	45 (mg/d)

Magnesium	400-420 (mg/d) males 3310-320 (mg/d) females	350 (mg/d)
Manganese	2.3 (mg/d) males 1.8 (mg/d) females	11 (mg/d)
Molybdenum	45 (mg/d)	2000 (mg/d)
Phosphorus	700 (mg/d)	4000 (mg/d)
Selenium	55 (mg/d)	400 (mg/d)
Zinc	11 (mg/d) males 8 (mg/d) females	40 (mg/d)

* *Concern with regard to lack of ability to handle excess amounts. Source of intake should be from food only to prevent high levels of intake.*

** *The maximum level of daily nutrient intake that is likely to pose no risk of adverse effects.*
Source: Institute of Medicine of the National Academies, Food and Nutrition Board. www.iom.edu/board.
Dietary Reference Intake Tables. 2004.

Dietary Reference Intakes

Dietary Reference Intakes (DRIs) for Nutrients can be found through the Institute of Medicine's Food and Nutrition Board. DRIs include Recommended Dietary Allowances (RDAs) and Adequate Intakes (AIs). These charts are fairly detailed and include recommendations for infants, children, males, females, pregnancy, and lactation. The charts are posted at www.nap.edu.

- Recommended Dietary Allowance (RDAs): The intake that meets the nutrient needs of almost all healthy individuals.
- Adequate Intake (AIs): A goal intake when sufficient scientific information is unavailable to estimate the RDA.
- Estimated Average Requirement: The intake that meets the estimated nutrient need of half the individuals in a specific group.
- Tolerable Upper Intake Level (Upper Limits): The maximum intake that is unlikely to pose risks of adverse health effects in almost all healthy individuals in a group.

Minerals

Minerals are naturally occurring, inorganic (do not contain carbon, hydrogen and oxygen), homogeneous substances. Minerals (as essential nutrients) are classified into two groups: The major minerals and trace minerals.

The major minerals are found in the body in amounts larger than 5 grams. The trace minerals are found in amounts less than 5 grams. The major minerals are no more important than the trace minerals. Relative deficiency in either causes body malfunctions and disease.

Minerals work as regulators of body processes, are components of various body cells, (i.e., the iron in red blood cells), or components of various structures (i.e. bone). The major minerals include calcium, chloride, magnesium, phosphorous, potassium, sodium, and sulfur. The trace minerals include iron, zinc, selenium, chromium, copper, molybdenum, manganese, boron, cobalt, nickel, and silium.

Like vitamins, oversupplementation of minerals can upset the normal balance of body processes. As with all drugs, when minerals are taken in drug quantities, one can expect to see side effects. Supplementation beyond the RDA should only be considered under a doctor's orders.

Water

Water is the single most important nutrient during exercise. While it is possible to go days, even weeks without food, this is not the case with water. Food is another source of water in the diet. Those who live in hot and dry conditions, hot and humid conditions, and those who exercise, will need to significantly increase their water intake in order to replenish water losses and prevent dehydration. Water and fluid replacement are discussed in more detail later in this chapter.

Toward a Healthy Diet

At this point, you've had an introduction to the nutrient classes and their general roles in the body. You may wonder how you can advise your clients to choose a diet that will meet their nutrient needs, maintain their health, control their weight, and lower the risks of developing various diseases. Although you may not be a dietitian and may not be trained to design individualized diets, especially for individuals with disease or other special needs, you can provide your clients with general information to guide their food choices. There are actually a number of tools that your clients can use to plan a healthy diet following the Dietary Guidelines for Americans developed by the U.S. Department of Agriculture (USDA) and the U.S. Department of Health and Human Services. (see table 13-3)

The intent of the Dietary Guidelines is to "summarize and synthesize knowledge regarding individual nutrients and food components into recommendations for a pattern of eating that can be adopted by the public." (4) The Guidelines are based on scientific knowledge and intended to help individuals lower disease risk and improve health. There are two examples of eating patterns based on the Guidelines; the USDA Food Guide and the Dietary Approaches to Stop Hypertension (DASH) Eating Plan. This manual will focus on the USDA Food Guide.

Table 13-3

Key Recommendations for Dietary Guidelines for Americans-2005*
ADEQUATE NUTRIENTS WITHIN CALORIE NEEDS • Consume a variety of nutrient-dense foods and beverages within and among the basic food groups while choosing foods that limit the intake of saturated and trans fats, cholesterol, added sugars, salt, and alcohol. • Meet recommended intakes within energy needs by adopting a balanced eating pattern, such as the USDA Food Guide or the DASH Eating Plan.
WEIGHT MANAGEMENT • To maintain body weight in a healthy range, balance calories from foods and beverages with calories expended. • To prevent gradual weight gain over time, make small decreases in food and beverage calories and increase physical activity.
PHYSICAL ACTIVITY • Engage in regular physical activity and reduce sedentary activities to promote health, psychological well-being, and a healthy body weight. 　■ To reduce the risk of chronic disease in adulthood: Engage in at least 30 minutes of moderate-intensity physical activity, above usual activity, at work or home on most days of the week. 　■ For most people, greater health benefits can be obtained by engaging in physical activity of more vigorous intensity or longer duration. 　■ To help manage body weight and prevent gradual, unhealthy body weight gain in adulthood: Engage in approximately 60 minutes of moderate- to vigorous- intensity activity on most days of the week while not exceeding caloric intake requirements. 　■ To sustain weight loss in adulthood: Participate in at least 60 to 90 minutes of daily moderate-intensity physical activity while not exceeding caloric intake requirements. Some people may need to consult with a healthcare provider before participating in this level of activity. • Achieve physical fitness by including cardiovascular conditioning, stretching exercises for flexibility, and resistance exercises or calisthenics for muscle strength and endurance.

FOOD GROUPS TO ENCOURAGE
- Consume a sufficient amount of fruits and vegetables while staying within energy needs. Two cups of fruit and 2 1/2 cups of vegetables per day are recommended for a reference 2,000-calorie intake, with higher or lower amounts depending on the calorie level.
- Choose a variety of fruits and vegetables each day. In particular, select from all five vegetable subgroups (dark green, orange, legumes, starchy vegetables, and other vegetables) several times a week.
- Consume 3 or more ounce-equivalents of whole-grain products per day, with the rest of the recommended grains coming from enriched or whole-grain products. In general, at least half the grains should come from whole grains.
- Consume 3 cups per day of fat-free or low-fat milk or equivalent milk products.

FATS
- Consume less than 10 percent of calories from saturated fatty acids and less than 300 mg/day of cholesterol, and keep trans fatty acid consumption as low as possible.
- Keep total fat intake between 20 to 35 percent of calories, with most fats coming from sources of polyunsaturated and monounsaturated fatty acids, such as fish, nuts, and vegetable oils.
- When selecting and preparing meat, poultry, dry beans and milk or milk products, make choices that are lean, low-fat or fat-free.
- Limit intake of fats and oils high in saturated and/or trans fatty acids, and choose products low in such fats and oils.

CARBOHYDRATES
- Choose fiber-rich fruits, vegetables, and whole grains often.
- Choose and prepare foods and beverages with little added sugars or caloric sweeteners, such as amounts suggested by the USDA Food Guide and the DASH Eating Plan.
- Reduce the incidence of dental carries by practicing good oral hygiene and consuming sugar- and starch-containing foods and beverages less frequently.

SODIUM AND POTASSIUM
- Consume less than 2,333mg (approximately 1 tsp. of salt) of sodium per day.
- Choose and prepare foods with little salt. At the same time, consume potassium-rich foods, such as fruits and vegetables.

ALCOHOLIC BEVERAGES
- Those who choose to drink alcoholic beverages should do so sensibly and in moderation- defined as the consumption of up to one drink per day for women and up to two drinks per day for men.
- Alcoholic beverages should not be consumed by some individuals, including those who cannot restrict their alcohol intake, women of childbearing age who may become pregnant, pregnant and lactating women, children and adolescents, individuals taking medications that can interact with alcohol, and those with specific medical conditions. Alcoholic beverages should be avoided by individuals engaging in activities that require attention, skill, or coordination, such as driving or operating machinery.

FOOD SAFETY
- To avoid microbial foodborne illness:
  - Clean hands, food contact surfaces, and fruits and vegetables. Meat and poultry should not be washed or rinsed.
  - Separate raw, cooked, and ready-to-eat foods while shopping, preparing, or storing foods.
  - Cook foods to a safe temperature to kill microorganisms.
  - Chill (refrigerate) perishable food promptly and defrost foods properly.
  - Avoid raw (unpasteurized) milk or any products made from unpasteurized milk, raw or partially cooked eggs or foods containing raw eggs, raw or uncooked meat and poultry, unpasteurized juices, and raw sprouts.

Dietary Guidelines for Americans is a document developed jointly by the USDA and the HHS. 2005.

The USDA Food Guide provides an excellent tool to help your clients follow the Dietary Guidelines for Americans. The servings listed in the Food Guide are the minimum amount necessary to meet the RDA for most adults, however they should be adjusted upwards to meet the energy and nutrient requirements of active adults, active adolescents, and pregnant and lactating women. These groups are advised to choose more servings of food from each group. Information about the Food Guide can be found in the Dietary Guidelines for Americans, 2005 (Publication HHS-ODPHP-2005-01-DGA-A) and can be found on line at www.healthierus.gov/dietaryguidelines. You can order copies of the Guidelines to distribute to your participants from the government bookstore. The Guidelines contain the following valuable information:

- Dietary Guidelines for Americans.
- Eating Patterns for various caloric goals with serving sizes and examples.
- USDA Food Guide.
- Discretionary Calorie Allowance in the USDA Food Guide.
- DASH Eating Plan.
- Calorie and Physical Activity Charts.
- Nutrient Intake Recommendations.
- Estimated Calorie Requirements.

Selections from the various food groups must be made with adequate guidance and knowledge. Make your participants aware of the Dietary Guidelines for Americans so that they can select properly from each group. Provide them with educational materials that give instruction on how to read labels to enable your clients to steer clear of high fat and high sugar foods. Low or no-cost materials are available from the American Dairy Council and the Wheat Foods Council. (Addresses are found at the back of this chapter under Resources.) Contact a Registered Dietitian to offer a healthy eating series of lectures to your clients. They will appreciate that you've taken a genuine interest in their health.

Preventive Nutrition

Although the term "**preventive nutrition**" is somewhat of a misnomer, it does convey the concept of eating well in order to stave off certain disease conditions. Actually, the more accurate term could be "risk-reducing nutrition" in that certain dietary patterns have been shown to reduce the risk of diseases such as atherosclerosis, certain cancers, hypertension and osteoporosis. For example, in the case of iron deficiency anemia, we can see that eating a high iron diet will in most cases prevent the condition. The role diet plays in iron deficiency, blood cholesterol levels, hypertension, and the risk for cardiovascular disease are discussed briefly below.

Iron Deficiency and Iron Deficiency Anemia

Iron plays a very important role in the body as it is a component of the proteins hemoglobin and myoglobin. Hemoglobin is found in the red blood cells that carry oxygen from the lungs to all of the cells throughout the body. Myoglobin carries and stores oxygen in the muscles.

Iron deficiency occurs when not enough iron is consumed and absorbed or through blood loss caused by injury, parasites, and ulcer. Menstruation also puts women at risk. Normally, the body absorbs 10 to 15% of dietary iron, including 33% from meat, but only 2-10% from plants and supplements. The absorption rate increases as iron stores become depleted or the need for iron increases in conditions such as pregnancy or intense growth.

There is a difference between iron deficiency and iron deficiency anemia. It is possible to become deficient without being anemic. Iron deficiency refers to depleted iron stores, although not necessarily the degree of depletion or the presence of anemia. Anemia refers to severe depletion of iron stores resulting in low blood hemoglobin. During iron depletion, the body is unable to make enough hemoglobin to fill its red blood cells. The red blood cells are smaller and pale as they contain less hemoglobin. As oxygen carrying capacity is compromised, cells no longer receive sufficient oxygen for energy breakdown, and the symptoms of iron deficiency occur. These symptoms include fatigue, tiredness, apathy, and a tendency to be cold.

Even before iron deficiency has progressed to anemia, the symptoms of diminished oxygen can be exhibited. Physical work capacity and productivity are affected and can keep people from being motivated to start an exercise program. Iron deficient children become restless, irritable, and unable to pay attention.

The RDA for iron is 8 mg a day for men and older women. Women of child bearing age have an RDA of 18 mg a day in order to replace the blood loss of menstruation. Pregnancy requires 30 mg a day in order to assure adequate iron stores for the mother and developing fetus. Although supplements are available, it is very important to eat an iron rich diet as the iron in food is more easily absorbed. Men, due to their higher food intakes, generally have less trouble meeting requirements compared to women, who must be much more selective in their food choices as they consume less food.

Iron occurs in two forms: heme iron and non-heme iron. Heme iron is found in the hemoglobin and myoglobin in meat, fish, and poultry. Non-heme iron is the form found in plants and also exists in animal flesh. Heme iron is much more readily absorbed than non-heme iron. Some foods that are high in both heme and non-heme iron are organ meats, beef, pork, chicken, fish, and oysters. Foods that are high in non-heme iron include raisins, greens, watermelon, strawberries, legumes, dried apricots, and prunes among others.

Fortunately, there are other factors in food that increase the absorption of non-heme iron. In addition to their heme iron, meat, fish, and poultry contain a factor (MFP factor) that increases the absorption of the non-heme iron in a meal. Eating lentil soup that contains even small chunks of meat would help to increase the absorption of iron from the lentils. Vitamin C in a meal also increases iron absorption. The salsa and/or hot peppers that are eaten with a bean burrito will increase the iron absorption of the beans. There are numerous other combinations that will increase iron absorption. Further, cooking in an iron pot or pan will add supplemental iron to food.

It is important to note that there are foods that impair iron absorption. These are tea, coffee, the calcium and phosphorus in milk, and the phytates and fiber in whole grain cereals. Phytates are compounds present in plant foods, particularly the whole grains that bind iron and prevent its absorption. As you can see, once again the concept of balance and variety must be applied to diet planning in order to assure the adequacy of all the essential nutrients.

Blood Cholesterol and Cardiovascular Risk

Cholesterol occurs in various forms in the bloodstream. The levels of certain types of cholesterol molecules, sometimes called total cholesterol, increase or decrease risk for atherosclerosis. As you know, cholesterol is a lipid and is insoluble in water. Therefore, in order for cholesterol and other fats to be transported in the blood, they must combine with proteins and phospholipids to form a molecule that will dissolve in water. These molecules are called **lipoproteins**.

There are four major classes of lipoprotein, three of which we'll mention here: **chylomicrons**, **low density lipoproteins** (LDL), and **high density lipoproteins** (HDL). Chylomicrons carry food fats from the intestines into the bloodstream and to the liver and other tissues. A blood test showing elevated chylomicrons simply reflects previous intake of a high fat meal. Although LDL and HDL carry lipids in the blood, they have different make-ups and different effects on atherosclerosis. LDL are lighter and more lipid filled. LDL carry cholesterol and triglycerides from the liver to the tissues. It is the cholesterol in LDL that finds its way into the plaques of atherosclerosis, and LDL cholesterol has been named the "bad cholesterol."

HDL are smaller, denser, and packaged with more protein. HDL act as scavengers and pick up excess cholesterol and phospholipids from the tissues and return them to the liver for disposal. HDL have earned themselves the labels of being "good cholesterol." High blood cholesterol levels, particularly a high ratio of LDL to HDL, are associated with cardiovascular disease.

Blood Cholesterol Guidelines	
Total Cholesterol Level	**Category**
Less than 200 mg/dL	Desirable
200-239 mg/dL	Borderline High
240 mg/dL and above	High
LDL Cholesterol Levels	**LDL Cholesterol Category**
Less than 100 mg/dL	Optimal
100-129 mg/dL	Near Optimal/ Above Optimal
130-159 mg/dL	Borderline High
160-189 mg/dL	High
190 mg/dL and above	Very High
Triglycerides Levels	**Triglyceride Level Categories**
150 -199 mg/dL	Borderline High
200 mg/dL or above	High
HDL Cholesterol Levels (good Cholesterol)	**HDL Cholesterol Categories (higher levels are better)**
< 40 mg/dL	Low- increases risk
≥ 60 mg/dL	High- decreases risk

Adapted from National Cholesterol Education Program. National Institutes for Health. US Department of Health and Human Services. Publication # 01-3290. May 2001.

Diet, weight management, and exercise are the keys to improving blood cholesterol levels. Research indicates that proper diet may not only slow the rate of atherosclerosis but may even reverse the process. Reducing saturated fats appears to be the most important dietary manipulation. Research has shown that diets should contain less than 10% of calories from saturated fat. Further, Americans are urged to hold their total fat intake to no more than 30% of calories and not to consume more than 300 milligrams of cholesterol a day. Other dietary changes of benefit include replacing saturated fats with monounsaturated fats (olive oil and canola oil) and by consuming more water soluble fibers, like those found in fruits, vegetables, legumes, and oat bran.

The Therapeutic Lifestyles Changes (TLC) Diet
This is a low-saturated-fat, low-cholesterol eating plan that calls for less than 7% of calories from saturated fat and less than 200 mg of dietary cholesterol per day. The TLC diet recommends only enough calories to maintain a desirable weight and avoid weight gain. If your LDL is not lowered enough by reducing saturated fat and cholesterol intakes, the amount of soluble fiber in your diet can be increased. Certain food products that contain plant stanols or plant sterols (for example, cholesterol lowering margarines and salad dressings) can also be added to the TLC diet to boost its LDL-lowering power.

Adapted from National Cholesterol Education Program. National Institutes for Health. US Department of Health and Human Services. Publication # 01-3290. May 2001.

Additional Dietary Considerations for Cardiovascular Disease Risk Reduction

Two omega-3 fatty acids found in certain cold water fish (eicosopentaenoic acid or EPA and docosahexaenoic acid or DHA), have been associated with a decreased risk of cardiovascular disease. Omega-3 describes the specific structure of the fatty acid. EPA and DHA seem to help control platelets so they don't form as many clots, thereby decreasing the risk of developing a thrombus or embolus.

Fish that are rich in omega-3 fatty acids include: European anchovy, blue fish, capeline conch, Atlantic and Pacific herring, mackerel, mullet, sablefish, salmon, saury, muroaji scad, Atlantic and common sturgeon, lake trout, white albacore or bluefish tuna, and lake white fish.

The antioxidant nutrients have been shown effective in lowering the risk of CVD. These nutrients which include vitamins C, E, selenium, and beta-carotene are found in fruits and vegetables. (Remember, over supplementation of any chemical can lead to side effects). It is thought that the antioxidants protect LDL cholesterol from oxidation which causes less injury to the arterial walls and less plaque formation.

Some research has linked moderate alcohol consumption, no more than 1-2 drinks per day, with decreased risk of cardiovascular disease. Although, considering the abundant research linking alcohol consumption with poor health, abstainers shouldn't be encouraged to consume alcohol.

Nutrition and Hypertension

Blood pressure is considered normal if it is ≤120 over 80. Above this level, the risk of heart attack and stroke increases in direct proportion to the increase in diastolic blood pressure. The risk factors for hypertension include age, family background (very highly associated), obesity, and being of African-American descent. Although there is not much one can do about genetics or ethnicity, exercise and dietary measures can lower blood pressure. (Your client's physician will determine whether hypertensive medication is warranted.)

Obesity and hypertension go hand in hand. In fact, in the obese, significant reductions in blood pressure can be seen with losses of as few as ten pounds. Physical activity, with or without weight loss, also effectively lowers blood pressure.

The minerals that affect blood pressure are calcium, potassium, and sodium. Potassium and calcium intake should be increased while sodium intake should be decreased.

While it is agreed that sodium restriction is beneficial for the treatment of hypertension, many are not so-called "salt sensitive", meaning their blood pressure doesn't respond to fluctuations in sodium intake. Still, minimal sodium needs are roughly 300 mg per day, while typical intake is closer to 3000 – 6000 mg, thus the general recommendation for everyone to reduce sodium intake is prudent. Foods that are especially high in salt or sodium include:

foods prepared in brine (pickles, olives, sauerkraut); salty or smoked meat (bologna, frankfurters, luncheon meats, saltpork, sausage, ham, smoked tongue); salty or smoked fish (anchovies, caviar, salted and dried cod, herring, sardines, and smoked salmon); snack items such as potato chips, pretzels, salted corn, salted nuts and crackers; certain seasoning (bullion cubes, seasoned salts, MSG, soy sauce, Worcestershire sauce, and barbecue sauce); fast foods; cheeses, especially processed types; and canned and instant soups.

Potassium intake is increased by consuming fruits and vegetables as directed by the USDA Food Guide. Nonfat or at least low fat milk products are encouraged to increase calcium intakes. The National Heart, Lung and Blood Institute's DASH diet for high blood pressure can be reviewed at www.nhlbi.nih.gov/health/public/heart/hbp/dash/.

5 a Day for Better Health Program

Another tools used to promote adherence to the Dietary Guidelines for Americans is the 5 a Day for Better Health Program. Approved by the Department of Health and Human Services, The National Cancer Institute, and the Centers for Disease Control and Prevention, this national nutrition education program encourages all Americans to eat 5-9 servings of vegetables and fruit each day. Unprocessed fruits and vegetables are the most nutrient dense of all foods, plus they're packed with phytochemicals (plant chemicals) that reduce disease risk.

Fluid Replacement

Although aqua exercisers are not at as great a risk for dehydration as land exercisers, they still need to consume plentiful amounts of liquid to avoid dehydration. Exercise in hot weather, especially for the instructor who is teaching outside from the pool deck, will require careful adherence to the following fluid replacement guidelines recommended by the Sports and Cardiovascular Nutritionists (SCAN) practice group of the American Dietetic Association.

In addition, water is strongly recommended. Increase water intake slowly to allow the body to adapt. Water is responsible for removal of metabolic by-products or toxins in your body. The more you exercise, the more you eat, the more you need water. Also, if you think about it, water is like oil for an engine. The engine, let's say your body, will not run

very well without oil, your daily water intake. With dehydration your metabolic functions will be slowed. Your organ systems may not work as efficiently. The liver is the central organ involved in fat metabolism. If the liver is sluggish, then fat metabolism may also be slowed. This is another important reason to tell students to drink more water.

Importance of Proper Hydration

Proper hydration is important to health and performance in the following ways:

- Chronic, mild dehydration, a constant 1 to 2 percent deficit of body weight caused by loss of fluids, can have a measurable effect on mental and physical performance, muscle growth, and long term health.
- Even a small loss of fluid or electrolytes will affect muscle strength and control. Muscle cell dehydration promotes protein breakdown and inhibits protein synthesis.
- Water dilutes and expedites the removal of body toxins.
- Proper hydration is essential in optimal brain function including arithmetic ability and short term memory.
- Fluid intake has a marked effect on all urinary risk factors.
- Research has linked fluid intake and certain cancers and mitral valve prolapse.

Adapted from American Dietetic Association. 1999. 99:200-206.

It is important to realize that water requirements change based on environment, sweat loss, body surface area, calorie intake, body size, lean muscle tissue, etc., leading to tremendous inter- and intra- individual variation. Each client's situation should be individually considered. Since thirst is triggered at about 1% dehydration, drinking when you are thirsty is a reasonable recommendation to maintain fluid balance for individual's in temperature-controlled environments who are sedentary and who have plenty of fluid readily available. For active individuals who engage in regular exercise, the recommendations for fluid intake and replacement are better defined. The guidelines given below should be used by exercisers before, during, and after an exercise session.

Fluid Replacement Guidelines

1. Drink a minimum of 1 quart (4 cups) of fluid for every 1,000 calories you eat every day.
2. Drink at least 5 cups of water every day.

3. Drink cool beverages.

4. For moderate exercise that lasts an hour or less, water is sufficient for replacing lost fluids.

5. Carbohydrate-electrolyte sports drinks are best if the exercise is intense and lasts for more than one hour, or if it's moderate and lasts for several (non-stop) hours. Otherwise, carbohydrate from food will amply replenish body carbohydrate stores.

6. Before exercise: drink 2 cups of fluid 2 hours before exercise.

7. During exercise: drink 4-6 ounces every 15 to 20 minutes.

8. After exercise: drink 16-20 ounces (2-2 1/2 cups) of fluid for every pound of body weight lost during exercise.

Adapted from American Dietetic Association. 1999. 99:200-206.

Supplementation

Contrary to popular belief, the regulatory standards for products labeled "dietary supplements" are meager when compared to those for foods, food additives, and over-the-counter (OTC) or prescription drugs. While manufacturers of food products are required to demonstrate their products' safety, no such standards exist for dietary supplements. In fact, as long as the dietary supplement's label avoids claims that the product prevents or treats any disease or condition, it can make statements unproven by science. These so-called function or structure claims are allowed without proof if they limit claims to those of normal body functioning. For example, the claim "improves memory" is exempt from requirements of proof, while "effective against Alzheimer's" (a disease) is not allowed on a label without passing the rigorous standards set for OTC and prescription drugs.

Historically, the Food and Drug Administration has attempted to establish standards of safety and effectiveness for nutritional supplements, but consumer protests against such regulation has always been strong. In response to consumer demand, Congress passed the 1994 Dietary Supplement Health and Education Act, which loosened the regulation of vitamins, minerals, amino acids, herbs, plants, or any concentrate or extract of any of these.

The most important thing you can share with your clients about the law is that proof of safety or effectiveness was essentially waived. Still clients will insist on taking supplements, and reliable information about many available supplements can be found through the National Institutes of Health's Office of Dietary Supplements (visit their site at http://dietary-supplements.info.nih.gov). A few independent organizations are good sources for consumer information, although, unfortunately safety and effectiveness testing is outside of the scope of tasks they perform. ConsumerLab.com evaluates products using four criteria: identity (does the product contain what it says it does?), strength (does it contain the amount promised?), purity (is it free from contaminants?) and availability (does it break apart so the body can use it?) Another organization, the United States Pharmacopeial Convention, Inc. consists of about 400 volunteers representing state associations and colleges of medicine and pharmacy; the federal government; national and international professional, scientific, and trade organizations; the pharmaceutical industry; and consumer organizations. They allow use of their USP-Verified mark for dietary supplements that meet standards similar to those of ConsumerLab.com.

Certain populations are more at risk for a nutrient deficiency, and a vitamin or mineral supplement would be appropriate therapy. Those with little sunlight exposure (many older adults) might need a vitamin D supplement; women of childbearing age need adequate folic acid to prevent a certain type of birth defect (neural tube defects); those who seldom eat dairy products might benefit from a calcium supplement; while those who eat no animal foods (vegans) must have a supplemental source of vitamin B12 (otherwise found only in animal products).

Still it's important to note that concentrated doses of nutrients in pill form, just like concentrated doses of any chemical, can induce side effects. While the minuscule amount of iron found in the body is critical for cellular oxygen delivery, excessive body iron leads to liver damage and diabetes induction. Vitamin A in normal amounts maintains mucous production of soft tissues and aids in bone growth, but excessive amounts taken by pregnant women can cause urinary malformations in their offspring. Vitamin D helps us absorb calcium, yet too much can lead to calcium buildup in soft tissues. The term "dietary supplement" leads consumers to believe these products are a key part of healthy eating, while for most chemicals found in dietary supplements, evidence of benefit is lacking. It's your job to be sympathetic to your clients' beliefs, then to steer them to their most reliable source of nutrients: a healthy diet.

Supplements tend to fall into the following categories:

- Meal replacements such as drinks and bars.
- Protein sources such as drinks, powders, and tablets.
- Amino acids such as glutamine and tyrosine.
- Carbohydrate sources such as sports drinks, energy drinks, bars, and gels.
- Pre- and prohormones that are enhancers of hormone production such as androstenedione and dehydroepiandosterone (DHEA).
- Biochemicals and energy metabolites such as creatine, hydroxyl metylbutyrate (HMB), pyruvate, and conjugated linoleic acid (CLA).
- Herbs such as ginseng, guarana, St. John's wort, etc.

Weight Management: A Controversial Problem

There are two commonly used terms in the process of weight management: **overweight** and **obesity**. Overweight is a condition where an individual's weight exceeds the population norm or average, which can be determined by height-weight tables based on gender, height, and frame size. Although a standard approach, weight/height measurements lack the ability to account for differences in muscle mass. A more accurate measure would be to determine percentage of body fat which takes into account individual differences in lean tissue mass, although such measurements are not as readily available, and thus are used less frequently.

Obesity is a condition where there is "an excess of body fat frequently resulting in a significant impairment of health," a level of 20% or more above your individual ideal body weight. When looking at percentage of fat, obesity is generally defined and accepted as above 25% body fat for males, and above 32% body fat for females, although you will see variances on the threshold for obesity for men and women in different sources. Some sources set the criteria at 20% body fat for men and 30% for women, where others consider men to be obese at 31% body

fat and women at 36%. The National Institute for Health at the website http://www.nhlbi.nih.gov/guidelines/obesity/obgdlns.htm provides federal guidelines (1998) for the identification, evaluation, and treatment of overweight and obesity.

Obesity assessment tools that use weight/height measurements include height/weight tables, rule-of-thumb methods, and Body Mass Index (BMI). Tools which assess body fat percentage were covered in Chapter 10.

In 1943, The Metropolitan Life Insurance Company formulated height/weight tables used in many doctors' offices based on *average* weights of young, white, middle class Americans who buy insurance (these were revised in 1983). Many have come to believe that these are medically-established *ideal* weights, which they are not.

Often rule-of-thumb methods for assessing weight are called methods for assessing *ideal* body weight. As these techniques only use weight and height measurements and make no adjustment for muscle mass, it's more accurate to say that the methods estimate *reasonable* body weight. (See the following box for one example of a rule-of thumb technique.)

Assessing Ideal Body Weight

For women, allow 100 pounds of weight for the first 5 feet in height. For each additional inch in height, 5 more pounds for an estimate of reasonable weight. For men, allow 106 pounds for the first 5 feet in height, and add 6 pounds for each additional inch in height.

If your client has a large frame size, allow for 10% more weight (i.e. if 160 has been determined as a reasonable weight for your large framed male, you'll add 16 more pounds (160 x .10) to the 160 to arrive at an adjusted reasonable weight of 176 pounds. For small framed clients, subtract 10% of the weight from the original reasonable weight value.

Once you've determined a reasonable body weight, you can compare your client's actual body weight to the weight you've determined is more reasonable. To do that: take actual weight and divided it by your calculated reasonable weight, then multiply this by 100 to arrive at a percentage. For example, I've calculated a reasonable weight of 130 pounds for my 149 pound client. 149/130 x 100 = 115%. My client weighs 115% of what I've estimated is reasonable for a person of her height (or 15% more than 130 pounds).

While BMI is an accurate tool for assessing obesity in populations, in individuals it only can assess "heaviness." As this tool only uses weight/height values, it does not assess internal muscle mass. Use it as a tool to screen obesity, then confirm your assessment by estimating body fat status (there's also a strong possibility that you can eyeball whether or not the heaviness is due to excess weight or excess muscle). The formula for determining BMI is located in Chapter 10.

Theories of Obesity

There are a number of obesity theories that have been set forth to explain why some people become overly fat while others remain a normal weight. These theories generally fall into one of two fields of thought, the inherited or genetic metabolic causes (inside-the-body causes) or behavioral factors (outside-the-body causes).

It is important to realize that these two views are not necessarily in conflict. Any one theory or a number of them can explain the cause(s) of obesity in a specific individual while other theories of obesity may explain the cause of obesity in a different individual. Behavioral tendencies may also have a genetic component. It is important to note that the etiology of obesity is both complex and not yet completely understood. In the meantime, familiarize yourself with the varying theories in order to help understand your clients and their needs.

Inside-the Body Causes of Obesity:

Set-Point Theory

This theory proposes that the body chooses a weight that it wants to be and defends that weight by regulating eating behaviors, hormonal actions, and its metabolism. Exercise and the consumption of certain foods have been theorized to favorably "reset" the set-point.

Enzyme Theory

Research has shown a strong link between fat storage levels and elevated concentrations of the enzyme LPL, or lipoprotein lipase. LPL enables the fat cells to store triglycerides. The more LPL, the more easily fat cells store lipid, which increases the risk of becoming obese.

Fat Cell Theory

The fat cell theory is based upon the premise that both fat cell number and size determine the amount of fat on an individual's body. Fat cell number increases during the growth years and levels off during adulthood. The development of an increased number of fat cells as a child may determine the onset of obesity.

Although is was previously thought that the increase in a fat cell number only occurred during childhood and adolescence, it has now been shown that a fat cell may also divide when it increases in size by eight to tenfold. As the fat cells of obese people also contain more LPL, the cells are likely to reach a large size quickly. Consequently, an obese person does not only have fat cells that are increased in size and number, but they are also more efficient. Unfortunately, when a person loses weight, they will decrease their fat cell size but not their number. This makes it more difficult for an obese person to lose and maintain weight loss, which demonstrates the importance of obesity prevention at any point of the lifecycle.

The Theory of Thermogenesis

Thermogenesis is defined as the generation and release of body fat associated with the breakdown of body fuels. The theory of thermogenesis addresses the relationship of a tissue, brown fat, to the body's metabolism. Brown fat is adipose tissue that is abundant in hibernating animals and human infants. Brown fat cells are packed with pigmented, energy-burning enzymes that give brown fat cells a darkened appearance when viewed under a microscope. Lean animals tend to have more brown fat than obese ones.

The theory is based upon the premise that an individual that has less brown fat or whose body burns off too little fat, will tend to store more white fat than other people. Although research has demonstrated that heredity plays a significant role in the development of brown fat in animals, the same relationship has not been clearly demonstrated in human obesity studies.

Outside-the-Body Causes of Obesity:

External Cue Theory

This theory proposes that people overeat as a response to their surroundings, such as the clock (eating just because the clock says it's time), a candy jar on a desk (triggers you to want food), or driving by your favorite donut shop. We learn to associate certain environmental cues with eating.

The Fattening Power of Fat

Excess dietary fat is stored more efficiently as body fat compared to excess dietary carbohydrate. A surplus of 100 carbohydrate calories requires 23 of those calories to convert the food into body fat, while a surplus of 100 fat calories requires only 3 of those calories to store it as body fat.

Exercise

Exercise has been called the single most important predictor for who will succeed at keeping weight off. Likewise, lack of exercise is a primary contributor to obesity. Not only does exercise significantly increase energy expenditure, it also elevates metabolic rate even after the exercise bout is done. The most beneficial forms of exercise for weight loss/maintenance are sessions of progressively longer duration (or several sessions to add up to the same long duration) and progressively increasing intensity over time.

Eating Disorders

"An eating disorder is an obsession with food and weight that harms a person's well-being." (1) Eating disorders seriously threaten physical and psychological well-being. The cause of eating disorders is unknown, but suggested causes include the belief that a person would be happier and more successful if they were thin, perfectionism, stress, over-commitment, feeling a need to be "in control", and the pressure society puts on people to be thin. Most often, eating disorders are found in teenage girls, but it can also occur in teenage boys, women, and men. Treatment often includes medical intervention, counseling or therapy, and in some cases, hospitalization.

Since eating disorders are psychological disorders, the role of a fitness professional does not include counseling for such. Only enough information will be presented on this subject to help you identify possible candidates. It is your responsibility to warn clients of the associated dangers and provide professional referrals (to a Registered Dietitian or a behavior specialist, such as a psychologist) to those who you suspect have an eating disorder.

Did you know?
- 8,000,000 or more people in the United States have an eating disorder.
- 90% of them are women.
- Victims may be rich or poor.
- Eating disorders usually start in the teens but may begin as early as age 8.

Source: National Association of Anorexia Nervosa and Associated Disorders.

Medical and psychological complications associated with eating disorders include:
1. Gastrointestinal (digestive) problems.
2. Cardiac arrhythmia's (irregular heart beat).
3. Hypotension (low blood pressure).
4. Hypothermia (cold intolerance).
5. Dehydration.
6. Amenorrhea/osteoporosis.
7. Sleep disorders.
8. Excessively dry sky.
9. Low self-esteem.
10. Depression, anger, anxiety.
11. Low frustration tolerance.
12. High need for approval.

Anorexia is a condition where a person is obsessed with being thin. Anorexics lose a lot of weight and are terrified of gaining weight. They don't want to eat and may constantly worry about how many calories they consume or how much fat is in their food. They may use diet pills, laxatives, and water pills to lose weight and may exercise too much. The warning signs of anorexia include:
- Deliberate self-starvation with weight loss.
- Fear of gaining weight.
- Refusal to eat.
- Denial of hunger.
- Constant exercising.
- Greater amounts of hair on the body or the face.
- Sensitivity to cold temperatures.
- Absent or irregular periods. (Amenorrhea)
- Loss of scalp hair.
- A self-perception of being fat when the person is really too thin.

Bulimia is characterized by a person who eats a lot of food at one time (binging) and then throwing up or using laxatives to remove the food from the body (purging). Some bulimics may fast or over-exercise after binging to keep from gaining weight. Bulimics may use water pills, laxatives, and diet pills to "control" their weight and usually stash food and hide binging behavior. They are usually around normal weight with fluctuations. The warning signs of bulimia include:
- Preoccupation with food (binges on carbohydrates, high fluid intake, eats fast and in large bites, can't waste food, somewhat aware of calories).
- Relentless pursuit of thinness, significant body dissatisfaction.

- Unusual eating habits and behaviors.
- Menstrual irregularities.
- Dental and gum disease.
- Swollen salivary glands.
- Gastrointestinal problems.
- Dehydration.
- Complications associated with diuretic and laxative use such as bloating, diarrhea, constipation, fatigue, muscle cramps, and decreased bone density.

Binge Eating Disorder, also called compulsive overeating, is characterized by eating unusually large amounts of food and often feeling guilty or secretive about it. People with binge eating disorder have a different relationship with food. At first food may provide sustenance or comfort, but eventually may become the focus of guilt or distress. People with this condition eat large amounts of food quickly and feel completely out of control as they do it. It is different than occasionally eating too much in that there is a sense in loss of control and a feeling that you cannot stop or control how much you are eating. It differs from anorexia and bulimia, as people with binge eating disorder are usually overweight. The most common health risks are the same as those that accompany obesity. The causes are unknown, but many people who binge eat say that it is triggered by feelings of anger, sadness, boredom, or anxiety. The warning signs of binge eating disorder include:

- Eating a lot of food quickly.
- A pattern of eating in response to emotional stress, such as family conflict, peer rejection, and poor academic performance.
- Feeling ashamed or disgusted by the amount of food eaten.
- Finding food containers hidden in the person's room or house.
- Possessing an increasingly irregular eating pattern, such as skipping meals, eating lots of junk food, and eating at unusual times (like late at night).

The diagnostic category of "eating disorder not otherwise specified" is used to cover persons who do not meet all criteria for anorexia or bulimia. This may represent combination eating disorders as well as persons who do not meet all criteria for diagnosis but who are on their way to developing a full-blown eating disorder. The significance of this is that people who do not quite fit into a profile can be identified and still obtain help.

Choosing Safe and Effective Weight Management Strategies

Unfortunately, for every good diet plan or book, there are ten or more misleading and/or dangerous alternatives. Use the Diet Rating Guide provided below to help you identify the alternatives so that through your awareness you can warn your clients to steer clear of misleading or wrong information.

A GUIDE TO RATING DIETS

Use this checklist to evaluate popular weight loss diets. If the answer to any of these questions is NO, beware of the diet. If it sounds too good to be true, it probably is.

- Is the author or counselor a reputable nutrition professional such as a Dietitian (R.D.) or physician (M.D.)?
- Does the diet plan include nutrition education and lifestyle changes you can live with for the rest of your life?
- Is regular exercise included?
- Does the diet provide at least 1200 calories daily for women and at least 1500 calories for men? If not, is the diet supervised closely by a physician?
- Does the diet include a variety of foods from all food groups to avoid monotony and provide adequate nutrients and a balanced intake?
- Is there a maintenance plan to keep weight off after achieving your goal weight?
- Does the diet avoid making sensational claims like "eat all you want," "works like magic," "melts away fat," "quick and easy results?"
- Does the diet promote a gradual, steady weight loss of 1/2 to 2 pounds weekly?
- Is the diet practical? Are all foods allowed? Are the recommended foods easy to obtain and prepare, affordable, and appealing?
- Is consultation with a physician advised before beginning the diet?
- Can the diet be followed wherever you eat: home, restaurant, cafeteria, office, parties?
- Are food portions realistic and satisfying?
- Does the diet exclude drugs, megadoses of vitamin/mineral pills, and appetite suppressants?
- Is the cost reasonable?
- Does the diet avoid claims that a single food or combinations of food will cause weight loss and must be eaten at specific times of the day?

Guidelines for Safe and Effective Weight Management

You may be your client's first professional exposure to the concept of total health. What sound guidelines should you give for clients wanting to manage their weight? The remainder of this chapter is devoted to giving practical advice that will make your responsibility to spread the word for healthy eating habits and proper nutrition easier.

Calorie/Fat Requirements

It is not recommended that you advise anyone to count calories, but it is wise to have healthy calorie recommendations and a sound eating plan for many reasons. As noted previously, specific fat, protein, and carbohydrate recommended intakes are based on a percentage of total calories. If someone already counts calories, you can compare your healthy recommendation to his or her actual intake. This is a great way to identify a possible case of starvation mode or even an eating disorder. And for overeaters, this may give them a general idea of how much they overeat to better help them cut back.

Calorie requirements are influenced by metabolism, activity, gender, age, and physical condition. To promote slow and safe weight loss (1/2 to 2 lbs. per week), women should not consume less than 1200 calories per day; men not less than 1500 calories due to the difficulty to receiving a nutritionally adequate diet and a significant drop in metabolic rate. Anyone attempting to follow a regimen of lesser calories should be medically supervised.

There are many different ways to determine calorie requirements. Two such ways will be demonstrated, one very simple and one more complex. There are many variations on the simple formula because it is not exact at all. It will only give you a rough estimate of needs, which may be all that is called for. This calculation simply asks you to multiply your current weight times ten, and that number represents your daily calorie needs to promote weight loss. For example, a 160-pound person would need approximately 1600 calories per day, but remember this is a rough approximation.

Current weight x 10 = Daily Calories
Example: 160 lbs. x 10 = 1600 calories/day

A more complex calculation is called the Harris Benedict Equation. This equation is referred to as the BEE because it approximates your calorie requirements for **basal metabolism** (the amount of energy needed by the body for maintenance of life when the person is at digestive, physical, and emotional rest). (see table 13-4)

Table 13-4

DETERMINING CALORIE REQIREMENTS WITH THE HARRIS BENEDICT EQUATION (BEE)
Conversions: Weight: Pounds to kilograms, divide pounds by 2.2 Height: Inches to centimeters, multiply inches by 2.54
BEE Equation: Male: 66 + (13.7 x weight in kg) + (5 x height in cm) - (6.8 x age in years) = BEE Female: 665 + (9.6 x weight in kg) + (1.8 x height in cm) - (4.7 x age in years) = BEE
Activity Factors: Sedentary — BEE x 1.2= Calories required Light Active — BEE x 1.3= Calories required Moderately Active — BEE x 1.4= Calories required Very Active — BEE x 1.5= Calories required Athletic — BEE x 1.6 or more Calories required
To determine IBW: Female: 100 pounds for every 5 feet, and 5 pounds added for every inch Above 5 feet Male: 106 pounds for every 5 feet, and 6 pounds added for every inch Above 5 feet

continued on the next page

To determine % of IBW:
> Actual weight divided by ideal body weight x 100

EXAMPLE:
A 36 year old woman who is 5' 6" and weighs 145 pounds. She goes to low-impact aerobics twice a week and enjoys going on walks with her husband on the weekend.

Conversions:
> 145 pounds divided by 2.2 = 65.9kg
> 66 inches x 2.54 = 167.6 cm

Female BEE Equation:
> 655 + (9.6 x 65.9kg) + (1.8 x 167.6cm) − (4.7 x 36) = 1,420 kcal.

Activity Factor:
> Estimated to be 1.4. 1,420 kcal x 1.4 = 1,988 Total kcal required per day.

To determine % of IBW:
> 100 pounds for the first 5 feet + (6 inches x 5 per inch) = 130.
> (145 pounds divided by 130 pounds x 100 = 112% of her IBW)

The BEE equation calculates the energy requirements per day for someone who wants to maintain their weight. If weight loss is desired, subtract 500 calories, thereby promoting one pound of loss per week (500 x 7 = 3500 calories = one pound). More than a 500-calorie decrease per day may promote starvation mode.

If a person is greater than 120% of their IBW (and you know they also have a high body fat) the equation must be adjusted to determine a more realistic body weight. These individuals should be referred to a Registered Dietitian. Remember that some people may be over 120% of their IBW because of extra muscle they carry. In this case, as long as this is a situation you feel comfortable with, there is no need for any adjustment to the equation or referral to a Registered Dietitian.

It is important when determining calorie recommendations, that current intake be taken into consideration. If a person does not know how many calories they take in, there are computer dietary analysis programs available (check online or with your local dietitian for this service) that will give you a good indication of average daily caloric intake. When someone maintains their weight at a particular calorie level that is different than what you calculate (but not by more than approximately 400 calories), it is safe to say that they are eating the right amount.

However, if someone is maintaining his or her weight at a significantly lower amount of calories than what you calculate, that person is most likely in starvation mode. These people probably have a slow running metabolism and usually represent quite a challenge. It may be necessary for them to see a registered dietitian who will often prescribe a diet higher in calories in order to stimulate weight loss. Food intake is usually increased very slowly, usually only 50-100 calories/day each week. Translated into food, this represents one extra serving from one of the food groups each day.

Beside calories, fat is a very important factor in weight loss. Because fat was discussed previously in detail, recommendations for daily intake will be added here. Counting fat grams can be a very eye-opening and valuable learning experience. Counting fat grams is recommended instead of looking at percentages of fat compared to total calories since this is a confusing concept for many people. In order to make gram recommendations, however, you need to take a percentage of total calories

The American Heart Association recommends that 30% or less of total calories come from fat. To calculate recommended fat grams, multiply the calories times 30% then divide by 9 (1 gram of fat = 9 calories). For example, for a 2000-calorie recommended intake, 67 grams of fat per day would be recommended. The equation looks like this:

(2000 cals x .30)/9 cals per gram = 67 grams of fat/day

It is a good idea to have a computer analysis done or have your clients keep a food/fat diary (more about this in the behavior modification section) for one week so you know where they are starting from. If someone averages a fat intake of 100 grams per day, cutting to 67 grams may be too drastic and uncomfortable.

Changes need to be made slowly, so there is time to adapt. This will insure better compliance for a successful outcome in the long run. The ultimate goal is to alleviate any feelings of deprivation. Remember this is a change you want this person to maintain for the rest of his or her life. It is not realist to say "No more cheesecake, it's too fattening." This is just like a diet. Why not recommend having the cheesecake, but having less of it, less often. The bottom line is to make the goodies fit into the recommended amount of fat for the day.

People with low calorie intakes must be told to watch fat only if it represents more than 30% of total calories, and then, only if they replace the cut-out fat calories with the equivalent number of calories from nutrient dense foods, i.e., not sugar calories.

Exercise

Unfortunately, when someone goes on a weight loss diet without exercise, the body doesn't receive information that muscular tissue is important (because the person isn't using muscles for exercise), so the body burns both fat and muscle for energy (still need energy to keep yourself alive). To compound matters, when the person goes off the diet-only weight loss plan and regains body weight, a greater percentage of regained weight is fat.

However, dieting plus exercise protects muscle tissue, since the muscle has been assigned a role (to perform during that exercise). Since fat is primarily a storage depot for calories, this fuel will be burned preferentially when exercising clients lose weight. Some clients will be afraid they will not lose enough weight if they exercise, or may be discouraged because, especially in the beginning, fat weight loss is often offset by muscle weight gain, resulting in no loss of scale weight. This is a good time to take out your tape measure and show them that increased muscle will result in lost inches, or an improved appearance that won't register on the scale.

When clients complain of diet-induced fatigue, there's a good chance that they're either under-eating or over-exercising. With inadequate calories, there is a negative effect on exercise performance, as inadequate fuel (food) means inadequate energy for that performance. Body building athletes often want to build muscle while losing weight. This takes careful planning, as you can't gain (build muscle) and lose weight at the same time.

The muscle loss effects are even worse with high protein, low carbohydrate, fasting, or extremely low calorie intakes. One of the body's most vital needs is brain function. The brain is primarily dependent on glucose but can use ketone bodies produced from **ketosis** (a condition in which ketones, or abnormal products of fat and protein metabolism, accumulate in the blood). A low carbohydrate intake jeopardizes the brain's glucose supply, which signals an even greater amount of muscle and fat breakdown than usual.

With initial starvation, **glycogenolysis** (the breakdown of glycogen) provides the major part of circulating glucose. As starvation progresses, **gluconeogenesis** (the formation of glucose from something other than carbohydrate) from amino acids becomes the primary source. In final stages of starvation, liver production of ketone bodies provides an alternative source of fuel for the brain, thereby sparing glucose and, indirectly, amino acids. This becomes very dangerous as ketosis indicates that body proteins (found not only in skeletal muscle, but also in essential organs) are being broken down for fuel.

Exercise programs of moderate intensity, long duration, and high frequency have been found to be the most beneficial for weight loss in women. A review of current research (5) indicates the following strategies for safe and effective weight loss and long term weight management. It appears that exercise intensity and duration may play a more significant role in fat loss than previously thought.

1. For optimal fat loss, encourage clients to progressively increase their exertion in classes. Include interval training segments and combination classes, which include safe moderate to high intensity (65-85% maximal heart rate, 11-13 or higher RPE) challenges for exercise participants. It is found that exercise intensity >60% VO_2 max helps to preserve muscle tissue and promote fat loss. This intensity level is slightly higher than the low intensity (40 - 60%)

exercise previously used in most weight loss and management strategies.

2. Check heart rate or rate of perceived exertion every 15 minutes during exercise to encourage participants to work at an intensity level that is optimal for weight loss.

3. Encourage clients to accumulate ≥200 minutes of aerobic activity in the course of a week. Emphasis has shifted more to accumulated time for exercise in weight loss programs.

4. Regularly incorporate resistance training into your client's work out to help preserve, maintain, and in some cases increase muscle or fat free mass.

5. Including a moderate dietary restriction (500 to 1000 kcal/day) and behavioral intervention is necessary for successful weight and fat loss.

The effectiveness of water exercise in weight management has been questioned in the past. Just as on land, there are several variables that affect caloric consumption during vertical water exercise. Variables include: 1) water depth (which affects weight bearing, control of movement and the amount of water resistance), 2) speed of movement (which affects the amount of drag and resistance), 3) the amount of force applied against the water's resistance, 4) the length of the person's limbs, and 5) environmental factors such as water temperature, air temperature, humidity, chemicals etc. Obviously, the client that "works the water" by applying more force is going to expend more energy, have a higher VO2, and therefore expend more calories. In any form of exercise, the harder you work, the more calories you burn.

Research clearly indicates that you do burn calories in a vertical aquatic workout. How many calories do you burn? In the proper conditions, with proper motivation to work, research indicates an estimate of approximately 400 to 500 calories per one hour session. (Shallow water class, armpit depth, water 83-86 degrees F, using arm and leg movements.) It appears that the water's resistance makes up for the loss of workload due to reduced weight bearing from the water's buoyancy. This is obvious when we see clients lose weight in aquatic workouts. Caloric expenditure and therefore weight loss is inevitable in the water as long as the client adheres to recommendations for intensity, duration, and frequency for exercise.

Recent research has shown that spurts of micro-exercise or increased activity in general can be beneficial to weight loss. Three to five minutes of any type of exercise done preferably in the later afternoon can "rev" up the metabolism just when it is starting to slow down for the day. This is great news for people who get discouraged when they can only do three minutes of exercise at a time. Although it may not have a huge impact on weight loss, any increase in physical activity is beneficial.

Exercise without dieting is also known to be an effective form of weight management. This is because the body has a chance to adapt to metabolic changes slowly, without drastic effects from dieting. Exercisers usually become aware of and modify their eating habits on their own.

Behavior Modification

Behavior modification is simply the changing of behaviors or bad habits. This is probably the hardest aspect of weight management, but at the same time, it is the most essential. Without change, anything you do to try to lose weight is temporary. After you've lost the weight and go back to your normal habits, the weight will come back as well. In other words, a program without behavior change is just another diet!

Encourage your clients to keep food diaries so they can monitor themselves. It is also a great reinforcement when they can see the proof of their change. A good food diary keeps track of the type of food and the amount, when the food was eaten, how much fat was obtained from the food, a check-list for the servings recommended from the Food Guide Pyramid, and a space to record behavior change and exercise habits. Not all records are this detailed. Actually, any record that helps your client become more aware of habits would be useful. Food record forms can be obtained from different sources, including dietitians.

Below is a list of additional behavior change ideas that you may want to pass on or "assign" to your clients. The most important thing to remember is to choose one or two changes to work on at one time. As has been already stated, change is a very hard thing to do. Habits that took a lifetime to develop won't permanently change overnight. Encourage your clients to be patient with themselves and realize that it may take a month or two to develop a new habit that sticks.

Behavior Modification Strategies

- Preplan your meals.
- Preplan snacks into your eating plan.
- Make out a shopping list and stick to it.

- Keep tempting foods out of sight.
- Store tempting foods in opaque containers or aluminum foil.
- Rearrange your refrigerator and cupboards.
- Turn packages so you can't see the picture.
- Don't taste while cooking.
- Cook when your control is highest.
- Preload your stomach with liquids.
- Drink ample non-calorie liquids during meals.
- Make eating important. Don't eat while reading or watching TV.
- Use smaller plates, bowls, and glasses, serving spoons.
- Do not keep serving dishes on the table.
- Put your utensil down between bites.
- Cut your food only as needed.
- Stop eating for a minute during the meal.
- Change your usual place at the table.
- Eat only at the table.
- Put leftovers away before you sit down to eat.
- Leave a little food on your plate.
- Remove your plate as soon as you've finished eating.
- Brush your teeth after every meal and use mouthwash.
- Let someone else clear the table and put leftovers away.
- Make leftovers less visible. If there is no good use for a leftover, throw it out.
- Celebrate in a nonfood, nondrink way.
- Order first in a restaurant so you are not influenced by others.
- Share a menu item instead of eating it all yourself.
- Change to non-binging friends.
- Practice relaxation exercises.

Motivation

Motivation is an important aspect of weight management success and is associated with behavior modificaiton. Without it, efforts will likely cease. This is especially true when you are promoting slow weight loss. Try to keep your clients motivated with things other than the drop in scale weight.

For instance, goal setting can be very motivating. Make sure that for every long-term goal, there are many short-term goals to reach along the way. Goals should be behavior oriented, measurable, and realistic. Avoid having clients set a scale weight goal. Instead, attempt to make it a body fat percentage goal if body composition assessment is available. "I need to cut back on Oreo cookies" is a very vague goal. It's hard

to know when you've actually reached that goal. A better example might be: "Within one week's time, I will decrease my Oreo cookie consumption to no more than three per day."

Positive feedback is another good way for fitness professionals to motivate their clients. Don't praise the person who loses the most amount of weight quickly, as this only reinforces the importance of scale weight and the speed of loss. Instead of saying, "You look great, you're so thin!" why not say "You're looking really healthy and lean; keep up the good work!" Also, pick out small things to praise that show habit changes. You should show concern for the student who loses weight too quickly and in large amounts, but these concerns should be addressed one on one, not in a group.

Support can be critical to anyone trying to make changes. Your clients will look at their family and friends for support. Without it, they will surely be de-motivated. Caution your clients that they will not always find support where they expect it, even from a spouse. Clients in this case can focus so much energy on getting support from their spouses that they lose sight of themselves and their efforts. Encourage your clients to identify their real supporters and to use them only. Offer yourself as a support figure and encourage influence from other motivators as well. Oprah Winfrey, Covert Bailey, Richard Simmons, and Susan Powter are just a few examples, but of course, excellent motivators are not necessarily educated practitioners.

Nutrition Education

Many people are never exposed to a Registered Dietitian. They rely on getting their nutrition information from the media, word of mouth, and you. Referrals can be made, and it is recommended that you have Registered Dietitians give a lecture series or even consult for your facility. But on a day-to-day basis, you'll probably have the most influence over your clients. The significance of your role in getting out sound nutrition information to your clients cannot be emphasized enough! You may want to have a Registered Dietitian review educational materials before giving them to your participants. An additional list of resources for educational materials is provided at the end of this chapter.

There are many ways for you to use these materials and educate your clients. One way is to make it part of your class or workout. Pick one topic each week and say a little something about it when you are doing toning or stretching work. Some fitness professionals like to start or end their class with a "did you know" statement. For example: "Did you know 95% fat free does not necessary mean a product has 5% of its calories coming from fat?" (It's usually much higher!) This usually peaks curiosity or starts conversations.

For the educational materials, pass out a handout that is relevant to the subject you've just talked about or have handouts available in a general location in your facility. The following is a list of some of the nutrition topics you may want to talk about and get handouts for:

Label reading	Increased fiber
Dining out	Fast food
Supermarket savvy	Salad bar surprises
Low-fat cooking	Recipe modification
Low-fat food substitutions	Sugar substitutes
Guilt-free eating	Different types of fat
Supplement needs	Protein needs
Weight-loss guidelines	Changing eating behaviors

This is just a partial list. Attend continuing education seminars to keep yourself updated with new information and materials. Keep reading as much as you can on the subject from professional references and hook up with nutrition professionals for additional information and referral sources.

Summary

1. The basic nutrients in the body are carbohydrates, fats (lipids), protein, vitamins, minerals, and water.

2. For a healthy diet, clients should be guided by the Dietary Guidelines for Americans (USDA and HHS), Nutrient Intake Goals, and the Food Guide (USDA).

3. Proper nutrition can reduce the risk of chronic diseases such as atherosclerosis, certain cancers, hypertension, and osteoporosis.

4. Proper hydration is important to health and performance. Adequate liquids should be consumed before, during, and after exercise to insure proper hydration.

5. Overweight and obesity are two common terms used in weight management. Obesity more accurately takes into consideration a person's lean body mass as compared to fat mass.

6. Theories of Obesity generally fall into two fields of thought: inherited or genetic metabolic causes (inside-the-body causes) or behavioral factors (outside-the-body causes).

7. Eating disorders fall into three common categories: anorexia (starvation), bulimia (binge and purge), and binge eating disorder.

8. Effective weight management strategies include creating a healthy eating plan, nutrition education, proper exercise, and behavior modification.

Review Questions

1. What function do nutrients perform in the body?
2. How many calories are found in one gram of carbohydrate, fat and protein?
    a. Carbohydrate 6, Fat 7, and protein 4.
    b. Carbohydrate 4, Fat 4, and protein 9.
    c. Carbohydrate 2, Fat 9, and protein 4.
    d. Carbohydrate 4, Fat 9, and protein 4.
3. Which type of cholesterol is considered to be good cholesterol because it helps lower the risk of plaque sticking in the arteries?
    a. Low Density Lipoprotein (LDL)
    b. High Density Lipoprotein (HDL)
    c. Triglycerides
    d. Fiber
4. It is prudent practice for an exercise professional to recommend supplements to their clients. (True or False)
5. Which condition is characterized by starvation and weight loss to alleviate fear of gaining weight?
    a. Anorexia
    b. Bulimia
    c. Binge Eating Disorder
6. Which type of exercise is commonly prescribed and effective for weight loss efforts?
    a. Resistance training only.
    b. High intensity, short duration aerobic activity with moderate resistance training.
    c. Moderate intensity, long duration aerobic activity with moderate resistance training.
    d. Moderate, short duration aerobic exercise only.

See Appendix E for answers to review questions.

References

1. American Academy of Family Physicians. (2003). *Eating Disorders: Facts for Teens*. Leawood, KS. Online and Custom Publishing-American Academy of Family Physicians. http://family doctor.org/277.xml

2. Beachle, T. and R. Earle. (2004). *NSCA's Essentials of Personal Training*. Champaign, IL. Human Kinetics Publishers.

3. Bernardot, D. (1992). *Sports Nutrition-A Guide for the Professional Working with Active People*. 2nd Edition. Chicago, IL. American Dietetic Association.

4. Dietary Guidelines Advisory Committee. (2005). *Dietary Guidelines for Americans*. Washington DC. U.S. Department of Health and Human Services and U.S. Department of Agriculture. www.healthierus.gov/dietaryguidelines

5. Freeman, V. and L. Kravitz. (2004). Women and Weight Loss: Practical Applications for Water Fitness Instructors. Nokomis, FL. *AKWA*. 18:3, pp. 26-30. Aquatic Exercise Association

6. Kleiner S. (1999). Water: An Essential but Overlooked Nutrient. *Journal of the American Dietetic Association*. 99, pp. 200-206.

7. National Heart, Blood and Lung Institute. (2005). *High Blood Cholesterol, What You Need to Know*. Washington, DC. Department of Health and Human Services. NIH Publication No. 01-3290. www.nhlbi.nih.gov/health/public/heart/chol/wyntk.htm

8. NIH Consensus Panel. (1993). Triglyceride, High Density Lipoprotein and Coronary Heart Disease. *Joural of the American Medical Association*. Chicago, IL. 269, pp. 505-510.

Resources

US Department of Agriculture
Center for Nutrition Policy and Promotion
1120 20th ST. NW
Suite 200, North Lobby
Washington, DC 20036-3475
www.usda.com

The National Center for Nutrition and Dietetics, The American Dietetic Assoc.
215 West Jackson Blvd. Suite 800
Chicago, IL
1-800-366-1655
(Educational materials & referrals to dietitians)
www.eatright.org

US Department of Health and Human Services
Public Health Service
National Heart, Lung, and Blood Institute
www.hhs.gov

American Cancer Society
1701 Rickenbacker Drive Suite 5B
Sun City Center, FL 33573-5361
(Educational material available)
www.cancer.org

Wheat Foods Council
5500 South Quebec Suite 111
Engelwood, CO
(303)694-5828
(Educational materials on Grains)
www.wheatfoods.org

Gatorade Sports Science Institute
P.O. Box 049003
Chicago, IL 60604-9003
1-800-884-2867
www.gssiweb.com

Nasco: Nutrition Teaching Aids
Fort Atkinson, Wisconsin
Modesto, California
1-800-558-9595

Dairy Council of Wisconsin
990 Oakmont Plaza Drive, Suite 510
Westmont, IL 60559
1-800-325-9121
www.wisdairy.com

Chapter 14: Exercise Behavior

INTRODUCTION

Recruiting and retaining clients for fitness programs can be a difficult challenge. Why do participants drop out and what can be done to keep them motivated? How can a fitness professional be effective at offering support and encouragement? These questions and more are answered as you increase your knowledge and awareness of exercise behavior.

Unit Objectives

After completing Chapter 14, you should be able to:
1. Identify personal, program, and other factors contributing to exercise dropout.
2. Define exercise behavior. List factors contributing to exercise behavior.
3. Define adherence and compliance. List factors that affect exercise adherence and compliance. Identify strategies to reduce dropout and increase compliance.
4. Understand how to reach individuals with various learning styles by incorporating different methods of instruction.

Key Questions
1. What is the rate of dropout for exercise programs?
2. What factors contribute to exercise dropout?
3. What is the difference between adherence and compliance?
4. What roles do beliefs and attitudes play in exercise compliance?
5. List five strategies to motivate a client to comply to an exercise program.
6. List four different learning styles and/or methods.

Exercise Dropout

Exercise program initiation and dropout are frustrating issues encountered by many health professionals, registered dieticians, and exercise professionals. The client knows a healthy lifestyle will bring about positive changes, yet may have difficulty adopting and continuing to practice the behavior. The factors surrounding this dilemma are very complex and very individual. If you understand the basic psychology behind health/exercise behavior, you may be better able to motivate individuals to successful long-term adoption of a healthy lifestyle.

"To understand why people sometimes lack the motivation for regular physical activity, one must first acknowledge a simple yet important fact: exercise is voluntary and time consuming." (2) Daily activities and commitments often interfere with a person's time or motivation to exercise. Dropout rates are usually highest within the first three months of initiating an exercise program, and statistics for dropout ranges from 9% to 87% depending on how exercise dropout is defined in the research study. Dropout rates after one year are typically around the 50% range. Similar dropout rates are found in weight management programs, with smoking cessation, and for medication compliance. (2)

Research has identified several variables that predict exercise dropout. These variables are divided into personal factors, program factors, and other factors. (see table 14-1 for a list of these factors)

Smoking tends to be one of the most prevalent indicators of exercise dropout. Drop out rate tends to be progressive, with the addition or accumulation of factors increasing the dropout likelihood. It may be important to consider additional education and intervention programs in order to reduce exercise dropout. Often, participants will discontinue exercise because initially, exercise is difficult. Beginner exercisers may experience muscle soreness and fatigue, which causes discomfort. Often it is difficult to get exercisers over that "hump" to where exercise feels good and they see results. For some, that state is not reached for several months.

Attributes and Psychology of Exercise Behavior

Exercise behavior can be defined as: Behavior that motivates an individual to initiate and maintain regular exercise. In addition, exercise behavior dictates how a person chooses to exercise.

An individual's tendency to initiate and maintain exercise is primarily determined by his/her "beliefs" and "attitudes." A belief is defined as "a state or habit of mind in which trust or confidence is placed in some person or some thing." Beliefs are very powerful in determining exercise behavior and should not be overlooked. If a person does not believe that exercise promotes health, is instrumental in weight loss, or makes a person feel better,

Table 14-1

Variables Predicting the Exercise Dropout		
Principal factors: cigarette smoking, blue collar employment, inactive leisure time, and inactive occupation. The noncompliance rate appears to increase progressively: 59% in the presence of smoking alone to 95% with all four of these variables.		
Personal Factors	**Program Factors**	**Other Factors**
• Smoker • Inactive leisure time • Inactive occupation • Blue collar worker • Type A personality • Increased physical strength • Extroverted • Poor credit rating • Overweight • Poor self-motivation • Depressed • Hypochondriacal • Anxious • Introverted • Low ego strength	• Inconvenient time and/or location • Excessive cost • High-intensity exercise • Lack of exercise variety • Exercising alone • Lack of positive feedback or reinforcement • Inflexible exercise goals • Low enjoyment ratings for running programs • Poor exercise leadership	• Lack of spouse support • Inclement weather • Excessive job travel • Injury • Job change and/or move *(From ACSM, 2000)*

there is little chance he or she will initiate and comply to an exercise program. There is no motivation to exercise if there is no belief that exercise is beneficial. On the other hand, a belief that exercise is beneficial will help provide the motivation needed to initiate and maintain a program of regular exercise.

An attitude is defined as "a mental position or feeling of emotion with regard to a fact or state." If a person has a preconceived negative attitude toward exercise or people who exercise, there is little chance that person will become a regular exerciser. For example, if a person feels that all exercisers are fanatics or health nuts, and does not wish to be labeled as such, he will choose not to exercise. If a woman who has muscle definition is viewed as unattractive, it would be difficult to convince a woman with that attitude to exercise.

Attitudes and beliefs are formed through family, social, and educational experiences. Many attitudes and beliefs are passed on through families. In addition, one person's attitudes and beliefs can affect another person's exercise behavior. For example, a spouse or parent can have influence over exercise habits.

The second part of the exercise behavior definition deals with how a person chooses to exercise. Exercise choices are affected by attitudes and beliefs, personal choices, and exercise education. Personal choice will dictate whether a person makes the decision to exercise alone, with a partner, or in a group setting. Some people are self-exercisers and prefer to exercise alone, some are partner exercisers and prefer to exercise with one or two other people, and some are group exercisers and thrive on the interaction and support of a group. It is important to respect each individual's exercise preferences to enhance retention.

Exercise education also determines how a person chooses to exercise. If a person was taught at some point that straight leg full sit-ups are the best way to train the abdominal muscles, this is the exercise the person will consistently choose. There may be inappropriate exercise habits or behaviors that need to be addressed and corrected.

It is critical to explore an individual's exercise beliefs and attitudes in order to reduce the risk of exercise dropout. This can be done through direct questioning and conversation, or with the aid of questionnaires or surveys. As an exercise professional, be careful not to impose your beliefs and attitudes about exercise on your client or students. Instead, be a good role model by living your beliefs, and be open to exploring and discovering your client's beliefs.

Exercise Adherence and Compliance

Adherence is defined by Webster as "steady devotion, allegiance, or attachment." Compliance is defined by Webster as "the act of conforming, cooperation or obedience, as in following orders." Although the two terms are very similar, there is a slight difference with respect to exercise behavior and the attainment of exercise goals.

An individual who adheres may do so in the "spirit of the law." If a client is directed to exercise 3 times a week, they may do so, but not as specifically directed. The "orders" may have been to exercise 3 times a week at 75% intensity for 30 minutes. They may be adhering by doing some type of exercise, perhaps 15 minutes 3 times a week, but not strictly following the program.

Compliance implies abiding by "the letter of the law." If you want your client to reach the goals you have set, then you must determine whether your client is complying. Simply asking the client if they are exercising 3 times a week may not provide the entire picture. However, asking the client to keep an exercise journal noting the day exercised, the intensity, and the duration will better reveal if the client is complying.

Adherence is helpful, but compliance is typically your goal with clients. If you are not certain of compliance, lack of adaptation may be wrongly attributed to the program as opposed to the individual's behavior. In order to properly track progression, adaptation, and make program adjustments, you need to be certain your client is complying or "following orders to the letter of the law," as opposed to merely adhering. If your client is not complying, it is important to find out why. Is it the individual's exercise beliefs, lack of enjoyment for the prescribed program, lack of support, or some other cause? Discovering the cause or causes will allow you and the client to systematically work through overcoming barriers to exercise compliance.

The Law of Cause and Effect

The law of cause and effect promotes the premise that internal thoughts are the cause of every effect or result. Positive expectations lead to positive results and negative expectations lead to negative results. It is important for a fitness professional to foster positive attitudes and beliefs about exercise and nutrition in order to promote positive results. This can be done through education, example, or from testimonies of others. If the client positively believes that barriers can be overcome and a program can be initiated and maintained, compliance will likely ensue.

The Law of Attraction

The law of attraction promotes that other people are drawn to your most dominant thoughts. It is critical for a fitness professional to be genuine and open with clients in order to draw and foster a positive belief system. Being positive opens positive relationships. Being genuinely open and caring will attract many people to your classes or exercise sessions who will continue to come back for the good feeling you foster in them.

Exercise Self-Efficacy

Exercise self-efficacy is a powerful predictor of exercise behavior, compliance, and dropout. Efficacy is defined as "the capacity for producing a desired result or effect." (Webster) Self-efficacy in turn means self-effectiveness. It will largely determine if someone will be effective at initiating and complying with an exercise program. It is important to have confidence that exercise is within your capabilities and will provide favorable outcomes.

Self-efficacy can be impaired by previous exercise experiences. If an individual has initiated exercise programs several times in the past and has dropped out, it may be difficult for that person to believe that a consistent exercise behavior can be achieved. Helping that client work through behaviors or reasons for drop out in the past may provide more confidence for present exercise behavior.

There are many techniques that an exercise professional can use to boost and enhance self-efficacy. Exercise education along with form and technique training can enhance confidence that exercise can be comfortable and effective. One of the benefits of a consistent exercise program is improved self-efficacy. Self-efficacy leads to exercise compliance which in turn leads to higher self-efficacy, therefore accomplishment has a huge impact on self-efficacy. Performance accomplishments boost self-efficacy as does verbal persuasion and encouragement from a respected source. Seeing other people accomplish goals can also motivate an individual to model positive behavior.

Locus of Control

Locus of control determines where a person perceives personal power to emanate from. **External locus of control** is where a person believes that other people and the environment control an individual's life and consequent outcomes. This is a very disempowering view, with the person feeling he or she has very little control over their own life or "fate." Individuals with strong external locus of control may never be prompted to initiate an exercise program, and, if exercise is initiated, may have high drop out and poor compliance.

A person who has an **internal locus of control** believes that he/she is responsible for what happens and the outcomes in their own life. This mind set is very empowering, leaving a person feeling in control of their life and "destiny." People who have internal locus of control tend to take responsibility for their lives and their health.

For many, exercise seems to foster and promote feelings of self-control and self-empowerment. Locus of control is brought to a more internal perspective, leaving exercisers feeling more in control and in charge of their lives. The feelings of accomplishment and subsequent physiological change that occur in the body empower exercisers and enable them to get more out of life as the direct result of a self-initiated behavior.

Motivation

Successful fitness professionals are skilled in motivational techniques. Motivation stems from reinforcement. Reinforcement can be intrinsic, extrinsic, or indirect.

Intrinsic reinforcement occurs when the activity itself is the reward. People who are intrinsically motivated to exercise do so because of enjoyment and the fact that it makes them feel good. The process itself is the reward, not the outcome.

Extrinsic reinforcement occurs when external incentives and rewards provide the motivation. These people like encouragement and recognition. They enjoy participation incentives and games. They continue their exercise program because they see results-results are important. The outcome provides the motivation, not the process.

Indirect reinforcement occurs from the person's surroundings. Overall atmosphere, a clean, well-lit facility, a good sound system, and a comfortable setting all contribute to indirect motivation. Make the atmosphere, facility, and exercise experience as pleasing as possible to entice these people back.

You can provide motivation for all three types of reinforcement, but ultimately, motivation must come from within the individual. Intrinsically motivated participants are typically most compliant. By discovering which kind of reinforcement is motivating to your client, you can facilitate the process. Offer T-shirts, free perks, or have drawings for those who reach compliance goals. Schedule a class or training time at your facility when the atmosphere and clientele are appealing. For instance, if a person likes a quieter, more relaxed atmosphere, schedule that client during a low attendance time at the facility. Take into consideration where your client likes to exercise. They may prefer exercising outdoors or at home. If you are a group fitness instructor, class motivation can take many forms. Use a variety of intrinsic, extrinsic, and indirect reinforcement to reach as many students as possible.

Communication skills are also important in motivating participants before, during, and after exercise. Be an "active" listener. Attempt to give participants your full attention when listening. Use terms like "you" and "your" when teaching as opposed to "we" and "our" to help students avoid feeling "talked down to." Learn how to effectively communicate form, transition, and motivational cues to make class progress smoothly. Strive to make the experience enjoyable so clients will want to come back and do it again.

Move participants toward **internalization** on the motivation continuum. Internalization occurs when the person is engaging in the activity for self-fulfillment. When internalization is reached, compliance is very likely to occur. You want clients to exercise for self-fulfillment, not because you are the instructor or trainer, or because a spouse wants them to exercise. They do it for themselves, and therefore adopt a permanent healthy lifestyle.

Personality and Exercise

You will encounter and deal with many different types of personalities in group exercise classes, personal training, or physical therapy. Understanding personality types will help you in motivating and encouraging a wide variety of individuals. A few personality types commonly found in the exercise setting are discussed below.

The "type A" exerciser is motivated by competition and intensity. This individual has a tendency to overdo and would actually risk injury to work at very high levels of intensity. These exercisers

benefit from cross training to offset psychological and physical burnout. They tend to be the overt exercisers in class that love using equipment, jumping higher, working harder, and coming to class every day.

The "type B" exerciser is into exercise for health benefits. This person exercises at a reasonable intensity level, drinks plenty of water, and is well versed on exercise information. The "type B" exerciser tends to be satisfied with working at moderate intensity levels to reduce risk of injury but tends to exercise often.

The "intermittent" exerciser comes and goes. These exercisers tend to wander in and out of programs for weeks or months at a time. They are often caught up in time constraints and family affairs and do not have regular exercise habits. They enjoy exercise, but just can't seem to make a commitment to attend regularly.

The Transtheoretical Model

The Transtheoretical Model, or readiness for change, is used extensively in considerations for health change behavior. It is believed that if you understand the present stage of change, you can better guide that client through the change process by moving them forward.

The Stages of the Transtheoretical Model are: (2)
1. Precontemplation. In the precontemplation stage, the individual expresses lack of interest in initiating an exercise program. Individuals can be persuaded through this stage with educational materials, by their physician, or by family members.
2. Contemplation. In the contemplation stage, the individual is "thinking" about starting an exercise program. Often an individual is moved through this stage by making them aware of the risks and benefits associated with making or not making the decision to change.
3. Preparation. In the preparation stage, the individual starts to do some type of activity, but not necessarily to the extent or degree that will make the desired health changes. Encourage any type of activity or exercise in the hopes that the individual will eventually be ready for the action stage.
4. Action. The action stage is where the individual is complying to the exercise program and working toward the intended goals. At this point reinforcement strategies will help the client remain motivated.

5. Maintenance. In the maintenance stage, the individual has been in action for 6 months or longer. This is a very rewarding stage for both the client and the exercise professional. At this point the individual should be moving toward internalization on the motivation continuum.

By knowing the present stage of readiness for change, you can apply the correct methods for moving the individual towards maintenance. Most clients or students who come to you already know the importance of exercise. Many of them will be in contemplation or preparation. Don't bore them with all of the reasons you should exercise, they already know. Instead, work on convincing them that the benefits outweigh the risks. If the potential client is dabbling with exercise, encourage them to continue, and work to convince them that their time will be more efficiently spent doing the recommended intensity, duration and frequency of exercise. If the person is in the action stage, use meaningful goals, intrinsic and extrinsic rewards, and other means to keep them going.

Exercise Dependency

Exercise dependency can take two forms. The first form deals with a participant's dependence on an instructor or trainer's encouragement and motivation. An individual may also become dependent on external reinforcement. This exerciser may drop out of the program if the instructor moves to another time slot or to another facility, or if external rewards are discontinued. There is a fine line between encouraging and supporting a participant and fostering dependence. An instructor should encourage participants to attend other instructors' workouts. Instructors should promote other instructors' classes and create an atmosphere where instructors work together for the participants' benefit. Trainers should help their client move toward internalization, and then continue to offer "technical" support through new exercise and workout options. Creating an atmosphere of competition between instructors and trainers only causes dissention and fosters dependence in participants. Fitness professionals should work together for the good of all participants.

The second form of exercise dependence occurs when a participant focuses on the exercise itself. Everyone has a need for stimulation and motivation. When a person reaches an ideal level of arousal, he or she enters a state known as "flow." Flow is that feeling you have when everything feels just right and you seem to float through the workout. Physically and emotionally, the individual is very serene and at peace or in a state of euphoria. This state is also referred to as the "runner's high."

This special emotional state is, in part, physiologically induced. The body produces hormones and other chemicals that promote or allow this state. It is important for an instructor or trainer to help participants reach these "good feelings" brought on by regular exercise and improvements in physical fitness. This is known as a positive "exercise addiction" and provides intrinsic reinforcement. It is also possible, however, for people to become dependent on the state exercise produces. They become obsessive about exercise and ignore other important facets of their lives. A person negatively addicted to exercise tends to be obsessive and unhealthy. If the obsession becomes self-abusive or takes over the individual's life, psychological counseling may be required.

Facilitating Behavioral Change

There are several factors or reasons that an individual may decide to initiate an exercise program. These motivators are often used in advertising or marketing to coax the non-exerciser to join an exercise program. Common motivators include:
- A desire for improved physical appearance (weight reduction, weight gain, toned muscles, muscle mass).
- A doctor's recommendation or the desire to improve health.
- Prompting from a significant other or parent.
- The desire to feel better and have more energy.
- Stress reduction.
- Rehabilitation from surgery, injury or disease.
- Seeing a friend or spouse participating.
- A desire to do something for oneself, or have time for oneself.
- Improve one's quality of life.

When attempting to start new programs or recruit clients, appeal to the positive motivators and downplay or solve negative excuses. Many facilities offer child care to eliminate the excuse of needing childcare as a reason not to attend. Help potential participants by solving problems that block participation while boosting the positive benefits of exercise.

There are many ways to retain members once they have joined your program. The challenge does not end once you have them in the door. You want to create a meaningful and enjoyable experience so they will want to come back for more. Maslow's Hierarchy of Human Needs is well accepted in psychology and can give insight into adherence tactics. If you give someone what they need, they will come back. Maslow's Hierarchy is as follows:

1. Physiological needs.
2. Safety and security needs.
3. Need to feel Loved and Accepted.
4. Need for Self Esteem.
5. Need for Self Actualization (fulfillment).

The needs for each level must be met in order from number one to number five. The needs for level one must be met before level two, which must be met before level three, etc. In most cases, the needs for food, clothing, and shelter, level one, are met. The instructor can get involved in the second through the fifth levels. It is important to provide an atmosphere that is safe and offers feelings of security for participants. If participants feel uncomfortable because of their size, appearance, for what they wear, etc., they may not return.

It is the ultimate goal of every fitness program to help participants reach the fifth level or fulfillment. It is difficult because participants are individuals and at different points in personal development. There are some general adherence tactics you can use to help fill a participant's needs and to help them feel safe and comfortable. These tactics include:

- Introduce yourself and other workers to make the individual feel comfortable.
- Introduce them to other participants in the facility or class.
- Make them feel like a part of the facility or class.
- Have other participants help you make the newcomer feel welcome.
- Make the exercise program fun and rewarding.
- Encourage interaction and support.
- Discourage ridicule and competition.
- Encourage input and sharing.
- Be personable, friendly, and accessible.
- Be supportive.

Behavioral Modification Strategies

Now that you understand several psychological factors that affect exercise behavior, how can you

help your client reduce the risk of dropout and comply in an exercise program? Fortunately, there are several strategies that have been developed and researched to promote behavior modification. Unfortunately, you may need to use trial and error to find a method that works best for each individual. Assess your participant's behaviors with an exercise interest survey or a questionnaire and then use that information to narrow and choose a motivational tactic to use. If that tactic doesn't work, pull another "rabbit out of your hat." Employing behavioral modification techniques may be the determining factor that keeps a beginning exerciser coming. Following are some strategies that have been used for behavior modification.

Setting Goals

Goal setting can be a very powerful behavioral change strategy. The success of goal setting hinges on several factors. These factors include:

- Identification of realistic and meaningful goals. This is achieved by working closely with the client to discover what is important to them. Education may be needed to help a participant bring an unrealistic or unhealthy goal to a more healthy option. Check to be sure the individual believes the goals are attainable.
- Working with the participant to set short term behavioral goals. This may include showing up to exercise three times/week, or to eventually be able to water jog for 30 continuous minutes.
- Building on the short term behavioral goals to develop long term achievement goals. Achievement goals are generally monitored through measurable outcomes. Set a measurable criteria to determine if the program is working.
- Prioritizing and attaching a time frame to long and short term goals. Goals should be put on paper.
- Periodically reassessing goals to determine if they are still meaningful and realistic. Set new goals if necessary.

Agreements or Contracts

Some fitness professionals will write agreements or contracts and sign them with their client. The contract may state that the person agrees to participate in exercise four times/week or to reach a certain goal. In essence the client gives their word to abide by the contract. Contracts or agreements can be very motivating for some individuals.

Provide Frequent Feedback

Feedback can be verbal or in the form of measured results. Provide feedback that is meaningful to your participant. If you have a person who is motivated by numbers and charts, provide ways to track or chart simple measures such as exercise intensity, duration, frequency, recovery heart rate, or blood pressure. If you have a client who is motivated by visual feedback, tune them into how a particular pair of pants fits every Friday as they progress through their program.

Schedule Appropriate Rewards

Rewards can be group participation drawings each month, or specific rewards such as putting a dollar into a jar each time you exercise through the course of the month. You then spend that money at the end of each month on something enjoyable. Schedule a reward that is meaningful and that the person will work to achieve.

Integrating Social Support

Integrate social support from fellow exercisers, family, and spouses. Develop social opportunities within a class setting such as going out to lunch, having pot lucks, or celebrating birthdays. Work with an individual client to discover who their primary support comes from and how to tap into that support.

Provide Prompts

Prompts can include little hints, nudges, or habits that help a client remember to exercise. Some people may need to schedule their exercise session just like a business meeting. Placing a reminder note on the bathroom mirror may serve as a daily reminder that motivates others. Some may need to put their gym bag by the front door each night before their scheduled exercise day.

Identifying and Modifying Self-Talk

It is fun and very effective to work with an individual to discover self-talk that may sabotage exercise. The self-talk may make good excuses not to exercise, or simply make the statement that the individual hates to exercise. Replacing negative self-talk is easy. Write down positive statements for the person to recite several times during the day. Have them identify negative self-talk and learn to replace it with positive self-talk.

Mental Imagery

Some people are highly motivated by mental imagery, or through visualizing relaxation, positive results, or improved quality of life. Have them mentally review or visualize any positive facet or outcome of exercise to reinforce positive behavior and a positive experience. Mental imagery can also be used to refocus a person's attention through a perceived difficult or unpleasant part of an exercise session.

Identify False Beliefs

Identifying and replacing false beliefs can be very motivating. As mentioned previously, beliefs and attitudes are the primary factors that shape exercise behavior. By eliminating or replacing negative or false beliefs, barriers to participation and compliance may be removed.

Minimize Procrastination

People are distracted by family, work, and social commitments. With today's fast pace life, it is easy to put exercise off until later and then have later never come. Days slip into weeks, and weeks into months. It can be difficult, but prove very useful to talk clients though time management, scheduling, and juggling family to make a decision to act. Eliminate excuses one by one until there are no excuses left. This may motivate a person to start and maintain exercise.

It is important to find, choose, and use a tactic that will work for each individual client. In the group exercise setting, use a variety of techniques to reach as many different personalities as possible. You may want to offer a group monthly drawing combined with a chart for tracking progress or participation. You can ask clients to find a pair of pants to use each week for a weekly "fitting" and have them report on their progress. The best tactic to use is the one that works.

Facilitating Exercise Knowledge

As stated above, exercise knowledge will greatly determine how a person chooses to exercise. Unfortunately, people have been exposed to many poor exercise habits and misinformation. Since time is a constraint for many people, teaching participants how to get the most out of their exercise program in the least amount of time is very beneficial. This is referred to as exercise program "effectiveness." Program safety and effectiveness are of utmost consideration for the fitness professional. If a person sees results and is working within a manageable time frame, he or she will most likely continue to exercise. The instructor must become knowledgeable and pass accurate and meaningful information on to participants. Education will positively affect motivation and adherence. Knowledge should be disseminated in a clear, concise, and effective manner. It is beneficial to understand the basics of learning.

There are three domains of human behavior as associated with learning. The first domain is the "cognitive" domain. In the cognitive domain, humans collect and process knowledge. Knowledge can have impact on beliefs and attitudes and therefore impact exercise behavior. Providing participants with knowledge will foster positive feelings about exercise and improve exercise adherence.

The second domain is the "affective" domain. This domain is where feelings and emotions reside. It is essential to foster feelings of support, acceptance, and caring for participants. It is helpful if these feelings emanate from other participants and support systems as well as the instructor.

The third domain is the "motor" domain. This domain represents all learning acquired through movements or through the physical body. In exercise, motor learning is primary. Participants learn to accept and have confidence in their bodies. Physical activity promotes physical health as well as self-respect and a positive body image.

People learn in different ways. If information is always presented in the same way, for example through an educational handout, you will only reach part of your participants. Some people are visual learners and are stimulated to learn primarily through visual input. Some are auditory learners and are stimulated to learn through spoken word, music, or other auditory input. Some people learn through their sense of touch. They have to feel it to learn. These tactile learners are stimulated to learn through trying the movement or "touching" the concept being learned. It is beneficial to provide educational stimulus through visual, auditory, and tactile means. You will reach more people with educational information.

Another theory in education deals with how people process information. Some learners must see the whole picture before they can visualize a concept's parts. This approach to learning is called the whole-part method. Some participants must see all the parts before they can visualize the whole concept. This would exemplify the part-whole method of learning. When working with individual clients, try different methods until you find one that clicks. Utilize different types of aquatic choreography when teaching a group fitness class. A whole-part learner would enjoy patterned choreography where the entire pattern is first learned then broken down. The part-whole learner would enjoy building block choreography where patterns are built by putting together and sequentially adding moves.

One final concept to consider is the way in which adults learn. They learn primarily based on their beliefs, culture, prior experiences, and knowledge. (2) It is easy for you to educate in the style in which you prefer to learn. In order to reach more people, be aware that additional learning styles, methods of processing information, and educational techniques exist.

Summary

1. Exercise dropout is a frustrating problem encountered by most exercise professionals. Exercise dropout is attributed to personal, program, and other factors.

2. Exercise behavior motivates a person to initiate and maintain an exercise program. It also determines what kind of exercise the individual is likely to pursue. Attitudes and beliefs are strong determinants for exercise behavior as well as personal choice and exercise education.

3. The psychology of exercise behavior is complicated and multi-faceted. Awareness of the Law of Cause and Effect, Law of Attraction, Self-Efficacy, Locus of Control, Motivation, Personality, the Transtheoretical Model, and Exercise Dependency will enable an exercise professional to best choose motivational techniques for individual clients.

4. Exercise behavior modification strategies include setting goals, making agreements or contracts, providing feedback, scheduling appropriate rewards, integrating social support, providing prompts, modifying self-talk, using mental imagery, identifying false beliefs, and minimizing procrastination.

5. Educational information should be disseminated in many forms to accommodate all types of learners and all styles and methods of learning.

References

1. Acton, M., L. Denomme and J. Powers. (2005). *Aquatic After Care Manual.* 2nd Edition. Venice, FL. Personal Health Trac.

2. American College of Sports Medicine. (2006). *Guidelines for Exercise Testing and Prescription.* 7th Edition. Baltimore, MD. Lippincott, Williams & Wilkins.

3. American Council on Exercise. (2000). *Group Fitness Instructor Manual.* San Diego, CA. American Council on Exercise.

4. Beachle, T. and R. Earle. (2004). *NSCA's Essentials of Personal Training.* Champaign, IL. Human Kinetics Publishers.

5. Howley, T and D. Franks. (2003). *Health Fitness Instructor's Handbook.* 4th Edition. Champaign, IL. Human Kinetics Publishers.

6. Pollock, M. and J. Wilmore. (1990). *Exercise in Health and Disease: Evaluation and Prescription for Prevention and Rehabilitation.* St. Louis, MO. W. B. Saunders Company.

7. Van Roden, J. and L. Gladwin. (2002). *Fitness: Theory & Practice.* 4th Edition. Sherman Oaks, CA. Aerobic & Fitness Association of America.

Review Questions

1. Exercise drop out after the first year averages about _____ percent.
   a. 20
   b. 30
   c. 40
   d. 50

2. Which is the most prevalent indicator of exercise dropout?
   a. Smoking
   b. Depression
   c. Exercising alone
   d. Poor exercise leadership

3. Which psychological concept promotes the premise that internal thoughts are the cause of every effect or result?
   a. The Law of Attraction
   b. The Law of Cause and Effect
   c. The Transtheoretical Model
   d. Self-Efficacy

4. List three common motivators that may serve as factors for initiating an exercise program.

See Appendix E for answers to review questions.

Chapter 15: Business Issues and Legal Considerations

INTRODUCTION

The purpose of this chapter is to give aquatic fitness professionals an overview of business issues and legal responsibilities in the industry. Key areas are labor status, insurance needs, risk management, standard of care, liability, negligence, and duty. Fitness professionals should be aware of important documents in relation to facility procedures, understand the legal aspects of music use, and be familiar with the Americans with Disabilities Act.

This chapter is intended as a resource only. AEA recommends that all aquatic fitness professionals retain appropriate counsel for individual needs or concerns as all states and countries vary in regulations. This chapter is not intended to be legal advice, but an informational resource only. All terms and definitions are based on United States terminology and definitions. Terminology may vary in other countries.

Unit Objectives

After Completing Chapter 15, you should be able to:

1. Define the different labor status or business categories of employee, independent contractor (subcontractor), sole proprietorship, partnership, limited liability company (LLC), and corporation. List the responsibilities of each with consideration to requirements for insurance, taxation, and business structure.
2. Identify the need for liability insurance required for fitness professionals.
3. Define legal terminology related to professional responsibility, negligence, duty, and liability. Identify factors that influence determination of liability and awarding damages.
4. Define Standard of Care for AEA certified fitness professionals with reference to an established code of ethics and understand the importance of proper education and training as it relates to legal and moral responsibilities.
5. Understand the need for risk management whenever services are provided to the public.
6. Understand the 1976 U.S. Copyright Act and your legal responsibility in regard to using music in fitness programs.
7. Understand the Americans with Disabilities Act.

Key Questions:

1. What differentiates an employee from an independent contractor?
2. What are the business and legal responsibilities for an independent contractor?
3. What is standard of care and how does it affect class leadership and participant safety?
4. What is the fitness professional's commitment as indicated in AEA's Code of Ethics?
5. What factors are involved in determining liability?
6. What is risk management?
7. How does the 1976 U.S. Copyright Act affect a fitness professional?
8. Why was the Americans with Disabilities Act put into place?

Labor Status

This section will define the labor status and business structures that are typical in the fitness industry. Two common terms associated with instructors/trainers are **employee** and **independent contractor** (some states also use subcontractor). It is important to recognize the differences between an independent contractor and an employee, as each has a unique definition, specific responsibilities, and liability differences.

Employee

An employee is a person who is hired to provide services to a company on a regular basis in exchange for compensation, and who does not provide these services as part of an independent business. If you are an employee, your employer/company is responsible for deducting federal and state required taxes from your compensation and all necessary reporting of such. You would be covered by the company's professional and general liability insurance when teaching in the company's facilities, or any time you represent the company and are receiving compensation. Other employee benefits, directives, and policies and procedures would be found in your employee handbook and/or incentive documentation.

Independent Contractor

A person or business that provides goods or services to another entity under terms specified in a contract, is referred to as an independent contractor. Unlike an employee, an independent contractor does not necessarily work on a regular basis for one company. An independent contractor is personally responsible for all federal and state taxes due on compensation received for services provided. The independent contractor is personally responsible for liability insurance, both professional and general, and may need to provide proof of coverage to each contracted entity. An independent contractor assumes all liability, financial obligation, debt, claim, or potential loss. Also important to note, an independent contractor is one who is hired to complete a specific service but who is free to do that work as he/she wishes, and set the schedule of duties or services as he/she wishes. An independent contractor cannot sue an employer for a wrongful act or injury suffered on the job, as they are not an employee. This individual assumes all risk and responsibility and generally works under contract for fitness facilities and/or in the private sector such as instructing in hotels, condominiums, etc. Some

independent contractors also utilize their own home pools and/or client home pools for exercise. It is important to be aware of the exact insurance coverage needed for each specific location. Most hotels, condominiums, and privately owned complexes will require proof of insurance and/or an insurance binder to verify that an independent contractor is appropriately covered in case of an incident.

With increased participation and public interest in exercise and better health, the fitness industry has shown growth in business ownership. Instructors may own and operate businesses that offer classes and programming as well as other industry related services. In this event, the business is typically established as a sole proprietorship, partnership, or a corporation.

Sole Proprietorship

A sole proprietorship is a business structure in which an individual and the company are considered a single entity for tax and liability purposes. A sole proprietorship is a company that is not registered with the state as a limited liability company or corporation. The owner does not pay income tax separately for the company, but reports business income or losses on his/her individual income tax return. The owner is inseparable from the sole proprietorship, and is therefore liable for any business debts.

Partnerships

Partnerships are also common in the fitness industry. A partnership is the relationship existing between two or more persons who join together to carry on a trade or business. Each person contributes money, property, labor, or skill, and expects to share in the profits and losses of the business. A partnership must file an annual information return to report the income, deductions, gains, losses etc., from its operations, but does not pay income tax. Instead, it "passes through" any profits or losses to its partners. Each partner includes his/her share of the partnership's income or loss on a personal tax return.

Most attorneys will suggest that the partnership operate under a legally binding partnership agreement. This agreement dictates parameters for participation, compensation, contribution, and what would happen if one or all parties decide to dissolve the partnership. Having this agreement written by a lawyer and signed by all partners is a sound business practice.

Limited Liability Company (LLC)

A Limited Liability Company (LLC) is a relatively new business structure allowed by state statute. An LLC business structure is a hybrid of a partnership and a corporation. Its owners are shielded from personal liability and all profits and losses pass directly to the owners without taxation of the entity itself. LLCs are popular because, similar to a corporation, owners have limited personal liability for the debts and actions of the LLC. Other features of LLCs are more like a partnership, providing management flexibility and the benefit of pass-through taxation. LLCs should be operated under a legally binding agreement as well.

Corporations

Corporations in the fitness profession are generally registered businesses/corporations and limited liability companies organized for the purpose of providing professional services. What services constitute professional services are defined by state law and differ from state to state. There are several types of corporations with different share holder and tax configurations. Your attorney and accountant can help you choose the corporation that is most beneficial for your business structure and personal needs. If the corporation has more than one share holder, it is prudent to operate under a legally binding share holder agreement. A share holder agreement will define the number of shares held, contribution, compensation, and involvement. The agreement will also determine how a shareholder is able to sell or dissolve shares in the company if they no longer want to be involved.

It is important for a fitness professional to understand his/her role and responsibility with regards to taxation, insurance requirements, legal responsibility and liability. Since professionals may have more than one labor status qualification (such as employee and business partnership), it is best to consult with an attorney, accountant, and the Department of State to ensure all requirements are met.

Insurance

Risk is inherent whenever professional services are provided to the public. The most common types of insurance associated with the fitness profession include, but are not limited to, those listed below.

- **General Liability** insurance protects your company in the event that a client is injured on your premises or if you or one of your employees injures someone or damages property at a client's location.
- **Professional Liability** insurance provides protection when you are held legally liable for how you rendered or failed to render professional services.
- **Property** insurance protects business property and inventory (assets) against physical loss or damage by theft, accident or other means - even if that property is removed from your place of business when it is lost or damaged.
- **Service Interruption** or **Business Interruption** insurance is a special type of insurance that covers indirect losses that occur when a direct loss (that results from a covered peril, such as fire) forces a temporary interruption of business. Dependent on policy structure, business interruption insurance reimburses policyholders for the difference between normal income and the income earned during the enforced shutdown period.
- **Worker's Compensation** insurance provides medical and disability coverage for employees who sustain job-related injuries. Generally, these worker's compensation insurance policies will cover an employee's medical expenses and reimburse him or her for some percentage of lost wages. Some states have a mandatory worker's compensation program in which you must participate, while other states require you to have coverage through a private broker. Either way, worker's compensation insurance is required by law and you are subject to penalties and fines if you do not hold a policy.

There are several types of insurance policies and it is best to consult an attorney and insurance agent to determine insurance requirements based upon business structure and services provided. It is also important to look at the amount of coverage recommended, or possibly mandated, by the state. There are several policies available through fitness organizations which offer lower group rates and coverage suitable for fitness professionals. It is important to read and understand your coverage. Call your insurance agency with questions if you conduct activities that are not clearly defined by your policy or if you are not sure of the extent of coverage. Review and renew your insurance policies every year or as indicated to insure that you avoid interruption of coverage.

Risk Management

Risk management is the process of measuring or assessing risk and then developing strategies to manage that risk. Risk management includes regulating and enforcing conduct and safety guidelines to ensure the safety of participants. Strict rules, guidelines, and potential risks should be posted for all exercise activities and areas. The rules should be visible to all participants and strictly enforced by the staff. Lack of appropriate risk management practices could lead to potential damages.

Examples of potential risks for aquatic fitness participants:

- Slippery deck surface
- Broken ladders, loose rails on steps into pool
- Chipped gutters
- Loose floor tiles (lap lane tiles) on pool bottom
- Improperly grounded electrical outlets
- Pool chemical and sanitation problems

The ability to identify existing and potential risk is important for fitness professionals. Create and implement policies with clear guidelines. Evaluate the guidelines on a regular basis to ensure the welfare of exercise participants.

Standard of Care

Standard of care is defined as the degree of care a reasonable person would take to prevent an injury to another. It is important to know the limitations and boundaries of a fitness professional and to develop a comfortable standard of care based on personal knowledge and skill. Do not exceed those boundaries and limitations. It is a professional responsibility to keep all certifications current and attend continuing education courses. Ongoing education is critical for a fitness professional to remain up to date with the latest knowledge and changes in the industry. Reading professional journals and researching reputable sources and organizations on the Internet will help you grow and gain fresh ideas for programming.

There are two sets of standards provided by the Aquatic Exercise Association. The first is AEA's **Code of Ethics and Conduct** which defines baseline standards that AEA certified fitness professionals are expected to follow. The code of ethics is listed below. The second is the AEA published **Standards and Guidelines for Aquatic Fitness Programming** which provides important information for professional leadership and application, environ-mental concerns, facility recommendations, and instructional issues for the overall safety of the participants serviced. Several of the standards and guidelines have been included in various places in this manual. The full list of Standards and Guidelines is available from AEA and is updated annually.

Aquatic Exercise Association
Certified Aquatic Fitness Professional Code of Ethics and Conduct

- I will maintain high standards of professional conduct at all times.
- I will remain aware of current AEA Standards & Guidelines for Aquatic Fitness Programming. I will not knowingly contradict current accepted industry standards.
- I shall maintain my AEA Certifications through Continuing Education to stay abreast of the industry. I recognize that a **minimum** of 15 hours of continuing education is recommended for each 2-year renewal period of my AEA Certification.
- I will maintain training & certification in Cardio Pulmonary Resuscitation (CPR) and will obtain training in the use of an Automatic External Defibrillator (AED) when possible.
- I will maintain recommended levels of training in First Aid and Water Safety.
- I will acknowledge my skills and limitations as an aquatic fitness professional. I will practice ethically and properly represent my qualifications.
- I shall maintain clear and honest communications with my clients and students and uphold confidentiality at all times.
- I shall respect and cooperate with all health care and fitness professionals to promote the betterment of the aquatic fitness industry.
- I will contribute to the health, safety, and welfare of my clients and students to gain continued respect for the aquatic industry.
- I shall uphold the standards, policies, and procedures as outlined by the aquatic facility for which I work.
- I shall dress in a professional and appropriate manner when representing the aquatic fitness industry.
- I shall refrain from using any mind-altering drugs, alcohol, or intoxicants when conducting classes or instructing clients.
- I shall provide the highest quality of service possible to my clients and students in conjunction with the standards, guidelines, and objectives of the Aquatic Exercise Association.

Liability

There is always a possibility of injury and/or damage when participating in fitness programs. As a fitness professional, you have the legal obligation and responsibility to ensure the safety of all participants. There are duties required of you from the facility where you work, as well as industry standards. To minimize liability, follow facility guidelines and protocol and be familiar with job role definitions and labor status.

There are five general factors that influence liability:
- Ignorance of the law: not knowing the law.
- Ignoring the law: doing something that you know is contrary to the law.
- Failure to act: you know that you should do something, but fail to act.
- Failure to warn: not making participants or supervisors sufficiently aware of inherent dangers.
- Expense: failing to budget or spend money to further safety objectives.

As mentioned in Chapter 10, it is important to follow your facility requirements with regard to reducing the risk of liability. AEA recommends that you should be properly qualified to perform health risk assessment and physical screening. Proper training and practice is required to become proficient at health risk appraisal, risk factor assessment, physical screening, and fitness assessment.

The following points can also help reduce liability: -
- Every participant should read and sign an informed consent and waiver of liability that is professionally drafted by an attorney in your area. This is further discussed later in this chapter.
- All participants should complete appropriate health screening forms. Please see Chapter 10 for more information and recommendations.
- Encourage participants to have fitness testing to identify initial fitness level and fitness ability. Follow recommended procedures for paperwork and policies for group fitness participants and personal training clients. Policies may vary for members, guests, and the type of services being provided.
- Follow facility procedures with regards to incident reports/injury reports; document all incidents and injuries.
- Avoid high risk exercises. Teach safe exercises with proper form and technique.

- Remain certified, educated, and up to date with industry practices.
- Check and ensure that the environment is safe and free of hazards.
- Determine that equipment is in good working order.
- Maintain adequate insurance protection.

Negligence

Negligence is defined as committing an act that a person exercising ordinary care would not do under similar circumstances. Negligence can also be defined as the failure to do what a person practicing ordinary care would do under similar circumstances.

Duty

Duty is the responsibility and moral obligation of the professional to perform the services following industry standards and guidelines. In a potential lawsuit or trial, the judge and jury would examine whether the individual (defendant) acted in accordance to avoid damage or acted in any way to promote damage. A fitness professional can be sued for doing something incorrectly, or by failing to act to prevent damage. All factors listed below must be confirmed to find an individual negligent. If any one of these factors is missing, liability/damage cannot be charged.
- Presence of the duty: was it your responsibility to provide the duty in question to the participant?
- Breach of duty: was that duty breached or compromised? Did you act inappropriately or fail to act to prevent damage?
- Cause of the injury: was your breach of duty the direct cause of the injury?
- Extent of the injury: what was the actual extent of the injury?

Injury Report Form

Injury reports are essential and should be properly filled out and documented for all accidents or injuries sustained by any participant or guest. You can be held responsible for damage for a few years and proper documentation is critical if the incident results in a law suit. It is irresponsible to try to rely on your memory-properly document and record all events. Regardless of your labor status, an injury report should be completed for any situation that has the possibility of damage. Below is a sample of an incident report. You may want to consult your insurance company for incident report forms. Many companies will provide them.

Sample Incident/ Injury Report

Facility Name: _____

Date of Incident: _____

Name of Injured/ Involved: _____

Address:_____ Phone: _____

Detailed Description of Incident: (use back of paper if necessary)

_____

_____

_____

_____

_____

_____

_____

_____

_____

_____

_____

_____

Signature of Injured/Involved: _____ Date: _____

Name of Witness: _____ Phone: _____

Name of Witness: _____ Phone: _____

Name of Witness: _____ Phone: _____

Name of Employee Present: _____

Name of Employee Present: _____

Name of person filling out this report: _____

Signature of Person filling out this report: _____ Date: _____

Additional Information: _____

_____

_____

Informed Consent

By legal definition, consent is *"a person's agreement to allow something to happen"*. It is important to inform all fitness participants of the risks and potential injury inherent in participation in exercise programming. An informed consent is often included in the initial contract and/or binding agreement of a participant for professional services provided.

Release/Waiver of Liability

A r**elease or waiver of liability** is commonly used in the fitness industry. This form is issued to protect the facility and/or individual from damages and potential lawsuits. The participant agrees that he/she is willingly using the facility and participating in the activity, and waives all rights to assign damage and/or negligence. Essentially, the participant is waiving his/her right for future lawsuits and damages that could result from participation.

In most cases, the informed consent and waiver of liability are combined into one form that must be signed by all participants. Signing this form should be mandatory before joining the program. For most facilities, members sign these forms in their initial agreement with the facility. If you have a guest or one-day participant, be sure to have a version of a waiver of liability and informed consent available and policies in place to have these participants sign the form. If you are a subcontractor, be sure to have an informed consent and waiver of liability form drafted by an attorney in your area to follow state or area guidelines. Periodically have your form reviewed and updated by your attorney. Be sure to have all participants sign the form before participating. Following is a sample of an informed consent/waiver of liability form.

Sample Informed Consent/Waiver of Liability

Name of Facility or Logo

"I, _____, have enrolled in a program of strenuous physical activity including, but not limited to, aerobic training, resistance training, deep and shallow water exercise, interval training, circuit training, and the use of various aerobic and conditioning machinery and free weights offered by (insert name of facility or business) and/or exercise equipment owned by _____ (client, homeowner).

I hereby affirm that I am in good physical condition and do not suffer from any disability that would prevent or limit my participation in this exercise program."

"In consideration of my participation in the (name of facility or business) program, I, _____, for myself, my heirs and assigns, hereby release (name of facility or business), its employees and owners, from any claims, demands and causes of action arising from my participation in the exercise program."

"I fully understand that I may injure myself as a result of my participation in the (name of facility or business) exercise program and I, _____, hereby release (name of facility or business), its employees and owners, from any liability now or in the future including, but not limited to, heart attacks, muscle strains, pulls or tears, broken bones, shin splints, heat prostration, knee/lower back/foot injuries, and any other illness, soreness or injury, however caused, occurring during or after my participation in this exercise program."

I hereby affirm that I have read and fully understand the above.

Signature: _____ Date _____

Printed Name: _____

Music Use in Fitness Programs

The US 1976 Copyright Act states, "...*the copyright owner has the right to charge a fee for the use of his or her music in public performance.*" Public performance is defined as "*a place open to the public or as any place where a substantial number of persons outside a normal circle or family and its social acquaintances is gathered.*" Under this definition, fitness classes and programs are considered to be a "public performance." In the United States, fees must be paid to appropriate performing rights companies by profit and non-profit organizations, health clubs, studios, churches, schools, etc., who use music in their fitness programs and/or throughout their facilities.

ASCAP (American Society of Composers, Authors and Publishers) and BMI (Broadcast Music Incorporated) are the two largest companies in the world that protect people making music. These companies help anyone using music for purposes other than personal enjoyment to comply with the U.S. copyright laws by issuing the required clearance (for a fee) to publicly use copyrighted music. Under the law, when a business or individual wishes to play music publicly, meaning outside a normal circle of friends or family, they must first obtain permission from the music's copyright owners. ASCAP and BMI services enable the fitness professional to access and use music through agreements, licensing procedures and the payment of fees without needing to contact each artist individually.

Many music companies and other businesses create and/or produce CDs and other products designed specifically for various exercise and fitness applications. Producers and performers are hired to create or recreate the music and the song tracks compiled for specific programming requirements, such as an aquatic, step, or interval format. These music products have appropriate counts, phrasing, adjusted beats per minutes, tempo range, rhythms and transitions that aid in teaching an effective fitness program. These businesses pay appropriate reproduction and mechanical fees for the right to produce, reproduce, sell or duplicate these products. When purchasing music from companies specializing in such formats, remember, public performance fees are not covered.

If you were to copy music from several original CDs onto one CD to use in class, this is acceptable as long as you and or the facility are paying public performance fees. If you were to sell and or distribute the CD you made, you would need to follow similar procedures as the music production companies mentioned above and pay the appropriate fees for selling and distribution purposes, even if you gave the CD away for free. Most fitness professionals don't want the hassle and want to abide by the Copyright Law. It is simpler and more professional to purchase music for fitness programming from the companies that specialize in this service unless of course you are a composer, publisher and/or producer.

Facilities using background music, classes using music, etc. must pay appropriate public performance rights licensing fees as these situations are considered public performance. It is the responsibility of the facility and/or professional to make sure ASCAP, BMI and/or other publisher fees are paid to ensure compliance with the Copyright Law. Under the law, the employer or the independent contractor is required to pay fees for the right to play the music for use in fitness programs. Typically these fees are structured based on the number of participants in class. In addition to paying fees for music used in programs, a facility must pay fees for music played over a speaker into the general facility, even if the music is from a local radio station. These fees are typically based on the number of speakers you have in the facility.

The law is simple, you play and you pay. Unless music used is original and in original format, or unprotected, or unless you have received written permission from the artist to use the music, it is illegal to use it for classes or exercise sessions until you pay the pubic performance fees.

For more information, go to the following websites.

www.ascap.com

www.bmi.com

If you would like to see more information on U.S. Music Copyright Legislation issues, please go to www.ascap.com/legislation.

For a good resource to understand many positions affecting the music industry, go to the Stanford University Libraries on line at http://fairuse.stanford.edu/index.html. This site provides condensed and extended versions of various laws throughout history.

Americans with Disabilities Act

The Americans with Disabilities Act was initiated and approved in 1990. The purpose of this act is *"to establish a clear and comprehensive prohibition of discrimination on the basis of disability."* The Americans with Disabilities Act (ADA) is a federal civil rights law that prohibits the exclusion of people with disabilities from everyday activities, such as buying an item at the store, watching a movie in a theater, enjoying a meal at a local restaurant, exercising at the local health club, or having the car serviced at a local garage. To meet the goals of the ADA, the law established requirements for private businesses of all sizes. These requirements first went into effect on January 26, 1992, and remain in effect for both profit and non-profit businesses or organizations.

Private businesses that provide goods or services to the public are called public accommodations in the ADA. The ADA establishes requirements for twelve categories of public accommodations, including stores and shops, restaurants and bars, service establishments, theaters, hotels, recreation facilities, private museums and schools, and others. Nearly all types of private businesses that serve the public are included in the categories, regardless of size.

If you own, operate, lease, or lease to a business that serves the public, then you have obligations to abide by the ADA for existing facilities, altered facilities, and new facilities. Existing facilities are typically not exempt by building code "grandfather provisions."

For small businesses, compliance with the ADA is not difficult. To help businesses with their compliance efforts, the US Congress established a technical assistance program to answer questions about the ADA. Answers to questions about the ADA are a phone call away. The Department of Justice operates a toll-free ADA Information Line (800- 514-0301 voice and 800-514-0383 TDD). In addition, tax credits and deductions are established that can be used annually to offset many costs of providing access to people with disabilities. For more information, you can go to The Department of Justice website at: http://www.usdoj.gov/crt/ada

Summary

1. It is important for professionals working in the fitness industry to understand the business issues, legal considerations, and potential liability when working with the public based on labor status or business structure.

2. The ultimate responsibility of fitness professionals is to maintain the highest standard of care in performance of duty, use proper risk management strategies, and to avoid negligence.

3. Fitness Professionals should carefully examine and recognize both personal and professional boundaries. It is important to receive certification and vital to maintain the most up to date industry information, education, publications, and training to ensure the safety of the public served.

4. It is necessary to understand and abide by associated government acts including the US 1976 Copyright Act and the Americans with Disabilities Act. Be aware that state and county laws will vary. For countries outside the United States, it is appropriate to follow applicable laws and recommendations as provided by respected organizations and authorized governing bodies.

5. AEA highly recommends all professionals secure legal council and business/accounting council to ensure and protect professional and personal liability.

References

1. Acton, M., L. Denomme and J. Powers. (2005). *Aquatic After Care Manual.* 2nd Edition. Venice, FL. Personal Health Trac.

2. American Society of Composers, Authors and Publishers. (2005). *Legislative History.* New York, NY. ASCAP. www.ascap.com/legislation

3. Broadcast Music, Inc. (2005). *Music Copyright: Do I need a License/ Frequently Asked Questions.* New York, NY. BMI, Inc. www.bmi.com

4. Herbert, D. and W. Herbert. (2003). *Exercise Standards and Malpractice Reporter, Full Series.* Canton, OH. PRC Publishing.

5. Internal Revenue Service. (2005). *Businesses.* Washington, D.C. Internal Revenue Service. www.irs.gov/businesses

6. Spezzano, M. (2004). *ISCA Personal Training Manual.* 2nd Edition. Miami, FL. International Sports Conditioning Association.

7. U.S. Department of Justice. (2004). *Enforcing the ADA: A Status Report from the Department of Justice.* U.S. Department of Justice, Civil Rights Division, Disability Rights Section. www.usdoj.gov/crt/ada/statrpt.htm

8. U.S. Small Business Administration. (1999). *ADA Guide for Small Business.* 4th Printing. U.S. Small Business Administration, U.S. Department of Justice, Civil Rights Division. www.usdoj.gov/crt/ada/smbustxt.htm

Review Questions

1. A(n) _____ is legally responsible for covering your liability insurance and paying federal and state taxes on your behalf based upon compensation paid to you.

2. Define negligence.

3. Duty is my _____ and moral obligation to my students and facility.

4. _____ is defined as the process of measuring or assessing risk and then developing strategies to manage the risk.

5. The 1976 U.S. Copyright Act provides protection for _____.

6. The Americans with Disabilities Act was established in _____ to protect the rights of _____.

See Appendix E for answers to review questions.

Chapter 16: Deep Water Exercise

INTRODUCTION

This chapter is devoted to deep water exercise – non-impact training that can offer a full range of exercise challenges. In the 1990's, several research studies explored the option of deep water exercise with favorable results. Aquatic programming in deep water has become very popular and continues to evolve with creative formats, effective equipment options, and target markets. Deep water provides an excellent training modality for all ages and abilities. Specialized programming can be geared toward older adults, individuals with back problems, obese participants, and marathon runners, to name just a few. Deep water is an enjoyable and effective aquatic cross-training medium for a full range of participants.

Unit Objectives

Chapter 16 is an in-depth study of deep water exercise. The information in this chapter will not be tested in the Aquatic Fitness Professional Certification. It is intended to be ancillary to the primary content of this manual and to be used in preparation for the Deep Water Certification. Preparation for the Deep Water Certification includes the study of Chapters 1-15 and Chapter 16. Objectives for the Deep Water Certification include topics in the following primary categories specifically related to deep water programming:
- The Aquatic Environment
- Physiology and Benefits
- Safety
- Equipment
- Movement Analysis
- Physical Laws
- Programming and Leadership

For a complete list of the Deep Water Certification objectives and to register for the Deep Water Certification, please contact the AEA at www.aeawave.com or 1-888-232-9283.

Key Questions:
1. What makes deep water exercise programs different from shallow water exercise programs?
2. Is safety a concern in deep water exercise?
3. Is it necessary to use equipment in deep water programming?
4. How are movements and transitions different in deep water as opposed to shallow water?
5. How do you alter intensity in deep water exercise?
6. What are typical program formats for deep water exercise?
7. How does an instructor teach deep water exercise?

Deep water exercise is traditionally defined as a fitness program performed suspended in water at a depth that is over the participant's head. Typically a flotation device is worn for neutral buoyancy, which allows the participant to concentrate on working against the drag properties/ resistance of the water as opposed to trying to stay afloat. Participants can move freely in all three planes of motion creating a total body workout, muscle balance, and a substantial challenge for the core muscles without impact stress to the joints.

Not all pools have water that accommodates true deep water training, but shallow water programs can be modified to include non-impact Level III movements. Working suspended in Level III, the hips and knees are flexed to perform the movement without touching the bottom of the pool. The participant works primarily against the horizontal drag forces of the water and typically shifts more of the workload to the upper torso. As Level III movements are considered a shallow water choreography option, shoes are generally recommended but neutral buoyancy equipment is typically not required.

Another circumstance where suspended movements may be used is for programs performed in transitional water depths, where water is too deep for traditional shallow water exercise and too shallow for traditional deep water exercise. Transitional deep water training is not considered traditional shallow water programming because the participant is not rebounding off the pool bottom. It is not considered traditional deep water exercise because the participant touches the bottom of the pool during some movements (similar to Level II movements but with less hip and knee flexion.) Thus the term "transitional" describes water exercise performed in pools with water depths between 4 and 6 feet (1 to 1.6 meters); flotation equipment may be utilized; and shoes are recommended since there will be some contact with the pool floor.

Physiology and Benefits of Deep Water Exercise

Deep Water Exercise Research

Deep water exercise matured as a training alternative in the 1980's and 1990's. Most of the research on deep water exercise compares land running/jogging/walking (road training or treadmill training) with deep water running/jogging/walking.

- Studies were conducted to investigate:
  - Comparison of heart rate responses.
  - Perceptual responses and rate of perceived exertion differences.
  - Running interval comparisons.
  - Maximal heart rate and oxygen consumption responses and comparisons.
  - Submaximal response comparisons.
  - Responses with and without neutral buoyancy.
  - Effects of deep water running mechanics on physiological responses.
  - Effects of deep water running on spinal shrinkage.
  - Physiological responses and gender differences.
  - Maintenance of VO_2max and leg strength in trained runners.
  - Maintenance of land-based running performance in rehabilitation of injury.
  - Comparisons in physiological responses in competitive and non-competitive athletes.
  - The effects of deep water running on land running performance.
- There is little replicated research. It is difficult to draw any firm conclusions because study methodology varies greatly in the subjects used, training methods and time formats, measurement techniques, and in the actual research question or goal. Investigators have found the cardiorespiratory responses to deep water training to be less than, similar, and greater than treadmill running on land.
- Published research on physiological responses for non-running/jogging/walking types of deep water aquatic fitness program formats is virtually non-existent.

Physiological Training Adaptations to a 14 Week Deep Water Exercise Program.
Rosalie G. Barretta, Ph.D.
University of New Mexico, 1993

Seventeen volunteers participated three days/week for 14 weeks in a deep water exercise

---

program with 4" ski belts and foam hand bars, offered as a physical education elective course. Music cadence was between 100 and 130 beats/min and the class consisted of a warm up, 20 minutes of cardiorespiratory work, resistance work with the foam hand bars, and a cool down.

Results showed significant improvements in VO₂max (measured with cycle ergometry), flexibility (modified sit and reach test), strength of shoulder flexion/extension, shoulder transverse abduction/adduction, thigh flexion/extension (Omnitron), and body composition (hydro-densiometry).

Application of Deep Water Exercise

Research does indicate that deep water exercise, when performed at the proper intensity and duration, will produce favorable health benefits and is a viable training option for improving physical fitness. In addition, the following benefits and specific training considerations for deep water exercise are indicated:

- Energy costs of treadmill walking and running versus matched speeds of deep water walking and running showed treadmill walking to expend 4.0 Kcal/minute, deep water walking 8.8 Kcal/minute, treadmill running 11.8 Kcal/minute, and deep water running 11.5 Kcal/minute. (Coad et al. 1987) Another study measured energy expenditure at 13.5 Kcal/minute for deep water running at 60% VO₂peak and 18.9 Kcal/minute at 80% VO₂peak. (DeMaere et al. 1997) It would be reasonable to assume caloric expenditure in deep water varies between 4.0 (lower intensity) and 18.9 (higher intensity) Kcal/minute for most cardiorespiratory class formats. Any form of exercise that elevates oxygen consumption and caloric expenditure is beneficial. Deep water exercise has been found to have favorable training responses, including the development of cardiorespiratory fitness, as measured by VO₂max improvements. (Kravitz et al., 1997 / Dowzer et al., 1999 / Whitley et al., 1987)
- Studies conducted using endurance-trained subjects have found deep water training to be successful in the maintenance of aerobic performance. (Bushman et al., 1997 / Hertler et al., 1992 / Wilbur et al., 1996 / Burns, 2001 / Rudzki, et al., 1999) Many athletes use the deep water to cross train or as a means to continue to exercise while

rehabilitating injuries. You may want to consider offering deep water running classes for the avid joggers/runners in your community as a cross training opportunity. Training should closely resemble intensity, duration and frequency of land based training or incorporate a similar training volume in the combination of land and water training.

- Several studies (Svedenhag et al., 1992 / Glass et al., 1995 / Frangolias et al., 1995 / Michaud et al., 1995) showed equivalent or higher blood lactate levels for water running/jogging trials as compared to land. It is hypothesized that working the arms and legs against the water's resistance may create more anaerobic energy use and explain the higher rating of perceived exertion (RPE) in both trained and untrained subjects. Heart rate responses were lower in the water as compared to land exercise. This is to be expected and is consistent with other aquatic research. (see Chapter 4 – heart rate responses) When teaching deep water classes, be aware of the increased perception of work (higher RPE) and the possible accumulation of lactic acid that may reflect as muscle fatigue. You may want to incorporate active recovery periods to allow for lactic acid removal; thus an interval format is one method that works well for deep water training. As submersion depth increases, so do the drag forces of the water. Deep water works the participant at neck depth, which allows for substantial drag forces. Additionally, aquatic adjustments need to be made for target heart rates in deep water exercise. It appears that when some participants are submerged to the neck, aquatic suppression of the heart rate is even greater than when submerged to the chest. (see Chapter 4 – Intensity of Exercise) Keep in mind that this response is individual.
- Vertical exercise form was found to contribute substantially to metabolic responses in deep water running. (Frangolias et al., 1995) Experienced deep water runners had VO₂max values on land and in water that were within 3.8 ml/kg/min, whereas the difference in the inexperienced deep water runners was 10.3 ml/kg/min. The lower aquatic metabolic values in the inexperienced runners were due primarily to vertical positioning. It is important in any deep water program to cue, correct, encourage, and program for proper, upright vertical posture. Familiarity with the deep water and proper form and technique can substantially affect metabolic responses and the effectiveness of the work out. This information also supports wearing a neutral

buoyancy device while performing deep water exercise. Neutral buoyancy allows the participant to work in a correct vertical position and thus have the potential to burn more calories. Wearing a flotation device can substantially add to the effectiveness of your deep water workout.

- An investigation with 8 male competitive runners running at a submaximal pace for 30 minutes showed deep water running incurred higher oxygen consumption values, respiratory exchange ratios, and RPE levels than normal treadmill or road running. (Richie et al., 1991) It was concluded that submaximal exercise at ACSM recommendations can be sufficiently and effectively completed in deep water.

- Blood pressure responses in deep water exercise are very similar to land exercise responses. Systolic pressure increases and plateaus with steady state exercise and diastolic pressure remains relatively unchanged.

- In a study conducted by Dowzer et al., 1998, it was found that deep water exercise decreased the compressive load on the spine when compared to shallow water and treadmill running. Implications include the use of deep water running/exercise for participants with chronic low back pain and rehabilitation of spinal conditions, keeping in mind that the participant must have adequate core strength to maintain vertical alignment. Successful back rehabilitation and back health programs are being conducted in the deep water.

Qualifying Participants

It is important to evaluate a participant's ability to participate in deep water exercise comfortably and safely. Basic abilities must be taken into consideration regardless of the intensity level of your deep water classes. The following guidelines will apply to your evaluation of each individual coming into your programs.

Will the participant be able to maintain a vertical body position in the deep water? A participant who wishes to take a deep water class must be able to achieve a vertical stance in the water utilizing their mid-body stabilizers. Generally, participants who are moderately active in their daily lives have an adequate level of abdominal strength to keep their legs underneath them.

Has the participant been doing any prior physical activity? If the participant is recovering from an injury, or has been sedentary, you may want to first observe him/her walking in shallow water to determine the ability to control the body's buoyancy and to maintain a vertical body position in the water.

Will the participant be able to enter and exit the pool independently? Assess basic physical condition, both leg and arm strength, by watching participants walk to class, shaking their hand as you greet them, asking a few questions about activities they enjoy, and looking for muscle tone in the arms and legs. If your pool only has vertical ladders for entries and exits, the client must be able to hold the handrails and stabilize on one leg as they push themselves up and out of the water.

Is the participant dealing with any heart or respiratory conditions? Ask if the participant is currently under a doctor's care for any health condition.

If a cardiac event has been experienced in the past 12 months, it would be prudent to determine more about current exercise levels. Individuals that have suffered a cardiac event in the last three months need to follow specific guidelines to begin an exercise program. The MET level (energy expended during activity) that is desirable for a cardiac rehabilitation patient, who is healed and able to exercise on land comfortably for a half-hour, is 5-6 METs. This represents a heart rate of about 30 beats above resting heart rate. As previously noted in Chapter 12, deep water typically produces an 11-13.1 MET level. Because of this, deep water exercise may not initially be the recommended program due to the high exertion level.

Participants with respiratory conditions sometimes find that the hydrostatic pressure and/or the flotation belt prohibit comfortable breathing during deep water exercise. In such cases, the individual may be more comfortable in a shallow water class or choose to put flotation on their arms or ankles to leave the mid-body free.

Is the participant nervous about being in water over his/her heads? It is important to be aware of a participant who is apprehensive about entering deep water due to lack of experience and/or swimming skills. Make sure that equipment is properly fitted, notify the lifeguard of his/her tentative status and instruct him/her to initially stay close to the side. Even though wearing buoyant support, the participant can still panic and have an unpleasant experience. Teach how to regain a vertical stance from both a supine and a prone position.

Following are various methods to help orient participants who are not ready to directly enter a deep water class.

- **Rehearse deep water activities in shallow water.** Introduce deep water moves with buoyant assistance in shallow water. "Controlled" opportunities to experience impact free exercise can help overcome fears while becoming familiar with moves and equipment.
- **Development of trunk stabilizer muscles.** Participation in shallow water exercise, or other core strengthening programs, can help strengthen the trunk stabilizers that will be required for a successful experience in the deep.
- **Empower individuals with self-rescue techniques.** Teach participants how to return to vertical from a back float and from a prone position. Explain how to control panic symptoms, i.e. lie back and relax until able to return to an upright position.

Managing the Environment

Pool Depth

Deep water exercise is most successful at a depth where a body can be suspended vertically and is free to move in any direction, at any speed, without experiencing impact or weight bearing stress. A pool depth of 6.5 feet or more provides the ideal environment for a deep water class.

Participant Workout Space

The optimum working space for deep water exercise is a little larger than shallow water, because deep water participants have a tendency to drift and float. Ideally, each deep water exercise participant should have 32-36 square feet of working space depending upon the level of the class, the type of programming, and equipment choices. Participants can create ample space by remaining vertical with arms abducted at the shoulders and turning in a circle. For an optimal situation, determine the maximum class size by calculating the square footage of deep water pool space and divide by 32-36. A beginner level class with predominantly stationary exercises will require

less space than an advanced workout that utilizes traveling exercises.

Water Temperature

Normal body temperature is 98.6 degrees F. Since water cools the body faster than air, the temperature of the water has a direct effect on the exercise intensity level that can be comfortably and safely maintained. The recommended temperature for a class that involves 20-40 minutes of aerobic activity is 83-86 degrees Fahrenheit (28-30 degrees Celsius). During the warm up and cool down phases of the workout, be mindful that the participant's body is 90% submerged and needs to continually move to keep from being chilled. The recommended temperature for a class that is slower paced with an emphasis on toning and stretching is 84-92 degrees.

Air Temperature

For the comfort of the exercise participant in the water, AEA recommends that air temperature be approximately 3-4 degrees higher than the water temperature. Otherwise, program modifications are necessary to maintain participant comfort and safety. If the air is warmer than the water temperature, the water will feel cool as the participant enters the pool. If the air temperature is cooler than the water, the water will feel warmer. In an outdoor facility, the air cannot be controlled, but it will offer similar sensory effects as in the indoor situation.

Also recognize that the instructor on deck must make appropriate modifications – clothing choices, adequate hydration, and teaching skills will influence comfort and safety. In an indoor situation, a strategically placed grounded fan on a dry deck will help dissipate heat while you are demonstrating moves. Make sure the fan does not blow across the water or it will chill the participants.

Pool Entry/Exit

There are a variety of entries and exits into pools depending on the age and configuration of the facility. If you are holding class in a deep tank that is separated from the shallow water pool, you generally find vertical handrails with steps carved into the pool wall or vertical ladders with handrails. These two options require a certain amount of upper body strength and also rely on a participant's ability to support his or her weight on one leg while pushing upward with the other leg.

If you have a deep water area connected to a shallow water area, participants may prefer entering the pool at the shallow end and walking into the deeper water. Pools with steps and handrails or gently sloping ramp entries provide access to a wider range of participants. There are also portable pool stairs for shallow water that allow for easier entry and exit.

> **A Note of Caution:**
> To avoid the potential for serious injury, participants should never jump or dive into the water wearing flotation or resistance equipment.

Returning to Vertical Position

As a pre-requisite for deep water exercise, participants should be tested for the ability to return to a vertical position. A participant may enter deep water and lose control of vertical alignment, ending up in either a supine or prone position. This can lead to panic and a distressed victim situation if the individual is not able to regain an upright posture quickly and efficiently. Some facilities offer a deep water orientation to acclimatize participants to the environment and teach vertical position recovery skills. Vertical position recovery skills include the following.

Regaining vertical stance from a supine position:

Have the participant draw the knees toward the chest while bringing the head and shoulders forward and pressing the arms forward/upward (shoulder flexion). The action of the arms assists in bringing the hips under the shoulders (reaction). Extend the legs toward the bottom of the pool to return to vertical.

Regaining vertical stance from a prone position:

If wearing a flotation belt, have the participant pull knees toward chest while pressing arms down in front to bring hips under the shoulders, then extend the legs toward the bottom of the pool.

If wearing flotation cuffs at the ankles, the participant should always roll over to a supine position first. Refer to "regaining vertical stand from a supine position." Note: it is easier to draw only one knee to the chest due to flotation equipment on the ankles.

Lifeguard

Teaching water exercise requires a lot of focus and attention. It is highly recommended that there be a lifeguard on duty during water exercise classes. This way the instructor can be focused on the workout and the participants' performance, and the lifeguard can be focused on the early warning signs of distress or health emergency. If a lifeguard is not on duty, you need to obtain skills for safely assisting participants in water emergencies (both deep and shallow) and you need to have a rescue tube near you at all times.

No one ever plans to panic. Panic is an overwhelming fear that inhibits the victim from thinking or reacting rationally. Panic can happen in deep and shallow water. In deep water, the danger level heightens because everyone involved is unable to stand on the pool bottom. A panicked victim generally requires assistance by a trained professional who can help him/her regain control.

Shoes

In deep water the participant is not coming in contact with the pool bottom during the workout. Water shoes are not required for deep water exercise, however they do add to the safety and comfort of participants as they walk the pool deck to and from class and climb in and out of the pool. Wearing shoes, in effect, adds a piece of resistance equipment on the foot, at the end of a long lever. Class content will determine if this is beneficial or adds unnecessary stress to the joints. As a potential plus, certain types of shoes provide additional weight that can assist participants with vertical alignment in this buoyant non-impacting environment.

Equipment Safety

Buoyancy equipment that requires an individual to hold on to the device, such as a noodle, kickboard, or hand bars, can create a false sense of well-being. The safest alternative for flotation (buoyancy assistance) in deep water attaches to the body of the participant, such as a belt, vest or cuffs. There is no potential for letting go of the buoyancy assistance device – even if the individual becomes panicked. During a typical recreational swim, the majority of aquatic facilities would not allow individuals to rely on kickboards or hand bars for flotation in deep water. The irony of this situation is that many of those same facilities invite adults, with limited skills, to participate in a deep water program using only hand-held flotation for buoyancy assistance. This practice can lead to a tragedy.

If you work in this type of situation you need to ask yourself the following questions:

- What if the participant panics and releases the hand bars?
- What if the participant lets go of the kickboard and then grabs another participant in an attempt to remain afloat?
- What if the participant tips backward on his/her noodle and is unable to regain vertical stability?
- What role do you play in the rescue and what is your professional liability?

There is another safety issue to consider when selecting equipment for deep water exercise. Suspending the body for extended periods of time with hand-held buoyant equipment can compromise joint integrity. Many participants lack adequate strength in the lower trapezius to keep the shoulder joint in a depressed position, thus leading to static overload of the upper trapezius, already a lifestyle activated over-used muscle group. Holding the buoyancy at the surface with arms abducted can cause impingement of the shoulder. Supporting with the buoyancy under the arms may create discomfort. When using buoyant equipment in a submerged position, a participant not only deals with the water's upward buoyant force, but also must compensate for the equipment's buoyancy and his/her own natural buoyancy. During dynamic movement, such as during aerobic conditioning, alignment runs an increased risk of compromise.

AEA makes the following equipment recommendations for deep water programs or shallow water suspended training to provide a safe and effective workout for the general population.

- AEA recommends that deep water exercise be performed with flotation equipment attached to the trunk of the body (flotation belt or vest) or attached to the upper arms (flotation upper arm cuffs specifically designed for water exercise). With proper progression and training, ankle cuffs may be an appropriate flotation option for some individuals.
- If hand-held buoyancy equipment is utilized for additional resistance, AEA recommends that options are provided for participants with special needs and that periods of training with the equipment submerged are limited and/or frequent breaks are incorporated. Maintain neutral alignment of the wrists and avoid tight gripping of the equipment. The instructor should carefully observe and cue to assure that proper alignment of the shoulder girdle is maintained.

- If hand-held flotation equipment is utilized for suspended training in shallow water, AEA recommends that options are provided for participants with special needs and that periods of suspended training are limited and/or frequent breaks from suspended training are incorporated. Avoid shoulder abduction beyond 90 degrees without external rotation. Scapular depression reduces the risk of impingement in the shoulder joint capsule. The instructor should carefully observe and cue to assure that proper alignment of the shoulder girdle is maintained.

Deep Water Equipment Options
Flotation Belts

The most common flotation device is a mid-body belt. There are numerous varieties of flotation belts in respect to size (width and thickness), shape, texture (soft or rigid foam) and overall buoyancy. It is important that the belt fits snugly and that the participant feels secure with the level of buoyancy provided. The flotation belt is designed to give buoyant support in the water so the exerciser can focus on using the water's resistance to achieve the desired intensity.

It is best to offer a variety of belts to accommodate a variety of individuals. The correct fit of the belt is dependent on the shape of the participant's body as well as body fat distribution. Some individuals may have enough buoyancy to maintain proper body position without a belt, but need the security of a flotation device when exercising in deep water. If a belt is too buoyant, then the participant may have difficulty maintaining a vertical body position. Inadequate buoyancy will bring the chin to the water's surface and have the participant in "survival mode," attempting to stay afloat the entire class. A participant that appears to pitch forward at the hips probably requires less buoyancy behind the body; a participant that appears to pitch backward or shows excessive arch of the lumbar area probably requires less buoyancy in front of the body. Consider a different type of belt, turn the belt around so the "front" is now behind the back, or distribute buoyancy differently if the belt design allows. A larger buoyant participant requires a belt with a longer strap, not a belt with increased buoyancy. A lean participant who continually needs to move his or her legs to stay at comfortable level in the water may require a more buoyant belt or a combination of belt and ankle cuffs.

The belt should be fitted at the waist below the breasts. If you try to fit the belt to the hips, the belt will slide up the body as soon as the participant submerges. When tightening the strap, hold the strap next to the belt with one hand and cinch the belt tighter by pulling the loose end of the strap with the other hand.

Flotation Vests

Flotation vests are worn on the upper body to provide neutral buoyancy and may provide a more comfortable alternative for some individuals. Proper fit is important for comfort and ease of movement. The shoulders of the vest should not ride up around the ears when the individual is submerged. The amount of buoyancy provided should also allow the participant to maintain correct vertical alignment during movement.

Flotation Upper Arm Cuffs

There are flotation cuffs that can be worn on the upper arm and may provide a more comfortable option for someone who feels restricted by a belt, for example a pre-natal or an asthmatic participant. The cuffs should be placed on the upper arm so the individual can rest his/her arm in a natural position to exercise. For some fearful participants, the cuffs on the arms feel more secure than a belt. The cuffs help an individual stay upright, whereas a belt can create more balance problems if they are lacking mid-body muscle tone. The cuffs should be made of foam and not be dependent on inflation.

Flotation Ankle Cuffs

There are flotation cuffs that can be attached at the ankle and provide buoyancy as well as added resistance for the workout. Buoyancy cuffs worn at the ankle require an individual to engage the trunk muscles to maintain a vertical body position. For this application, care should be taken to teach participants how to regain a vertical stance from both a supine and a prone position. For most participants, AEA recommends that a flotation belt/vest initially be worn with the ankle cuffs to provide adequate safety until the individual becomes comfortable and proficient training with lower body buoyancy.

Foam Logs

Foam logs are very popular for deep water workouts as well as transitional water exercises. The log provides flotation assistance, but is not attached to the participant, so is not considered as secure as a belt, vest, or arm cuffs. Logs are typically placed around the back or the front of the torso (under the arms while maintaining the shoulder girdle in neutral position) or between the legs.

Resistance Devices

There are a variety of equipment options for increasing resistance in the deep water. Upper body resistance equipment can be used safely if the participant is utilizing a flotation device for support. Options include webbed gloves, hand bars, hand-held drag equipment, and foam logs.

Lower body resistance equipment can be used safely if the participant is utilizing a flotation device for support. There are winged devices that attach to the ankle or lower leg and increase the surface area of the limb. There are shoe-like devices that increase the resistance below the ankle. Ankle cuffs can provide both increased surface area and needed buoyant support.

It is important that as an instructor you are well versed on how to use the equipment you choose to offer your classes. Equipment choices may affect cadence and exercise selection; prepare your program with the equipment in mind. (see Chapter 7)

Deep Water Technique and Alignment

Total Immersion

The most basic principle for the deep water instructor to remember is that the body is immersed in a predominantly unnatural environment. Total immersion is not a normal placement for the body, and yet it is the very first part of the deep water experience. Immersion, the effects of buoyancy, resistance, drag, hydrostatic pressure, and temperature all impact the way a person will be able to cope with the exercises that you choose and link together. Everything slows down; the body takes longer to begin a movement pattern, sustain repetitions, and make any kind of change. The ground is missing and neurological processes have to find new pathways for successful completion of tasks, from the simplest one of staying vertical to the potentially complex movement patterns of the exercises. Instructors should not ignore the moment of immersion. It is the first step into deep water and it factors in the teaching of deep water alignment and exercise technique.

Humans are bipedal and the erect stance is fundamental to function. Regardless of exercise modality, improved functional capacity on land must be at the top of the list of goals. By placing the body in a vertical position in water, it maintains a familiar organizational strategy for spatial orientation. Head above shoulders and shoulders above hips is 'normal' human body organization. This familiar placement helps the body deal with the other unfamiliar characteristics of deep water immersion – lack of contact with the ground and the diminished effect of gravity.

When cueing 'head above shoulders, shoulders above hips', reference is being made to the five bony landmarks of neutral postural alignment. (see Chapter 10) Instructors rarely call out 'mastoid process over acromion process.' Instead, the anatomical language is replaced with everyday words that will help participants achieve the same result. Instructors will say 'ears in line with shoulders, shoulders in line with hips.' In deep water, the vertical working position should reflect the exact same alignment, but typically the positioning is taught in a dynamic, rather than static, setting. The legs will be moving in an alternating jogging action, so the instructor needs to cue the placement of the legs so that they maintain the vertical alignment. For a stationary jogging action, cues will include:

- Raise each knee toward the chest in front of the body.
- Bend the knee so that the ankle is posterior to the knee.
- Fully extend each leg so that it returns to the vertical line.

Common mistakes to look for and correct include:

- Collapsing the chest towards the hips. Practice elongating the body and give cues for maximum space between the pelvis and the ribcage.
- Kicking the heels up behind the body, which may cause a compensatory anterior pelvic tilt and resultant low back arch because the body will be falling forwards. Correct this by asking for a higher lift of the knees in front and placement of the ankle posterior of the knee but not behind the body.
- Lifting the knee with the foot forward of the knee and not returning each leg to the fully extended position under the body. In this scenario the participant will feel that they are falling backwards, and will probably curl forward and project the chin to compensate. Although the degree of hip flexion is good, cue more knee flexion so that the heel is posterior to the knee. Reinforce hip and knee extension so that the body returns to the vertical line with each repetition.

These alignment issues are unique to deep water because the feet do not touch the pool bottom. In shallow water, it is easier to maintain alignment because participants will naturally bring the foot down under the body, just as they do on land.

Dynamic Stabilization

Dynamic stabilization is the body's ability to maintain neutral, or near neutral postural alignment (a stable position) while moving. In the majority of activities performed, a structurally safe position for the core of the body is attempted before overload is added. Neutral postural alignment is a position that places the spine in its strongest, safest alignment. This vertically aligned position in deep water allows a centering from which other movements are possible without causing injury. The lack of contact with the ground in deep water causes the body to use a totally new strategy to achieve this neutral postural alignment.

On land the proprioceptive mechanism by which you know if you are standing upright and balanced is primarily through the ankle joints and actual contact with the ground. From a standing position, the brain receives continuous messages through the ankles. These messages to the central nervous system initiate a loop of proprioceptive feedback to control muscle tone and generate reflex responses. In simple terms, sensory receptors in the muscles, joints and connective tissues gather information about the body's position, process that information, and enable the central nervous system to make the appropriate response. For example, when you are falling, proprioception allows the brain to know that the fall is occurring, to activate the correct strategies to regain balance, and to actually send the messages to the muscles to contract and avoid the fall. The muscles in the legs and feet will contract to adjust positioning and regain balance.

In deep water you can no longer use this strategy of proprioceptive feedback. The body now has to utilize a different system to know if the body is vertical and balanced. The messages to the brain no longer come through the feet and ankles. Instead, engagement of the stabilization muscles of the core occurs – the abdominals, erector spinae, and intercostals contract. These core postural muscles play a key role in the new strategy for balance and correct alignment of the body. These muscle groups are active 100% of the time in deep water. Their activity is discreet, but constant. This continuous contracting of core muscles is the main reason why such good postural improvements are seen in people who regularly attend deep water classes. Core stabilization also occurs in shallow water, but it is much more dynamic in deep. An understanding of this dynamic stabilization process is essential for the instructor teaching deep water exercise.

This process translates into the following guidelines for the instructor:

• At the beginning of class allow time for the body to establish the dynamic stabilization strategy through the postural muscles. This means offering non-traveling exercises at the start of class and giving postural corrections to achieve neutral alignment.
• Frequently revisit neutral postural alignment, especially before a very challenging exercise where high intensity resistance is loaded on any of the limbs.
• Use neutral postural alignment for transitions. Pass through 'center' on the way to another exercise.
• Make sure that the flotation belt or other equipment does not hinder a participant's ability to achieve neutral postural alignment.

Center of Buoyancy and Diminished Gravity

The diminished effect of gravity also plays a vital role in achieving good alignment for deep water exercise. Remember that the force of gravity is still present - otherwise the water would not stay in the pool. For the moving body this means that we still have a center of gravity (the center of a body's mass) through which the body maintains equilibrium. On land, the body's center of gravity tends to stay in the pelvic area. In shallow water classes, participants can still maintain a base of support and keep the center of gravity low and within the base. As the water gets deeper, center of buoyancy (the center of a body's volume) starts to influence equilibrium and balance more than center of gravity. We no longer have the

feet in contact with the ground or that base of support.

Center of buoyancy is located in the chest region close to the pockets of air created by the lungs. In deep water, there is interplay between center of gravity and center of buoyancy. Gravity is a downward force and buoyancy is an upward force, so when a body is immersed in water there are two opposing forces acting on that body. If you entered deep water and did nothing at all, center of buoyancy and center of gravity would most likely place the body horizontal, face down. When participants are asked to be in a vertical working position, center of buoyancy and center of gravity move into vertical alignment. As they line up, there is a feeling of balance and equilibrium. It is important for instructors to watch participants carefully as they make these alignment adjustments. Look for anything that might be causing difficulty for a participant; for example, body composition, placement of flotation equipment, and/or the type of flotation utilized.

Archimedes' Principle

Following Archimedes' Principle, there is a direct relationship between the weight of the submerged part of the body and the amount of fluid displaced by that part of the body. This principle determines if the individual floats or sinks. When the weight of the submerged body is equal to the weight of the fluid displaced, the center of gravity and center of buoyancy will be in vertical alignment. If this equation is not equal, center of gravity and center of buoyancy will not be vertically aligned causing the body to roll and turn until it finds a place of equilibrium. Participants will struggle to stay vertical. Fat and air have greater water-displacement volume than lean tissue. So, although a participant with more body fat may float easily, he or she may have difficulty staying in alignment. In the opposite situation, a very muscular body will sink because the body is not displacing enough water to allow the participant to float.

Placement of Buoyant Equipment

A key issue in all of these alignment considerations is the placement of buoyant equipment on the immersed body. Additional buoyancy will affect equilibrium. Too much buoyancy will mean that the weight of the submerged body is no longer equal to the weight of the fluid displaced causing the body to shift away from vertical, struggling to find a place of equilibrium. Although a flotation belt is generally recommended for deep water exercise, each participant needs individual evaluation. Remember that the belt has its own center of gravity and center of buoyancy. Wearing a belt could alter neutral postural alignment.

A scuba diver performs a buoyancy check with each dive that includes hanging motionless and vertical while holding a normal breath. This test can be applied to vertical water exercise – a well-fitting flotation belt will allow an individual to maintain the appropriate level in the water with the head above the water while in a motionless vertical position. During inhalation and exhalation, the body will naturally rise and fall as air pressure changes within the lungs. Upon inhalation the body rises slightly, and sinks slightly upon exhalation. When proper neutral buoyancy is established, this change in level will be minimal. Also, the more relaxed a person remains, and the more evenly and consistently one breathes, the easier it is to maintain the proper level in the water. By then engaging core stabilization and proper breathing patterns, proper alignment can be achieved more effectively.

This translates into the following guidelines for the instructor:

• Flotation belts will be suitable for the majority of deep water participants.
• Facilities should have a selection of belt styles.
• The participant with higher body fat reserves may not need a belt for flotation, but may need assistance with proper alignment.
• The muscular participant may need a belt and additional flotation.
• Consider altering location of buoyancy to accommodate body fat distribution.

In a similar way, the addition of equipment like submerged buoyant hand bars for upper body strengthening exercises, will also upset the established equilibrium. The equation is altered and the body will try to adjust to this change in displacement and find a new place of equilibrium. Alignment could be compromised; therefore additional equipment requires extra cues from the instructor.

Body Mechanics

Balance

Balance is key in deep water movement. With no anchor points for the feet on the bottom of the pool, each movement still needs an end point. When you do a cross-country ski, how do the legs know when to change direction? They are limited by personal range of motion and controlled by the instructor showing a specific demonstration and rhythm (musical or otherwise). If each leg is placed equidistance in front and behind the body, the movement feels balanced. Symmetrical exercises are easier to perform because both sides of the body match. Hence a deep water jack feels comfortable because both legs do the same movement pattern at the same time. Symmetrical alternating exercises like running and cross-country are also easy because they are balanced through each side of the body doing the same action. Asymmetrical moves are more challenging because the uneven placement of the limbs in deep water will often cause the trunk to shift away from vertical.

For example moguls, where both legs are placed to one side of the body and then switched across to the other side, are more challenging to perform because the movement is asymmetrical. When the legs push to one side, the body will naturally lean to the opposite side. As the participant feels the body going off-balance, an attempt to maintain the vertical working position is made. This will make the postural muscles of the trunk work harder. An instructor can offer asymmetrical exercises specifically with the intention of core strength development. However, compromised body alignment is obviously discouraged, so care must be taken to select exercises appropriate for the population. The less accomplished mover will react to the loss of control by jerking and flailing to regain equilibrium, potentially overstressing the postural muscles, particularly in the low back.

Evaluate each exercise for postural integrity and decide if the move is suitable for beginners or if it should be considered a more advanced exercise. Deep water instructors need to carefully plan all exercises so that balance can be maintained and additional challenges remain safe and effective. Controlled and precise movements at an appropriate tempo will assist in maintaining balance as well as proper alignment.

Muscle Balance

Deep water should address the basic principle of training all opposing muscle pairs. A balanced workout provides opportunities to strengthen and stretch all the major muscle groups to help gain and maintain good posture, joint integrity, and healthy functional capacity. Fortunately, deep water training encourages muscle balance as the body is immersed so all movements meet the resistance of the water in all directions. However, the instructor must still consciously plan for exercises in all movement planes. There is a tendency to focus movements anterior of the body; lateral exercises can be overlooked and posterior moves are often limited because our eyes are in the front.

Posterior movement is harder in terms of designing exercises. Instructors need to remember that movements like shoulder and hip hyperextension have limited range of motion. As you think about muscle balance, remember that activation of the opposing muscles begins as soon as the movement changes direction. For example, the leg has swung forward in a cross-country ski (hip flexion). As soon as the leg changes direction and starts the hip extension, the hip extensor muscles are engaged. The leg swings from its forward position all the way past neutral and into full hyperextension. This is a large deep water movement with plenty of time to achieve good strengthening of all the muscles involved in hip extension. Full range of motion with muscle balance is an excellent benefit of deep water exercise. No movement needs to be cut short because the foot was placed on the pool floor.

Planes and Axes

Achieving good muscle balance also requires knowledge of movement planes and axes. There are three basic types of axes. They are positioned at right angles to each other. If we imagine a line from the top of our head running vertically to the feet, this is known as the **longitudinal axis**. Another line from the front of the body to the back (anterior to posterior) is called the **sagittal axis**. The third one extends horizontally from one side of the body to the other side and is the **frontal axis**.

It is difficult to discuss movements around the axes without including their relationship to the planes. There are also three planes. Their reference is derived from the dimensions in space – forward/backward, up/down, side to side. The planes are also at right angles to each other. The **sagittal plane** is vertical and extends from front to back, dividing the body into right and left halves. The **frontal plane** is vertical and extends from side to side. We can think of this plane like a 'door' because it is easy to visualize if you stand in a doorway. It divides the body into an anterior and a posterior portion. The **transverse plane** is horizontal and divides the body into upper and lower

portions. Think of this one like a 'table', because transverse movements would be similar to moving on a table that was all around the body. (see Chapter 3)

The movements of abduction and adduction take place around the sagittal axis and in the frontal plane, for example, opening and closing the legs to the sides (jacks). Flexion and extension take place around the frontal axis in the sagittal plane. An example would be bending forward at the waist. The movements of medial and lateral rotation and horizontal abduction / adduction take place around the longitudinal axis in the transverse plane. Envision this as wrapping both arms around yourself in a hug.

The importance of axes and planes to the water exercise instructor is that by defining the essential directions and planes of movement, you have another choreographic tool. This knowledge helps the instructor provide a totally balanced movement experience.

Planes and Axes of Rotation		
Movement	**Plane**	**Axis of Rotation**
Flexion, Extension, and Hyperextension	Sagittal	Frontal
Abduction and Adduction	Frontal	Sagittal
Rotation	Transverse	Longitudinal
Transverse Abduction and Adduction	Transverse	Longitudinal

Transitions

Deep water transitions should be carefully planned to add to the flow of class, help maintain vertical posture, and to avoid injury. A **transition** occurs when there is a change from one move to another. Changing from a knee-high jog to a front kick is a transition. Turning right from a forward run is a transition. Putting 4 counts of centered jogging between a straddle jog and a cross-country ski is a **transition move**. It is important for an instructor to know how to teach smooth, safe transitions and recognize when a transition move is required.

In Chapter 9, there were three type of transitions discussed in shallow water choreography: a basic transition which passes through neutral alignment, an intermediate transition which requires a little more core strength and coordination to pass through neutral alignment, and an advanced transition which requires a lot of core strength and coordination to maintain postural control. Transitions provide smooth links and make for safe, effective sequencing. Transitions should keep reestablishing vertical posture and allow participants to feel balanced. Lack of good transitions can throw a participant off-balance and make the sequence disjointed. Poor transitions can also interrupt the energy of the class.

Remember that reaction time in water is slower than on land. In deep water it will be slower still, mainly because the participant cannot push off the pool bottom to assist with the transition. The body is totally suspended, so it has to be feasible to flow from one move to the next without any additional leverage. This is the reason why you cannot do rocking–horse in deep water. The rocking motion requires transfer of weight from the front foot to the back foot while the body leans forward then backward. In shallow water, you push off the pool bottom with one foot in order to rock to the other foot. In deep water, there is nothing solid from which to push off, so the movement is not possible.

In the deep water, transitioning from one move to the next can be more forgiving than in shallow water. Injury is more likely to occur when the body is impacting when out of alignment. Without impact in the deep water, injury potential is reduced. It is possible to hold the upper torso in alignment and make transitions with the lower torso in deep water that would be more awkward in shallow water. This of course would require a degree of core strength. Because of this difference, deep water transitions fall into three primary categories. These three categories are; a basic transition (T), a transition move (TM), and a tempo transition (Tempo T).

Consider this deep water sequence: knee high jog, to cross country ski, to vertical flutter kicks, to front kicks, to inner thigh lift, to straddle jog, to knee high jog – which brings you back to the initial move of the sequence. This sequence utilizes basic transitions (T) to maintain a safe and effective progression:

- Knee high jog
- (T) Cross-country ski
- (T) Vertical flutter kick
- (T) Front kicks
- (T) Inner thigh lifts
- (T) Straddle jog
- (T) Knee high jog

Transition moves are not required because you can flow from one move to the next, holding the upper torso stable while repositioning the legs. The knee high jog can go straight into cross-country ski; the ski action passes right through the position for flutter kick, so an easy transition; flutter kick is a good position to go into front kicks, etc.

Now consider this deep water sequence: knee high jog, to straddle jog, to cross-country ski, to running backwards, to running sideways, to front kicks. This sequence, needs several transition moves (TM).

- Knee high jog
- (T) Straddle jog
- (TM) - Knee high jog
- Cross-country ski
- (TM) - Knee high jog
- Running backwards
- (TM) - Knee high jog
- Running sideways
- (TM) - Knee high jog
- Front kicks

Why are the transitional moves more appropriate in this sequence? The straddle jog is in the frontal plane and cross-country ski is in the sagittal plane, so this change required a transition move. A cross-country ski into backwards running would also be awkward because two things are occurring: a change of exercise plus the addition of travel. Running backwards to running sideways involves two different directions, not to mention that running backwards in deep water is challenging. An immediate switch to sideways travel could compromise alignment. Although an accomplished deep water exerciser could manage these changes without a transition move, when working with a mixed level group, the safest teaching method will add the transition move. Running sideways involves travel in the frontal plane, changing to front kicks involves a stationary sagittal exercise with a completely different movement pattern. A safe transition would be to stop the travel, reestablish the neutral postural alignment, and then begin the kicks. This would assure that all participants are neutrally aligned as they pass through the transition.

There are many transitional methods that result in well-designed movement patterns. In addition to a basic transition, and a transition move, you can use a tempo transition (Tempo T). Just as in shallow water, you can use 1/2 Water Tempo movements in your deep water choreography to aid in smooth transitions. In the deep, a one-count return to the center position (neutral postural alignment) or a pause center, can replace the bounce center. A 1/2 Tempo kick that returns to center will fluidly transition in to a deep water jack, and a deep water jack will then transition fluidly into most other moves because the ending position is centered in neutral postural alignment. You can also incorporate "doubles" as a method of 1/2 Water Tempo in deep water training. Following is an example of how to use tempo transitions to move through neutral alignment to make transitions.

Combination:	Consider a More Fluid Transition:
8 Cross Country Skis to 8 Front Kicks	• 6 Cross Country Ski • 1 Cross Country Ski, 1/2 Tempo (Ski pause center) • 4 Front Kicks, 1/2 Tempo (Kick pause center)
8 Moguls to 4 Deep Water Jacks	• Moguls in 3 (R,L,R) – Center Tuck Hold • Moguls in 3 (L,R,L) – Center Tuck Hold • 4 Deep Water Jacks
8 Hurdles to 8 Leg Curls	• 7 hurdles • Shoot legs down to center • Leg curl single/single/double (R,L,RR) • Leg curl single/single/double (L,R,LL)

Well-planned transitions in the deep water will certainly add to the quality and effectiveness of your deep water workout while reducing the risk of injury. Having a variety of transitional methods will enhance your movement combinations as well as your teaching skills. If the instructor does not teach good transitions, the movements will feel awkward and disjointed. Participants may attempt to make adjustments because the body can feel that something is missing or the movements do not flow. The instructor should teach safe, effective transitions rather than allowing the participants to self-correct. Here are some general guidelines:

- When changing the plane of motion, a transition move is usually needed unless the body comes back to neutral postural alignment within the movement repetition. Straddle jog to cross-country ski requires a transition move. Cross-country ski (1/2 Tempo-ski pause center) to jacks can be a straightforward transition. Instructors need to follow the pathway of the exercise to see if the limbs can go directly to the next move or if there needs to be a transition move inserted.

- When continuing travel in the same direction, a transitional move is typically not needed. For example, deep running forward to traveling cross-country ski forward is an easy transition.

- Changing direction of travel (backward to forwards and vice versa, or sideways right then left) will be facilitated by a transitional move. Remember the inertia of the water and depth of submersion. If alignment is being compromised, it is better to add neutral knee high jogging before starting the new direction of travel.

- When the legs stay the same but the arms shift to a different plane of motion, consider using a transition. For example, you are performing a cross-country ski with an alternating arm swing in the sagittal plane and you would like to maintain the ski pattern for the legs but change the arms to horizontal abduction/adduction. It would be smoother if the legs come together and perform 4 counts of flutter kick while the arms are repositioned. Then begin the cross-country ski again with the new arm pattern.

- Beginners benefit from transitions in a centered alignment; accomplished deep water exercisers can typically handle sequences with less transition moves. As always, alignment should not be compromised.

Intensity Alterations

Intensity alterations require theoretical and practical knowledge of the physical laws. (see Chapter 6) An instructor needs a clear understanding of "how to work the water" before this information can be passed on to the participants. Although deck instruction is recognized as the preferred method for leading deep water programs, it is also important to see how the exercise feels by spending time practicing in the water. In deep water instruction it is important to remain connected to the water.

Deep water exercise can achieve very high levels of intensity, mainly because the whole body is immersed and the majority of the exercises are systemic. If the instructor knows how to effectively utilize the properties of water, a deep water workout can accommodate all levels of fitness and ability. Do not assume that everything will feel the same when transferring from shallow to deep water; there are differences because your feet are not in contact with the pool bottom.

Overload and Adaptation

In deep water as with all exercise, gradually increase exercise volume allowing time for technique improvements. Participants can easily exhaust themselves if deep water exercise technique is poor. Deep water exercise is typically not about complicated choreography. Classes can use less movement changes and incorporate more traveling, changes in lever length, and acceleration. A good deep water cardiorespiratory workout may comprise fewer base movements with each exercise sustained for longer periods. When the participant is ready for extra challenges, elements of travel, arm variations, and intensity variables can be incorporated.

Remember to reinforce alignment. Do not push participants to work harder if it means that they lose control of form and technique. Increasing fitness levels is not just about cardio and strength, but proper form and technique and improving posture as well.

Law of Inertia

One way of using inertia to increase intensity is to decrease the number of repetitions and change direction when traveling. In shallow water inertia is effectively utilized by creating a sequence such as:
- jog 4 (R,L,R,L) forward,
- 4 backward,
- 4 to the right,
- 4 to the left, and
- 8 in your own circle.

In deep water exercise, there would be too few repetitions and the directional changes would likely be too quick to effectively utilize the inertia of the water and maintain correct alignment. So this sequence would work better in deep water if it was:

- jog 8 forward,
- 1/4 turn R and jog 8 forward,
- 1/4 turn R and jog 8 forward,
- 1/4 turn R and jog 8 forward back to where you started.

The same goal of overcoming inertia multiple times to increase intensity within one movement pattern has been achieved, but with repetitions and directional changes that are more manageable in deep water. Remember that traveling may be too challenging for some participants and they may need to return to a stationary equivalent. Combining moves also utilizes the law of inertia. A cross-country ski combined with deep water jacks uses additional energy to change from the sagittal plane to the frontal plane.

Law of Acceleration

The Law of Acceleration in the aquatic environment, whether shallow or deep, is primarily about force as opposed to speed of execution. By putting more or less force into a movement, the intensity of that exercise can be increased or decreased. In shallow water, one of the ways to apply the law of acceleration is by pushing harder against the pool floor. This is obviously not an option in deep water. Instead, acceleration is utilized by pushing harder against the water's resistance with the arms and legs. The instructor may cue "power this move" to achieve an explosive movement as more force is applied. Force can be utilized in all directions and can be added to a traveling move. More force means more resistance. The amount of force will vary for each individual, but any increase in force will definitely be an increase in intensity.

If the direction of the force is downward, we call this **elevating** the deep water move. The body will lift or "pop up" in the water. This is the same principle as for shallow water, but will look and feel different because the participant cannot use the downward force against the pool bottom. Elevation in deep water is a great example of the Law of Action/Reaction (see next section) as well. Although we provide a specific explanation of each law or principle, in reality we utilize them concurrently.

Law of Action/Reaction

For every action or move in the water, there is an equal and opposite reaction. In deep water this law can be used for refining exercise technique. For example, to achieve the reaction of traveling forwards, the participant needs to know exactly how to move the legs (action) to achieve the desired reaction (forward travel). In shallow water, we can simply push down and backward against the pool floor to propel ourselves forward. In deep water, you have to push back with the arms and legs to propel the body forward.

Participants that are new to deep water exercise, in particular those with limited swimming skills, may need instruction on how to perform the recovery phase, as well as the power phase, of a movement. For example, if a participant is not able to travel forward while jogging with breaststroke arms, this person may be pushing in both directions (no movement), or the wrong direction which would result in backward movement. To travel forward with breast stroke arms, the recovery phase of the movement is when the arms come forward, so forward arms need to be sliced and minimized. The power phase of the breast stroke arms is when the arms pull back so you want to increase the lever length, surface area, and pull forcefully.

Frontal Resistance

The horizontal resistance of the water is very noticeable due to water's viscosity. As you walk through shallow water, you immediately feel this frontal resistance, even with only half of your body submerged. In the deep water, with all of body's surface area (except the head) submerged, frontal resistance is even more prevalent. Remember, you have to travel for the body to encounter frontal resistance.

What becomes important is vertical body position. By maintaining vertical position against the line of intended travel, the body can present maximum surface area against the water. With traveling movements, the combination of surface area and frontal resistance offers the participant a simple way to increase exercise intensity. A good example is deep water running. The participant is often tempted to lean too far forward and streamline the body to go faster and make the movement easier. Cue corrections in body position (the body leans forward only 5-10 degrees from vertical) to maintain maximum frontal resistance, and then offer the speed variable to further increase intensity. As indicated by research, maintaining proper vertical alignment in the deep water definitely affects energy expenditure.

The surface area of the body can be manipulated even more to further increase intensity. A straddle jog projects a wider surface area than a knee front jog, as does holding the arms out away from the sides. Adding equipment like webbed gloves or fins increases surface area as well. The opposite would decrease surface area for participants requiring lower intensity. For most participants, traveling sideways instead of forward or back would create less surface area and less frontal resistance.

Hand Positions

The hands are primarily under the water in deep programming. They play a vital role in maintaining stability and balance, form and technique, as well as upper torso training. The position of the hands should always be defined and clearly demonstrated by the instructor whenever possible. Hand and arm movements help participants get from point A to point B. You need to be scooping or pressing water to move.

The shape of the hand determines the level of resistance; use slicing for less intensity and cupped for more intensity. It is popular to add webbed gloves to the hands to make the surface area even larger. Provide options for hand positioning and encourage participants to modify as needed.

Levers

Changing lever length will have the same effect in deep water as in shallow. Remember to use this simple principle in deep water to increase or decrease intensity when needed. Without the pool bottom to interfere with leg movements, long levers and full range of motion movements can blend to make deep water a very powerful training option.

Buoyancy

Most of the time, the water's resistance provides work in the water environment. Depending on equipment use, body composition, or the type of movement, buoyancy may offer resistance as well. Buoyancy is resisted toward the pool bottom, and assisted toward the surface of the water. Use of buoyant equipment in deep water makes this effect much more obvious. Pulling a buoyant hand bar down under the water using elbow extension will elicit a greater overload for the triceps as opposed to just using the arm.

Speed

The most effective way to train a muscle is through full range of motion. Although speed is very easy to cue and very effective in terms of increasing intensity, the down side is that it compromises range of motion. If the instructor is urging participants to go faster, they will often chose to reduce range of motion to keep up, rather than add more force and maintain range of motion. So a knowledgeable instructor will keep a careful balance between increasing speed and still working the full range of motion. In deep water, when you jog faster, an instructor may use the term "power jog" so that the emphasis is on force more than speed. As the jogging action gets faster the instructor continues cuing for full range of motion and the participant should relinquish speed when his/her range of motion is compromised. It is better to focus on strong powerful movements with good technique and full range of motion.

Drag

Drag is the force you feel that opposes your movements in water, so you experience drag with every movement. Frontal surface area of the body and/or its moving parts affects the amount of drag you experience. The velocity of the moving body and its shape also affects this resistance. As previously explained, we can alter the shape and surface area of our bodies and our limbs in order to change the exercise challenge. Drag also factors into the way we move participants around the pool. If 20 people deep water run across the pool together, drag "shielding" will occur and the people behind the first runners will feel much less drag and work less. By letting deep water exercisers travel all over the pool in individual pathways, the level of effort will be more uniform.

A knowledgeable instructor uses the full selection of intensity variables to create a safe, effective, and enjoyable workout for participants of all abilities. Use inertia and acceleration for deep water running; add impeding arms or legs for further challenges. Use lever length and acceleration for a cross-country ski. Use speed and elevation for deep water flutter kick. Use range of motion and impeding legs for front kicks traveling forwards. There are so many variations to use with your deep water movement library.

Deep Water Programming and Leadership

As an instructor, you will need to learn a new set of skills to effectively teach deep water exercise. Class format, exercise selection, movement tempo, and equipment choices will differ somewhat from shallow water programming. Although deck instruction skills are similar to shallow water, leading deep water requires the ability to demonstrate an entire class of suspended patterns, often with longer levers, to accommodate full range of motion at the leg. For example, a vertical flutter kick cannot be performed in shallow water programming, but is a popular movement for deep water training. It is challenging to precisely demonstrate a vertical flutter kick from deck.

Class Formats

Class formatting in the deep water has evolved through the last decade. Developing safe, effective, and enjoyable deep water programs will require careful attention to specific pool conditions (temperature, size, wall design, etc.), the goals and abilities of the target population, and the teaching style preferred. To expand your deep water offerings and therefore your clientele, consider some of the following program formats.

Traditional "Aerobic" Deep Water Training

This popular format typically provides a 5-10 minute warm up followed by 20-60 minutes of cardiorespiratory training, an optional muscle conditioning segment often targeting upper body and core muscles, and a final 5-10 minute stretch and relaxation segment. As you will note, this follows the general recommendations for class components found in Chapter 9 and represents a continuous training format.

Remember to use movement patterns specific to deep water, follow ACSM guidelines to promote an adequate training response, and incorporate the physical laws and properties of water for intensity variations. The instructor has many options for choreography, style of movement patterns (sport, dance, callisthenic, etc), music choices, and equipment selection to make the program unique.

Deep Water Interval Training

Interval training works very well in the deep water due to the build up of lactic acid. Interval training automatically incorporates recovery cycles to facilitate lactic acid removal. As with shallow water, deep water interval training is comprised of a series of work cycles that alternate between "work" and "recovery". The work and recovery cycles can vary in intensity and duration depending upon the needs and goals of the particular exercise session. Cycles often follow specific work to recovery ratios set by the music or by the instructor.

Interval training is becoming popular because it can provide a challenging workout option for a variety of ability levels and allows participants to work through training plateaus. There are many combinations to consider for deep water interval training with some focusing only on cardiorespiratory training. In group exercise, the recovery period is most often a form of active rest – as opposed to true rest where all activity is ceased. A very challenging workout focused on cardiorespiratory improvements might include a short duration anaerobic work cycle followed by a longer duration aerobic recovery cycle. A less intense format – and thus applicable to a varied group of participants – could utilize an energetic aerobic work cycle followed by a recovery cycle of contrasting exercise techniques. Some deep water interval programming suggestions are included in the following table.

Deep Water Interval Options	
Work Cycle	**Recovery Cycle**
Anaerobic movement patterns.	Aerobic movement patterns.
Traveling cardiorespiratory movements.	Stationary trunk and core exercises.
Resistance training exercises with high repetitions and low resistance.	Dynamic stretching patterns.
Traditional deep water choreography.	Flowing Yoga or Pilates movements.

Combined Deep and Shallow Water Training

Combining deep water training with shallow water training can add variety and challenge to your program. If you have a pool that gradually goes from deep to shallow, you have an ideal environment to try this programming. The participants commonly use neutral buoyancy equipment and travel back and forth between the deep and shallow areas. You can start in the shallow water for a length of time and then finish class in the deep water. You can start class in the deep water for a length of time and then finish in the shallow water. You can also alternate moving back and forth between the shallow and deep water, incorporating the transition as part of the workout. For example you can do a 4-move pattern in the shallow water, flutter kick to the deep water, and then do a 4-move pattern in the deep water. It is important to carefully plan all exercises and transitions dependent upon the type of equipment being utilized. You are only limited by your own imagination and may never run out of ideas for combined deep and shallow water programming.

Transitional Deep Water Training

As mentioned in the beginning of this chapter, transitional deep water training provides opportunities for suspended exercise in pools with transitional depths. In addition, participants who are not comfortable in the deep water, but could benefit from suspended exercise, may be more successful in a transitional depth. Suspended movements and movements touching the bottom are combined to add to the choreography component possibilities. You can use a highly choreographed format, a calisthenics format, an interval format, or any other format your students may enjoy. All exercises must be viable options for both touching and suspended movement alternatives, with appropriate cues given for safety and proper execution.

Deep Water Circuit Training

Circuit training works well in both shallow and deep water programming. There are two primary options available for leading a circuit during group exercise:

- Self-Guided or Stations – Specific stations are designated, usually at the pool walls. Each station has visual information regarding the exercise to be performed, type of equipment needed, and technique tips. Participants move as individuals or small groups from station to station in a uniform manner, with or without bouts of cardiorespiratory group training in the center of the pool.
- Instructor-Guided Group Circuit – In this method, the entire group performs the same exercises simultaneously by following the instructor's cues. Again, there is the option to intermix the muscle-conditioning exercises with bouts of aerobic training. All participants will need to have the same type of equipment for each exercise.

Without the cardiorespiratory segments the focus of a circuit program is muscle conditioning, similar to training in the weight room by moving from machine to machine. With the cardio segments, the program blends aerobic training with muscle conditioning for a total body workout.

Instructors can use a variety of traditional aquatic equipment or stations/exercises that do not require equipment. Be aware of certain organizational elements that are crucial for a smooth and efficient circuit workout in deep water.

- Station Cards, if used, must be easy to read from within the pool and positioned at deck level.
- Equipment at stations must be easily accessible by the participant in the water; consider the amount of freeboard (space from water surface to pool deck) at the pool.
- Avoid additional equipment choices that require fitting. Equipment must be picked up, utilized at the station, and put back without losing the flow of the workout.
- Make sure that the initial flotation equipment (i.e. belt) can remain on the body for all exercises/stations.

Mind-Body Deep Water Programs

Mind-body programs have become mainstream in the 21st century and are a leading fitness trend, both land and water. Deep water is an excellent environment for this format because mind-body programs focus on increased postural awareness and body alignment skills. The deep water elements of core stabilization, freedom of movement, suspension, and joint mobility can all be integrated into exploration of body awareness and postural improvements. Instructors often incorporate movements from several philosophies such as Yoga, Tai Chi, Pilates, NIA, Feldenkrais, Graham Technique and various martial art disciplines. In this class format, you might see a mix of training such as the power of Karate, the grace of Tai Chi, and the spontaneity of ethnic dance.

Deck Instruction

As a group fitness instructor or personal trainer, your primary goal is to lead participants through a designated exercise session while providing education and motivation. Your goal, and therefore your purpose for teaching, should not be to get a personal workout.

AEA recommends that most deep water classes be taught from the deck. It is very difficult for participants to see what you are doing if you teach from in the water. Unless your class is very experienced and is familiar with your moves and program format, you have little choice but to teach from deck. It is also difficult for you to observe your class participants if you are in the water with them; this is important both for body alignment and exercise technique issues as well as general water safety concerns.

When leading from deck, you must always be aware of your personal safety as well. It is not necessary, nor recommended, to perform every repetition of every movement while on deck. An experienced deck instructor will develop a variety of low impact or non-impact exercise options to effectively demonstrate exercises. Also, use verbal cues, hand signals, cue cards, body language, and facial expressions to replace or reinforce actual demonstration.

Safe and effective deck instruction requires not only practice, but also specific training for strength, flexibility, balance, coordination, and movement execution. An instructor must develop skills that will minimize risk for personal injury.

Deck instruction for deep water exercise programming is particularly challenging because you are trying to demonstrate suspended movements on deck where gravity does not allow you to be suspended. Effectiveness is an important consideration as well. The better you show the moves from deck, the easier your class will catch on. There are techniques you can use to enhance your deck instruction.

Some instructors will suspend by holding the rails of the pool ladder to show deep water movements. Although visually very effective for suspended positioning, you need to be vigilant for shoulder overuse and injury as well as the possibility of falling. If you are teaching outdoors in the sun, the metal rails can become extremely hot.

Many instructors use a chair for deep water suspended moves that are difficult to show when one foot is in contact with the ground. Using a 24" or 36" stool instead of a chair may better approximate the movement you want your students to perform in the pool. A stool allows movements in all directions, including turns from side to side or front to back. You can show the movements with less hip and knee flexion when your body weight is supported on the edge of the stool. You can lift both feet off the ground at the same time and show moves that just have to be suspended to make sense. A chair or stool can also be helpful for balancing while on deck, as when demonstrating a single leg hamstring stretch. Be sure the stool is sturdy and is on a non-slip surface.

If your deep water program incorporates hand held equipment, it is helpful to utilize this in your deck instruction so that participants are clearly aware of proper positioning and technique. For example, you might choose to wear a webbed glove on one hand to show whether the palm, the back of the hand, the fist, or the thumb is leading the movement. Or, if your program incorporates buoyant hand bars, consider holding one hand bar for demonstration purposes. Leaving one hand free allows you more options in non-verbal cueing, such as counting down for a transition.

A teaching mat is quite beneficial for deck instructors of both shallow and deep programs. Not only does the mat provide shock absorption when impacting, but can prevents falls on a slippery deck surface. A mat provides comfort when demonstrating any supine or prone exercises.

Cue cards are another instructional aid that can make deck teaching easier, safer, and more enjoyable. Laminated cards with larger print can be helpful in clarifying an exercise, giving directions, altering intensity and adding motivation.

Remember when leading from deck that you are mirror imaging your class participants. Thus, when you want the participants to move right you will cue or demonstrate to your left. Practicing in front of a mirror is a great way to rehearse this teaching skill while also analyzing your movement demonstrations.

Music & Tempo

As water depth increases, tempo of movement needs to be proportionately decreased. Drag forces increase considerably from chest depth to neck depth. In addition to the changes in drag forces, deep water requires you to manipulate from your center of buoyancy as opposed to your center of gravity. Proper adjustment in music tempo is crucial to effective programming.

AEA Standards & Guidelines for Aquatic Programming recommends a cadence of 100-130 bpm for most deep water training formats; this is typical of step-tempo music created for the fitness industry. As with shallow water programming, most movements and exercises will be performed at Water Tempo (i.e. every other beat of the music). Some moves, such as a

knee high jog, can be performed to the beat of the music (Land Tempo) while maintaining full range of motion. Other moves can only be performed to the beat of the music with a limited range of motion. This is acceptable for short periods of time if the participant is able to maintain vertical body alignment and control. As mentioned previously, 1/2 Water Tempo movement variations can also be performed in deep water training.

Target Market

Deep water programming can appeal to the needs of a broad market including special populations as well as athletic and fit participants. Marketing opportunities include:

- The average adult who wants to train in the water, cross train in the water, or combine water and land exercise. Participants wanting to train specifically for core strength.
- Athletes such as endurance runners who want to reduce the volume of weight bearing conditioning; non-impact cross training can prevent overuse injuries while maintaining performance levels. Also, athletes who want to maintain fitness while recovering from an injury or surgery can benefit from deep water rehabilitation and training.
- Obese participants benefit from the non-impact environment. Utilize appropriate flotation equipment to maintain proper vertical alignment at a correct water depth (between the top of the shoulders and the bottom of the chin).
- Older adults will enjoy and benefit from deep water training as long as proper aquatic adaptation is provided. Keep in mind that some senior participants may not have had an opportunity to learn to swim and therefore may not initially be comfortable exercising in deep water. Practice returning to vertical from a horizontal position, maintain a strong focus on alignment and posture, and use extreme caution with additional hand held buoyancy as this may provide too much stress to the shoulder girdle.
- Deconditioned participants who have the core strength to maintain a vertical body position can benefit from non-weight bearing conditioning and the multi-directional resistance of the water.
- Persons with arthritis that need to avoid weight bearing activities and spinal compression. The Arthritis Foundation offers a specialized instructor

training program for deep water exercise programming.

- Individuals with Osteoporosis can derive significant benefits from water exercise. Deep water may be most appropriate for those who have suffered from a bone fracture(s) and need a non-impacting environment. Otherwise it is suggested to include shallow water movements to provide impact stress to the skeletal system – in a safe and controlled environment – to maintain performance in land based activities and daily living skills. When deep water training is included, the following formatting suggestions will enhance the safety and effectiveness of the program. It is recommended that if the pool has both shallow and deep water, finish the class in the shallow area so participants gradually return to the impacting environment. If the pool only has deep water but has a submerged step/ledge, then incorporate some weight bearing movements here prior to exiting the water. If there is no step or ledge and deep water is the only option, at least include movements where the feet touch the pool wall before exiting. For example, facing the pool edge and walking/jogging the feet up and down the wall.

- Participants with low back syndrome, or those recovering from back surgery or rehabilitating from a back injury.

- Pregnant women who prefer or require a lower impact exercise alternative. The suspended position will alleviate spinal compression, the reduced gravity will assist in returning the normal curvature of the spine, and the resistance of the water will allow for training of postural muscles in a vertical position. Many women will feel comfortable exercising with a flotation belt as long as the material and sizing is appropriate. The position of the belt should not restrict breathing during exercise and may need to be adjusted as the pregnancy advances. Options for Upper Arm Cuffs can be offered.

Summary

1. Research for deep water exercise provides a base of good practical application opportunities.

2. Safety for deep water exercise includes qualifying participants, teaching proper entry and exit from the pool with equipment, and proper recovery from supine and prone position to vertical position.

3. A variety of belts should be made available to accommodate different body compositions and provide proper neutral buoyancy.

4. Proper vertical alignment and neutral postural alignment are key to the safety and effectiveness of a deep water work out.

5. Basic transitions, transitions moves, and tempo transitions can be used for deep water programming.

6. There are a variety of training formats that work well in deep water exercise.

7. Utilize the physical laws and properties of water to effectively increase and decrease intensity in the deep water.

8. Teach deep water primarily from deck, keeping in mind personal safety and effective movement demonstration.

9. Deep water formats can be adapted to a wide number of target markets.

Review Questions

1. _____ is greater in deep water because of depth of immersion.
   a. Frontal resistance
   b. Music tempo
   c. Lever length
   d. Air temperature

2. A _____ in deep water exercise is when you insert a move to regain vertical alignment.
   a. basic transition
   b. transition move
   c. tempo transition

Continued on next page.

References

1. Aquatic Exercise Association Staff. (2005). *Deep Water Techniques.* Instructor Training Workshop. Nokomis, FL. Aquatic Exercise Association.

2. Ashlie, D. (2004). *Aqua Hearts® Instructor Training Manual.* Instructor Training Workshop. Vancouver, WA.

3. Ashlie, D. (2000). V.I.P. Populations Section 1. Nokomis, FL. *AKWA* 14:6, pp. 33-34. Aquatic Exercise Association.

4. Dowzer, C., T. Reilly and N. Cable. (1998). Effects of Deep and Shallow Water Running on Spinal Shrinkage. *British Journal of Sports Medicine.* 22, pp. 44-48.

5. Dowzer, C., T. Reilly, N. Cable and A. Nevill (1998). Maximal Physiological Responses to Deep and Shallow Water Running. *Ergonomics.* 42, pp. 275-281.

6. Kravitz, L. and J. Mayo. (1997). *The Physiological Effects of Aquatic Exercise: A Brief Review.* Nokomis, FL. Aquatic Exercise Association

7. Rudzki, S. and M. Cunningham. (1999). The Effect of a Modified Physical Training Program in Reducing Injury and Medical Discharge Rates in Australian Army Recruits. Linthicum, MD. *Military Medicine.* September. 164:9, pp. 648-652

8. Slane, L and YMCA Staff. (1999). *YMCA Water Fitness for Health.* Champaign, IL. Human Kinetics Publishers.

9. Sova, R. (2000). *AQUATICS: The Complete Reference Guide for Aquatic Fitness Professionals.* 2nd Edition. Pt. Washington, WI. DSL, Ltd.

10. Stuart C. and P. Ivens. (2004). *HYDRO-FIT® Hand Buoy Owner's Manual.* Eugene, OR. HYDRO-FIT, Inc.

11. Stuart C. and P. Ivens. (2003). *HYDRO-FIT® Buoyancy & Resistance Cuff Owner's Manual.* Eugene, OR. HYDRO-FIT, Inc.

12. Stuart C. and P. Ivens. (2003). *HYDRO-FIT® Wave Belt Pro Owner's Manual.* Eugene, OR. HYDRO-FIT, Inc.

Review Questions Continued

3. Deep water is beneficial for clients with back conditions because of:
   a. the hydrostatic properties of the water.
   b. increased tempo of movement.
   c. reduced compression load on the spine.
   d. reduced stress entering and exiting the pool.

4. Shoes are mandatory for deep water exercise. (True or False)

5. Applying more force against the resistance of the water with the arms and legs to increase intensity in deep water exercise is an example of _____.

See Appendix E for answers to review questions.

Appendix A:
Shallow Water Exercise

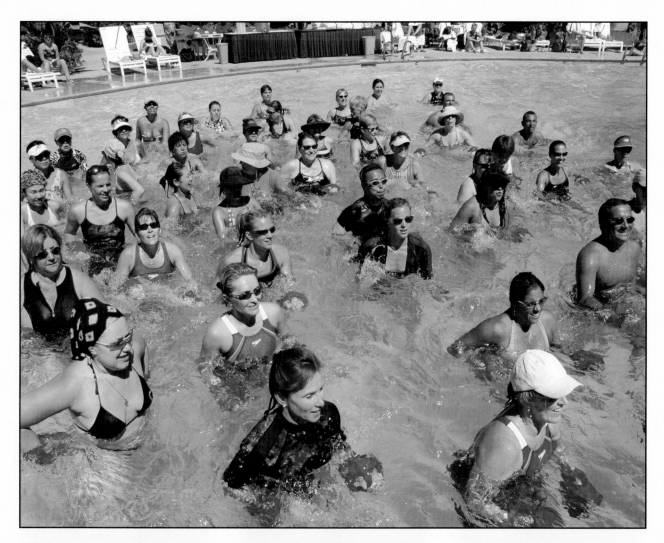

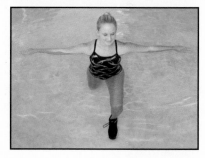 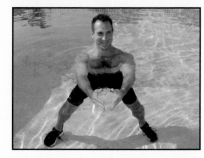 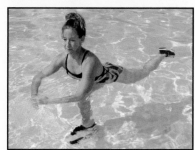

The exercises shown in this appendix represent techniques designed for the average healthy adult.
Special populations and/or medical conditions may warrant exercise modifications.
Some techniques are advanced and should be practiced with caution.

Shallow Water Impact Levels — Jumping Jack Example

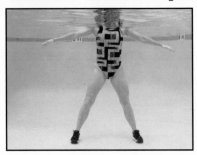 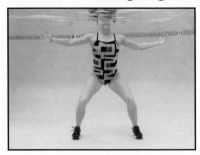 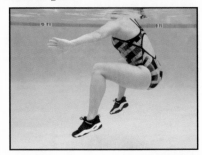

Level I: Level I movements are performed in an upright position with water level at waist to armpit depth. The degree of rebound (impact) can be altered with various methods.

Level II: Level II movements are performed by flexing at the hips and knees to submerge the body to shoulder depth while executing the move. A low-impact option.

Level III: Level III movements are performed without touching the pool bottom (suspended). A non-impact option.

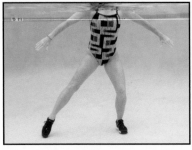 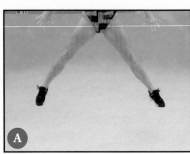 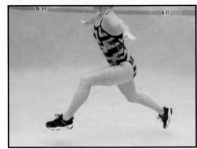

Grounded / Anchored: Grounded moves are performed with one foot in contact with the pool bottom at all times. The variation pictured is a Side Tap. A low-impact option.

Propelled / Elevated: Photo A shows a movement Propelled up and out of the water – plyometric-type training (high-impact). Photo B shows an Elevated tuck or power jump (can be from Level I or II, so impact varies but intensity is increased either way).

Shallow Water Impact Levels — Cross Country Ski Example

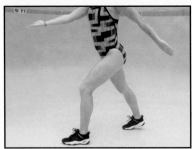 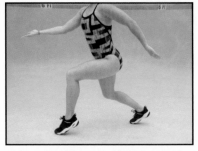 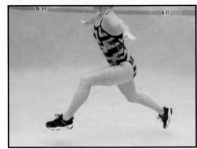

Level I: Level I movements are performed in an upright position with water level at waist to armpit depth. The degree of rebound (impact) can be altered with various methods.

Level II: Level II movements are performed by flexing at the hips and knees to submerge the body to shoulder depth while executing the move. A low-impact option.

Level III: Level III movements are performed without touching the pool bottom (suspended). A non-impact option.

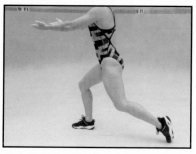

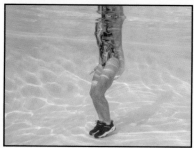

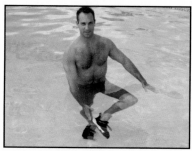

Grounded / Anchored: Grounded moves are performed with one foot in contact with the pool bottom at all times. The variation pictured is a Tap Behind. A low-impact option.

Propelled / Elevated: Photo A shows a movement Propelled up and out of the water – plyometric-type training (high-impact). Photo B shows an Elevated tuck or power jump as the legs switch leads (can be from Level I or II, so impact varies but intensity is increased either way).

Shallow Water Cardiorespiratory Exercises

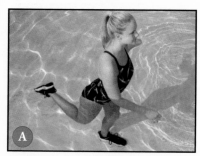

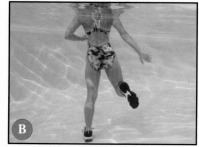

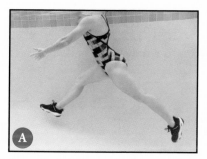

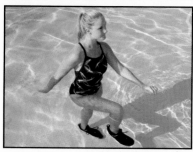

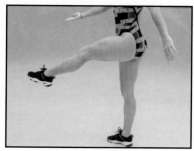

Bounce: Jumping with both feet. A common transitional move, the bounce can be performed in place or traveling; alternating front to back or side to side; or with many variations such as a twist (rotating the body from side to side) or a tuck (pulling knees toward the chest).

Knee Lift / Knee High Jog: Alternately lift the knees in front of the body while shifting the weight from one foot to the other. A low-impact alternative would be a march where the body does not rebound off the pool bottom.

Inner Thigh Lift / Ankle Reach Front: Variation of the Knee Lift / Knee High Jog where the hip externally rotates as the knee lifts; opposite hand reaches toward the ankle.

Leg Curl / Hamstring Curl / Heel High Jog: Alternating knee flexion (photo A). Lift heels behind to about knee height (see underwater view, photo B); bringing heels up to the buttocks may cause stress to the knees. Compared to the Knee Lift / Knee High Jog, this move focuses more on the posterior leg muscles.

Kick Front – Straight Leg: Kick forward of the body by flexing at the hip; knee is extended but not locked. Focusing on the pull downward (hip extension) will place more focus on the gluteal and hamstring muscles.

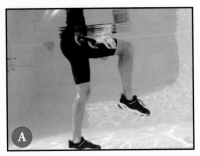
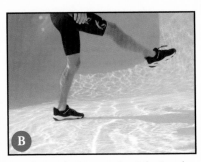
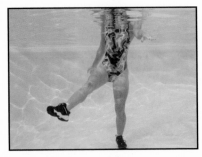

Kick Front – Karate: This move differs from the Kick Front – Straight Leg by involving movement at the knee **and** hip joint. The leg has four positions – knee and hip flexion (photo A), knee extension (photo B), knee flexion (photo A), and return to start.

Kick Corner: This move is a variation of the Kick Front – Straight Leg where the leg kicks toward the outside corner rather than straight ahead.

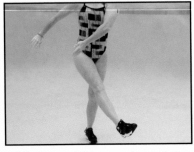
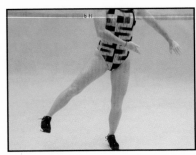
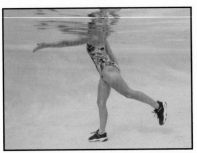

Kick Across: This move is a variation of the Kick Front – Straight Leg where the leg kicks across the front of the body rather than straight ahead. *Because this move crosses the body's midline with the legs, it is not recommended for most participants with hip replacements.*

Kick Side: Kick laterally by abducting at the hip; knee is extended but not locked. Avoid rotation of the hip; the toes should face forward not up toward the pool's surface. Variation: Kick Side – Karate.

Kick Back: Kick behind the body. Keep kick low enough that lower back (lumbar) does not hyperextend during the move; movement is at hip joint. Bringing one or both arms forward will also assist in maintaining spinal alignment. Variation: Kick Back – Karate.

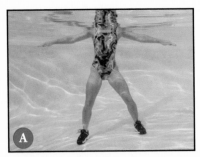
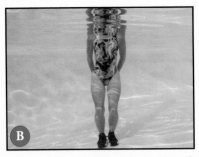
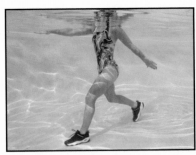

Jumping Jack: Jump with the feet apart into straddle position (photo A) and then jump bringing the feet together (photo B). There are many variations of this movement including Jumping Jack with Ankle Crossovers (alternately cross one foot in front of the other) and other variations using tempo, impact and arm patterns.

Cross Country Ski: Jump with feet apart into a stride position (one leg forward, the other leg behind) and then jump to switch leg positions. There are many variations of this movement using different tempo, impact and arm patterns.

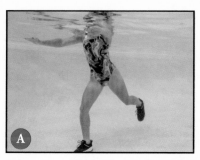
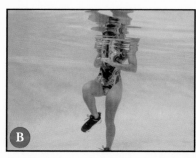
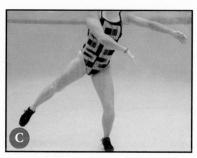

Leap: Jump forward with the right leg, letting the left leg trail behind (photo A). Jump again bringing the left leg to meet the right; by shifting the weight to the left foot, the right leg is ready to repeat the movement (photo B). Repeat several times and change to the left lead. Variation: Perform the leap laterally (photo C).

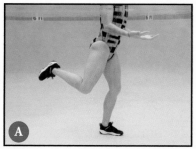
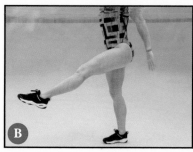
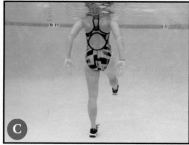

Jazz Kick - Front: Lift one heel behind the body (photo A). Swing the leg forward (hip flexion) and extend the leg at the knee (photo B). Alternate legs, avoid hyperextending the lower back (lumbar) and over extending the knees. Arms pressing back as the leg kicks forward to assist with balance (photo C).

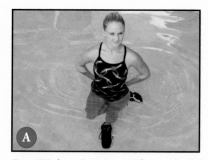
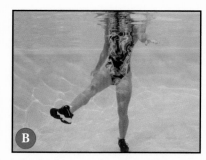
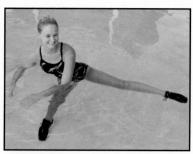

Jazz Kick - Corner: Lift one heel behind the body toward opposite buttock. Swing that leg diagonally (to the outside corner) forward (hip flexion) and extend the leg at the knee. Alternate legs, avoid hyperextending the lower back (lumbar) and over extending the knees.

Pendulum: Bounce on the right foot and lift the left leg laterally (hip abduction). Pull the left leg toward the midline (hip adduction) and bounce on left foot while lifting the right leg laterally. Shift the weight from side to side like a pendulum.

301

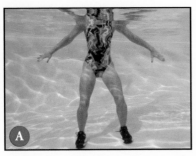
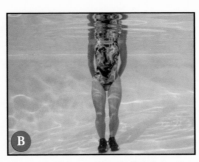
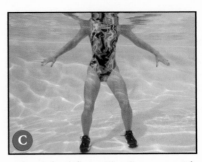

Wide Steps / Side Steps: Step right leg out to side (photo A). Pull left leg in to meet the right (photo B). Step out with right leg again (photo C) and continue to travel laterally the desired distance. Repeat with opposite lead.

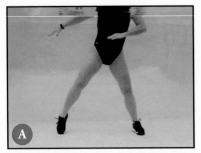
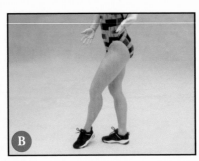
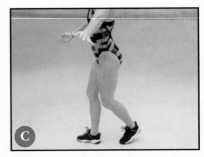

Step and Cross: Step right leg out to side (photo A). Step left leg across the right – alternate crossing in front (photo B) and then behind (photo C). Repeat with opposite lead. *Because this move crosses the body's midline with the legs, it is not recommended for most participants with hip replacements.*

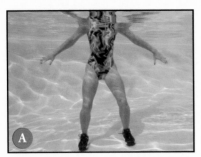
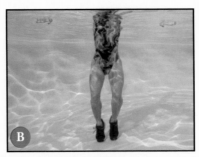
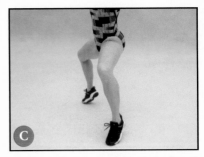

Slide: Similar to the Wide Step, but involves a rebounding action and the rhythm is syncopated. More emphasis is placed on the lead leg and dragging (sliding) the trailing leg in to meet the lead leg. Level II variation on the toes with hips externally rotated – Glide (photo C).

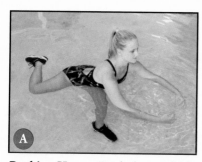 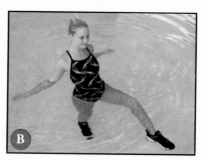 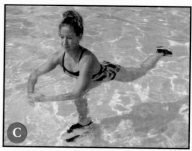

Rocking Horse: Rock the weight forward onto the left leg while lifting the right heel up behind the body (photo A). Rock backward onto the right leg while lifting the left knee up in front of the body (photo B). Alternate the rocking motion several repetitions before changing the lead. Variation: Long levers with the legs will increase intensity (photo C).

Shallow Water Toning Exercises (Muscle Conditioning)

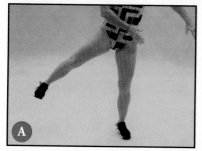 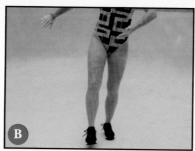 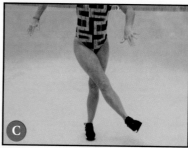

Hip Abduction & Adduction – Hip Abductors & Adductors: Lift the leg to the side with toes facing forward (photo A) and pull back down to center (photo B). Crossing the midline is acceptable (photo C) *unless participant has had hip replacement surgery.*

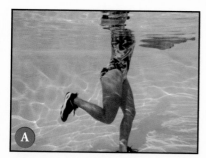 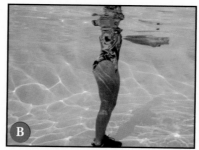 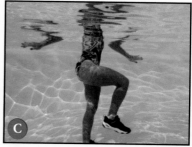

Knee Flexion & Extension – Hamstrings & Quadriceps: Lift the heel toward the buttocks (photo A) and then return to the extended position (photo B). Variation: begin with hip flexed (leg lifted in front of body) – bend the knee (photo C) and then straighten the leg.

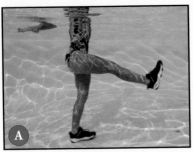
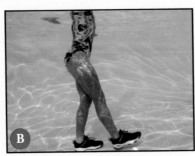
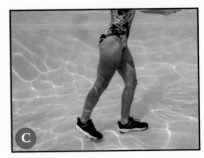

Hip Flexion, Extension & Hyperextension – Iliopsoas & Gluteals: Flex leg at the hip (photo A). Extend at the hip by pulling the leg down (photo B) and then slightly to the back of the body into hyperextension (photo C).

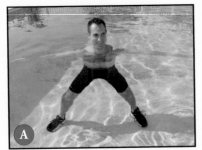
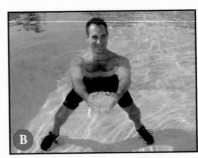
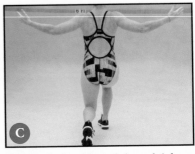

Transverse Shoulder Abduction & Adduction – Pectoralis & Middle Trapezius: Begin with shoulders abducted (photo A). Arms pull forward parallel to pool bottom (photo B) and then return to start position (photo A) while retracting the scapulae – squeezing shoulder blades (photo C).

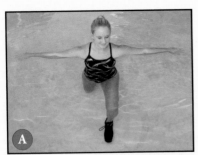
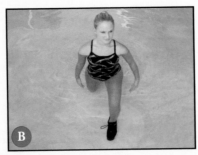
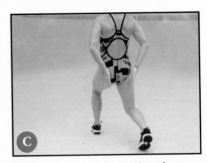

Shoulder Abduction & Adduction – Deltoids & Latissimus Dorsi: Lift arms laterally – abduction (photo A) and return to the sides – adduction (photo B). Avoid lifting above shoulder height. Variations: pull the hands down behind (photo C) or in front of body.

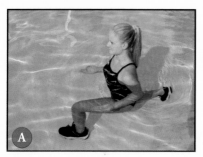
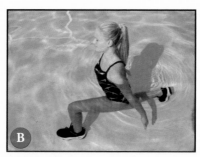
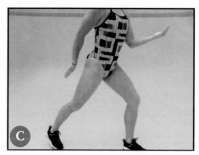

Elbow Flexion & Extension – Biceps & Triceps: Bend or flex at the elbow (photo A) with hands pulling forward. Then straighten or extend the elbow (photo B) with hands pressing down and back.   Variation: Alternating arms (photo C).

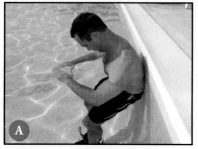
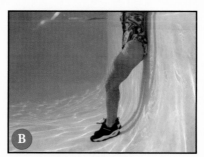
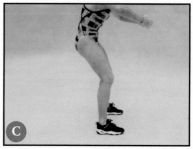

Standing Spinal Flexion & Extension – Rectus Abdominis & Erector Spinae: Flex the spine forward bringing rib cage toward hip bones (photo A); movement is along the spine not at the hips. Extend the spine returning to upright position (photo B). Note: the wall is a good reference point but exercise can be performed mid-pool (photo C); equipment is optional.

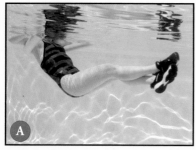
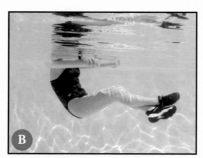
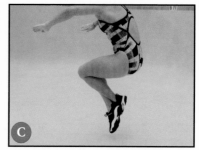

Supine Spinal Flexion & Extension – Rectus Abdominis & Erector Spinae: Performed suspended in a modified supine position (photo A). Flex the spine forward bringing rib cage toward hip bones (photo B). Variation: suspended but in vertical position, rather than supine (photo C).

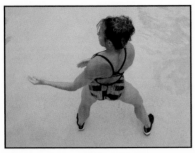

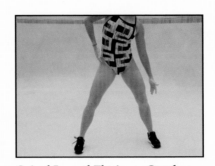

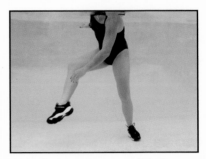

Spinal Rotation – Internal & External Obliques: Perform rotational movement from the spine making certain that hips remain forward. Repeat opposite side.

Spinal Lateral Flexion – Quadratus Lumborum & Rectus Abdominis: Lean the body to one side remaining in the frontal plane, i.e. do not lean to the front or to the back. Repeat opposite side. Visualization cue: slide hand down side of leg.

Spinal Rotation & Flexion – Obliques & Rectus Abdominis: Combine forward flexion with rotation; bring shoulder toward opposite hip bone. Many variations; standing vertical position is shown. Repeat opposite side.

Shallow Water Stretches

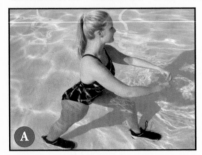

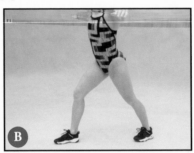

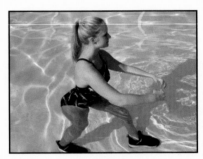

Gastrocnemius: Basic stride position with one leg forward and knee bent, other leg back and knee extended with toe facing forward (photo A). Variations: One hand on wall for balance (photo B) or facing wall with both hands on wall. Repeat both sides.

Soleus: Beginning from Gastrocnemius stretch, slightly bend the back leg, keeping the heel down, to stretch the Soleus. Repeat both sides.

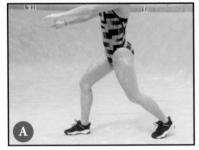

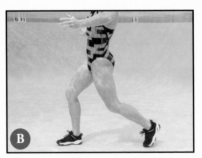

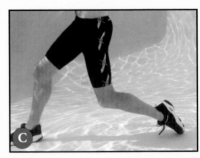

Quadriceps & Iliopsoas – Stride Position: From a stride position, lower the knee and allow heel to lift (photo A); tilt the pelvis and push the back hip forward (photo B). Variation: The top of the foot, dorsal surface, can be positioned toward pool bottom to incorporate a stretch for the tibialis anterior (photo C). Repeat both sides.

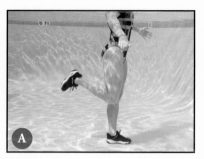 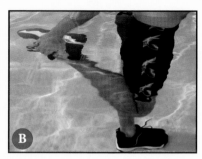 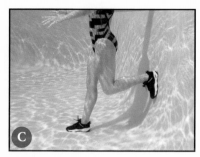

Quadriceps & Iliopsoas – Elevated Foot Position: Lift one foot up behind the body with the knee pointed down and the pelvis tilted (photo A). If range of motion allows, the foot can be held with the hand (photo B). Option: foot can be placed on the pool wall (photo C). Repeat both sides.

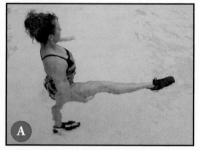 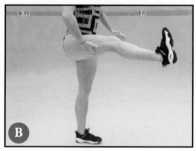 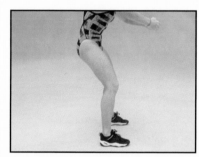

Hamstrings & Gluteus Maximus: Lift one leg up in front of the body (hip flexion with knee extension). Hold under the thigh for support if range of motion allows (photo A). Dorsi flexing the ankle will increase the stretch through the Gastrocnemius (photo B). Repeat both sides.

Lower Back: With the arms forward tilt the pelvis (posterior), tuck the tail bone and round the lower back.

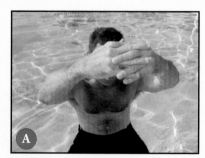 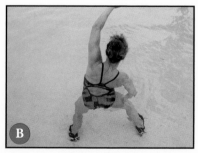 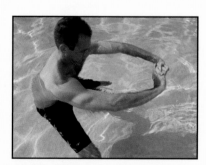

Latissimus Dorsi: Raise both arms overhead and lift the rib cage upward. Remind the students to keep the arms slightly forward of the head to maintain proper alignment (photo A). Fingers can be interlocked or hands apart. Variation: One arm stretch (photo B).

Middle Trapezius: Press both arms forward "opening" or "rounding" the upper back. The stretch can be slightly intensified by lowering the chin toward the chest.

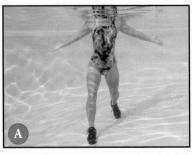
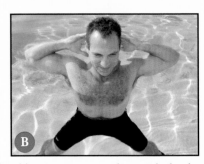
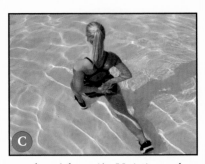

Pectoralis & Anterior Deltoid: Abduct shoulders in transverse plane with the thumbs turned up (photo A). Variations: place hands behind head and open elbows wide (photo B); grasp hands behind the back with shoulders pulled down and back (photo C).

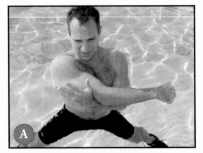
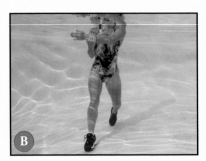
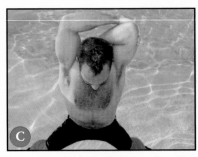

Triceps & Posterior Deltoid: Bring one arm across toward the opposite shoulder at mid-chest. Gently pull with the other hand above the elbow (photo A) or at the forearm (photo B). Variation: Drop one hand behind the head and push gently with other hand above the elbow (photo C). Repeat both sides.

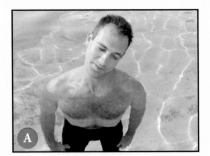
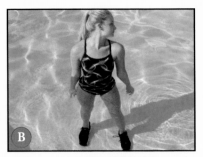
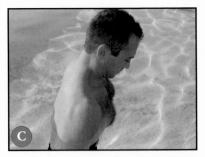

Upper Trapezius & Neck: Tilt the head laterally to the right and left (photo A); rotate the head to look to the right and left (photo B); flex the neck forward (photo C) and extend the neck to look up – limit range of motion to comfortable position.

Appendix B:
Deep Water Exercise

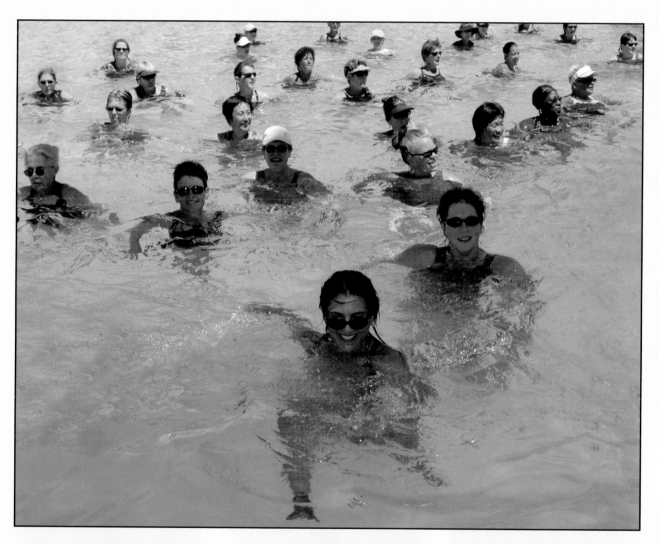

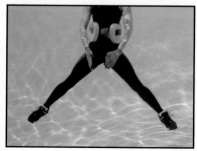 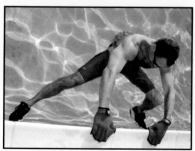 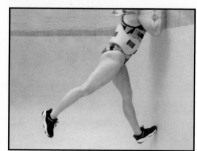

The exercises shown in this appendix represent techniques designed for the average healthy adult.
Special populations and/or medical conditions may warrant exercise modifications.
Some techniques are advanced and should be practiced with caution.

Deep Water Alignment

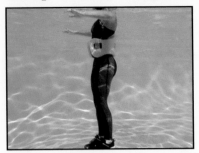

Proper Alignment: Correct vertical position with proper amount of flotation and belt positioning.

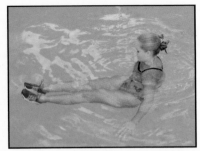

Incorrect Alignment: The legs are flexed at the hips (seated position) rather than hips extended with the feet under the hips as in proper vertical position.

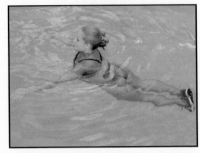

Incorrect Alignment: Inability to maintain upright vertical alignment may be caused by improper placement of flotation – adjust the position or amount of buoyancy as needed.

Deep Water Cardiorespiratory Exercises

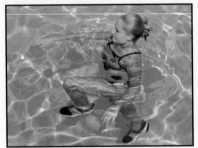

Knee High Jog - Stationary: As the hip is flexed, the knee is flexed with the foot positioned slightly posterior to the knee (side view). Emphasize the flat foot pressing down as the hip and knee extend. This is NOT a bicycling motion.

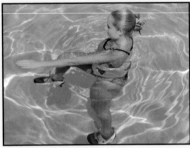

Knee Lift: Differs from Stationary Knee High Jog in that the move is more like a "march" with the foot directly under the knee (side view) when the hip/knee flex.

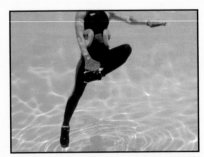

Inner Thigh Lift / Ankle Reach Front: Variation of the Knee High Jog where the hip externally rotates as the knee lifts; opposite hand reaches toward the ankle. Alternate side to side.

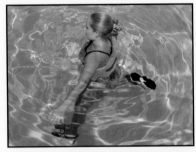

Leg Curl / Hamstring Curl / Heel High Jog: Alternating knee flexion. Lift heels behind to about knee height. Compared to the Knee High Jog or Knee Lift, this move focuses more on the posterior leg muscles.

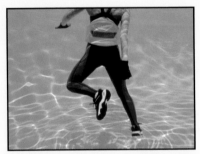

Heel Reach Behind (opposite hand toward heel): This move is a variation of the Leg Curl, where the hip externally rotates as the knee flexes; opposite hand reaches toward the heel behind the body. Alternate side to side.

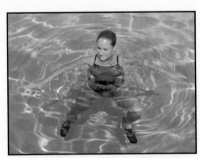

Wide Jog / Straddle Jog: Jogging with the legs in a slightly abducted position (legs apart); may be done with knees high or heels high.

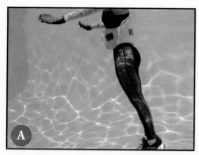 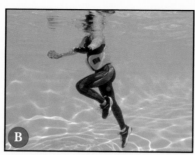 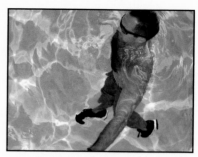

Deep Water Running: This is a traveling movement. Lean the body forward 5-10 degrees from vertical (photo A). The leg action drives down and slightly diagonally backward to achieve the forward run (photo B).

Vertical Flutter Kick: Maintain correct vertical alignment and contract the core muscles. Legs perform alternating, small ROM, hip flexion and extension with the knees soft. Pointing the toes (plantar flexion) lengthens the lever.

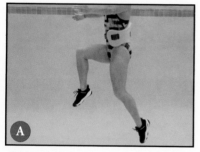 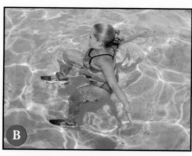 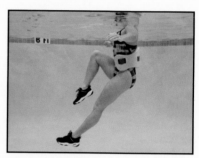

Backward Jog: The leg movement is similar to riding a bicycle backwards but body remains vertical. The feet 'pedal' down and back, scooping the water forward with the front of the leg/foot (photo A). Assist by adding a symmetrical arm action like reverse breaststroke (photo B).

Biking: Body positioned as seated on a bicycle with some flexion at the hips; legs perform pedaling motion slightly in front of the body. Travel can be forward or backward by changing the focus of the pull with the legs.

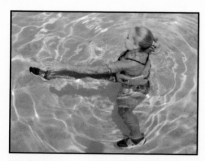 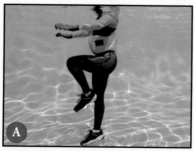 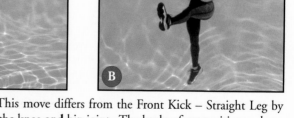

Kick Front – Straight Leg: Kick forward of the body by flexing at the hip, knee is extended but not locked. Opposite leg should remain vertical and aligned under the hips. Arms move in opposition to legs.

Kick Front – Karate: This move differs from the Front Kick – Straight Leg by involving movement at the knee **and** hip joint. The leg has four positions – knee and hip flexion (photo A), knee extension (photo B), knee flexion (photo A), and return to start.

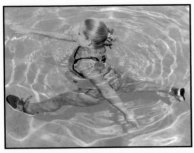

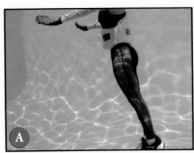

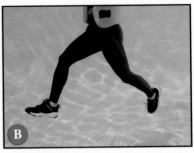

Cross-Country Ski – Stationary: The torso remains centered and vertical. The legs swing equidistance front and back. Both legs remain straight (slight knee flexion).

Cross-Country Ski – Traveling: Lean the body slightly forward (photo A). The knee is slightly flexed while swinging forward (photo B), and then straightens as the leg moves backward into hip hyperextension to propel the body forward.

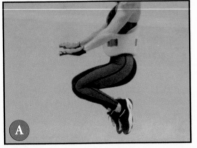

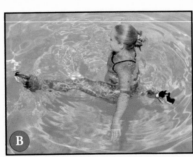

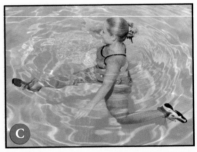

Modified Hurdle: This move initiates from a tuck position (photo A). One leg shoots forward and straightens at the knee (without locking) while the opposite leg pushes behind and the knee remains bent (photo B). The back leg does NOT externally rotate (photo C) as in a true hurdle motion on land.

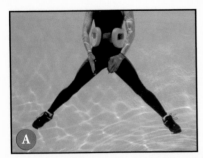

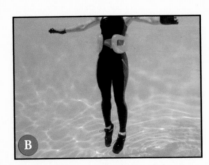

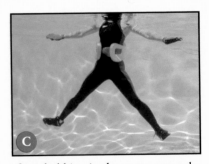

Deep Water Jack: Hip abduction (photo A) and adduction (photo B). In order to keep from bobbing in the water, move the arms in opposition to the legs (photo A). Arms can also move in synchrony with legs (photo C). Many variations are available and options include tempo, knee tuck and arm patterns.

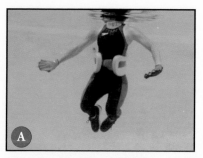
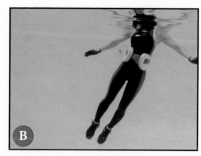
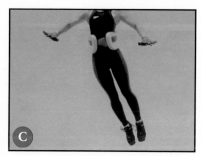

Moguls / Small ROM Side-to-Side Tuck: Tuck the knees (photo A), then shoot both legs to one side of the body, diagonally downward, while maintaining spinal alignment (photo B). Tuck and repeat to opposite side (photo C). Use arms as needed for balance and stabilization.

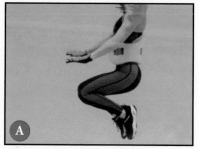
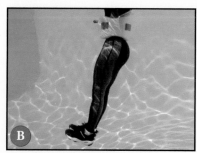
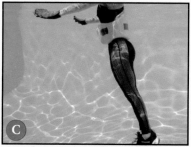

Log Jump / Small ROM Forward and Backward Tuck: Tuck knees (photo A), then shoot both legs forward of the body, diagonally and downward, while maintaining spinal alignment (photo B). Tuck and repeat behind the body (photo C). Use arms as needed for balance and stabilization – arms in opposition to the legs often is best.

Deep Water Suspended Stretches

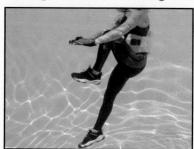
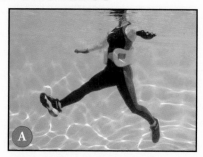
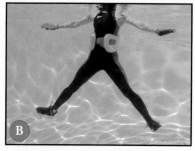

Lower Back: Lift one knee toward the chest focusing on rounding the spine forward. An option is to support with the hand under the thigh. Scull with the free arm to maintain balance. Repeat other side.

Quadriceps / Iliopsoas and Hamstrings / Gluteus Maximus: Slow-motion cross-country ski with a hold at full range of motion and then switch lead leg; arms maintain balance (photo A). Four-Point Variation – abduct legs to jack position (photo B) between the cross-country strides.

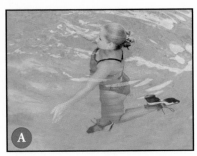

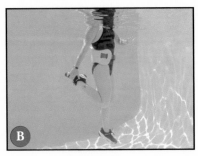

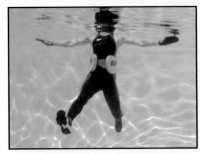

Quadriceps - One-leg: Flex one leg at the knee, lifting the heel toward the buttocks (photo A). If flexibility allows, hold the foot or ankle with the hand on the same side of the body, i.e. right hand to right foot (photo B). Scull with free arm to maintain balance. Repeat other side.

Gastrocnemius - Rhythmical Option: Perform a slow cross-country ski, dorsi-flexing the ankle as the leg swings forward. Repeat other side.

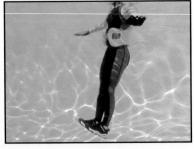

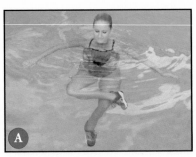

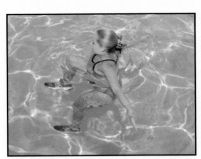

Gastrocnemius - Stationary: Dorsi-flex ankles with extended knees and hips while vertically suspended; arms sculling to maintain balance.

Outer Thigh: Cross ankle over opposite knee (Tailor Stretch); arms sculling or use hand bars to maintain balance (photo A). Maintain vertical alignment of the spine (photo B). Repeat other side.

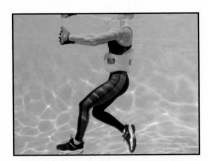

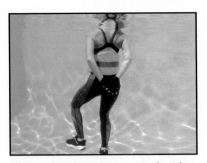

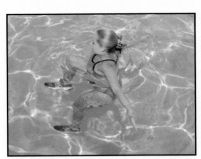

Middle Trapezius: Press both arms forward 'opening' the shoulder blades or 'rounding' the upper back. Perform a slow Jog or Biking action to maintain vertical body position.

Pectoralis / Anterior Deltoid - Stationary: Hands grasp behind the back with the shoulders pulled down and back to 'open' the chest. Perform a slow Jog or Biking action to maintain vertical body position.

Pectoralis / Anterior Deltoid –Traveling: Both arms abducted, shoulders rotated with thumbs up, and scapula retracted. Travel forward with a Deep Water Run to enhance the stretch.

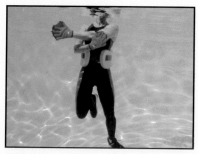

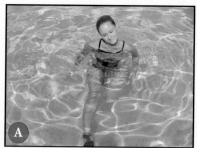

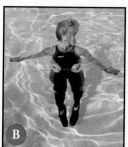

Triceps / Posterior Deltoids: Bring one arm across the body at mid-chest; assist the stretch by gently pulling with the opposite hand above or below the elbow. Keep the shoulders pressed down and back. Perform a slow Jog to maintain vertical body position.

Upper Trapezius / Neck: Tilt the head laterally to the right and left (photo A). Rotate the head to look right and left (photo B). Perform a slow Jog or Biking action to maintain vertical body position.

Deep Water Wall Stretches

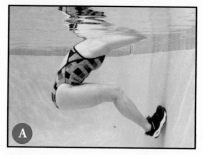

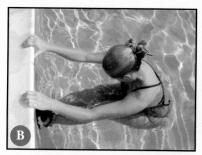

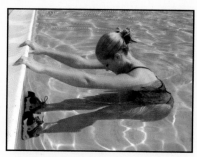

Lower Back: Face the wall, place both feet close together on the wall with the knees bent (photo A). Both hands hold the pool edge (photo B). Round the spine forward (photo A demonstrates without the belt for better view of spinal flexion).

Hamstrings: Begin in the Lower Back wall stretch and slowly extend the knees, but do not hyperextend or 'lock' the knee joint, to stretch the back of the thighs.

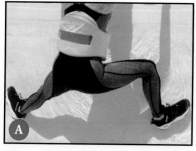

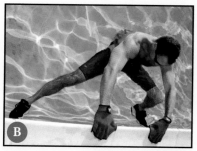

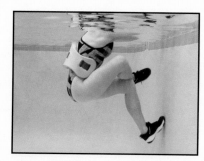

Inner Thigh: Begin in the Hamstring wall stretch and move legs to a straddle position. Lean to the right side by bending the right knee, focus on pressing the left inner thigh toward the pool wall (photo A, underwater view); (photo B, above water view). Repeat other side.

Outer Thigh: Cross the right ankle above the left knee and place left foot on the wall, with knee bent. Visualize sitting in a chair with leg crossed. Repeat other side.

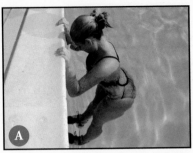

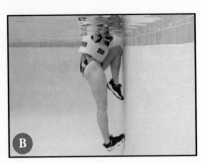

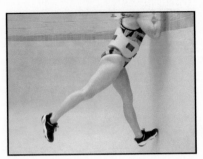

Gastrocnemius: Face the wall with the body long and vertical. Both hands hold the pool edge and the balls of the feet rest against the wall (photo A). Press the heels toward the pool bottom (dorsi-flex ankles). Variation: One leg and alternate sides (photo B).

Iliopsoas: Face the wall with the body long and vertical. Both hands hold the pool edge and the balls of the feet rest against the wall. Extend one leg behind the body to stretch the iliopsoas and rectus femoris of the quadricep. Repeat other side.

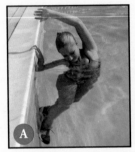

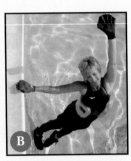

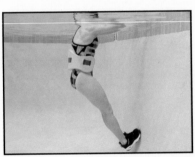

Latissimus Dorsi: Position right side toward wall with right arm holding pool edge (2 options shown). With the feet braced against the wall, allow the body to lean away from the wall. Extend left arm above head with the arm against the ear, and then stretch toward the right upper corner. Repeat opposite side.

Middle Trapezius: Face the wall with the body long and vertical. Both hands hold the pool edge and the balls of the feet rest against the wall. Protract ("open up") the scapulae. To intensify, lower the chin toward the chest.

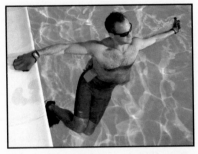

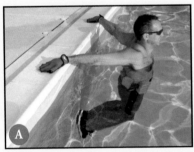

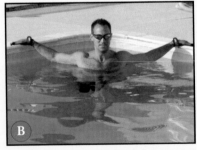

Pectoralis / Biceps – Single Arm: Hold pool edge with right arm, right side to wall. Brace feet against wall, and lean away from the wall. Left arm is abducted; stretch the left arm back to "open" the chest. Repeat other side.

Pectoralis / Biceps – Double Arm: Face away from the wall with the feet resting on the pool wall for support. Hold the pool edge with both arms behind the body (photo A). Lean the body away from the wall, or move the arms closer together to enhance the stretch. Visualization cue: 'bust on a boat.' Photo B shows an option for the stretch at the corner of the pool.

Appendix C:
Pure Movement, Land Movement, and Submerged Movement Muscle Action Chart

Pure Movement

"Pure movement" is muscle action void of gravity, water, or equipment. If you were in outer space, there would be no environmental impact, and your movement would be caused by the contraction of the muscle(s) that move that joint.

Land Movement

Land movement is affected by the downward vertical vector of gravity. Any movement performed away from the center of the earth is gravity resisted, and any movement performed down toward the center of the earth is gravity assisted. Isotonic land movement typically consist of concentric and eccentric muscle actions of the same muscle.

Submerged Movement

Submerged movement is affected by the environmental conditions imposed by the water. The primary force affecting movement in the water is the water's viscosity/ resistance/ drag. Because the water surrounds you and affects movement in every direction, every movement in every plane is resisted in the water. Since it takes muscular contraction in both parts of the muscle pair to flex and then extend a limb, the muscle action is typically concentric for both parts of the muscle pair.

Muscle Actions for Common Exercises for Pure Movement, Land Movement, and Submerged Movement			
Exercise	**Pure Movement**	**Land Movement**	**Submerged Movement**
Biceps Curl Flexion of the forearm Extension of the forearm	Biceps brachii Triceps brachii	Concentric Biceps brachii Eccentric Biceps brachii	Concentric Biceps brachii Concentric Triceps brachii
Leg Curl Flexion of the lower leg Extension of the lower leg	Hamstrings Quadriceps	Concentric Hamstrings Eccentric Hamstrings	Concentric Hamstrings Concentric Quadriceps
Lateral Arm Raise Abduction of the arm Adduction of the arm	Deltoid Latissimus	Concentric Deltoid Eccentric Deltoid	Concentric Deltoid Concentric Latissimus
Lateral Leg Raise Abduction of the leg Adduction of the leg	Abductors Adductors	Concentric Abductors Eccentric Abductors	Concentric Abductors Concentric Adductors
Transverse Arm Adduction and Abduction Transverse Adduction Transverse Abduction**	Pectoralis/ A. Deltoid P. Deltoid/ Infraspinatus/ Teres Minor	Primarily isometric deltoids to hold the arm up at shoulder height Primarily isometric deltoids to hold the arm up at shoulder height	Concentric Pectoralis/ A. Deltoid Concentric P. Deltoid/ Infraspinatus/ Teres Minor
** Squeeze the shoulder blades together on Transverse Abduction to contract the Middle Trapezius			
Front Arm Raise Flexion of the arm Extension of the arm	A. Deltoid/ Pectoralis/ Biceps brachii P. Deltoid/ Latissimus/ Triceps	Concentric A. Deltoid/ Pectoralis/ Biceps brachii Eccentric A. Deltoid/ Pectoralis/ Biceps brachii	Concentric A. Deltoid/ Pectoralis/ Biceps brachii Concentric P. Deltoid/ Latissimus/ Triceps
Front Kick Flexion of the leg Extension of the leg	Iliopsoas/ Rectus femoris Gluteus Maximus/ Hamstrings	Concentric Iliopsoas/ Rectus femoris Eccentric Iliopsoas/ Rectus femoris	Concentric Iliopsoas/ Rectus femoris Concentric Gluteus Maximus/ Hamstrings

Appendix D:
Muscle Actions with Weighted, Buoyant, Drag, and Rubberized Equipment

Buoyant Equipment

Buoyant equipment is relatively specific to the aquatic environment. Any movement toward the bottom of the pool with a buoyant object is buoyancy resisted and is usually a concentric muscle action. This movement goes against the object's tendency to float or be supported by the water's buoyancy. Any movement toward the surface of the water is buoyancy assisted and is usually an eccentric muscle action. The muscle has to generate force as it lengthens to control the upward movement facilitated by buoyancy.

Weighted Equipment

Muscle action for weighted resistance in the water is very similar to land. Although the effects of gravity are diluted in the water, as long as the weighted resistance is denser than water and sinks, it will be affected by gravity. Any movement performed upward against the forces of gravity are gravity resisted and usually create concentric muscle actions. Any movement performed downward is assisted by the forces of gravity usually create eccentric muscle actions.

Drag Equipment

When you introduce a piece of drag equipment, you are just increasing the drag forces of the water. The muscle equation becomes the same as the equation for moving in the water without equipment, however the resistive force has been magnified. You are back to using primarily concentric contractions in any direction of movement.

Muscle Actions for Common Exercises Using Buoyant, Weighted, and Drag Equipment			
Exercise	**Buoyant Equipment**	**Weighted Equipment**	**Drag Equipment**
Biceps Curl Flexion of the forearm	Eccentric Triceps brachii	Concentric Biceps brachii	Concentric Biceps brachii
Extension of the forearm	Concentric Triceps brachii	Eccentric Biceps brachii	Concentric Triceps brachii
Leg Curl Flexion of the lower leg Extension of the lower leg	Eccentric Quadriceps Concentric Quadriceps	Concentric Hamstrings Eccentric Hamstrings	Concentric Hamstrings Concentric Quadriceps
Lateral Arm Raise Abduction of the arm Adduction of the arm	Eccentric Latissimus Concentric Latissimus	Concentric Deltoids Eccentric Deltoids	Concentric Deltoids Concentric Latissimus
Lateral Leg Raise Abduction of the leg Adduction of the leg	Eccentric Adductors Concentric Adductors	Concentric Abductors Eccentric Abductors	Concentric Abductors Concentric Adductors
Transverse Arm Adduction and Abduction Transverse Adduction	Primarily isometric Latissimus/ Lower Trapezius to hold the buoyancy under water. Concentric Pectoralis/ A. Deltoid from the drag resistance	Primarily isometric deltoids to hold the arm up at shoulder height. Concentric Pectoralis/ A. Deltoid from the drag resistance	Concentric Pectoralis/ A. Deltoid
Transverse Abduction**	Primarily isometric Latissimus/ Lower Trapezius to hold the buoyancy under water. Concentric P. Deltoid/ Infraspinatus/ Teres Minor from the drag resistance	Primarily isometric deltoids to hold the arm up at shoulder height. Concentric P. Deltoid/ Infraspinatus/ Teres Minor from the drag resistance	Concentric P. Deltoid/ Infraspinatus/ Teres Minor
** Squeeze the shoulder blades together on Transverse Abduction to contract the Middle Trapezius			
Front Arm Raise Flexion of the arm	Eccentric P. Deltoid/ Latissimus/ Triceps	Concentric A. Deltoid/ Pectoralis/ Biceps brachii	Concentric A. Deltoid/ Pectoralis/ Biceps brachii
Extension of the arm	Concentric P. Deltoid/ Latissimus/ Triceps	Eccentric A. Deltoid/ Pectoralis/ Biceps brachii	Concentric P. Deltoid/ Latissimus/Triceps
Front Kick Flexion of the leg	Eccentric Gluteus Maximus/ Hamstrings	Concentric Iliopsoas/ Rectus femoris	Concentric Iliopsoas/ Rectus femoris
Extension of the leg	Concentric Gluteus Maximus/ Hamstrings	Eccentric Iliopsoas/ Rectus femoris	Concentric Gluteus Maximus/ Hamstrings

Rubberized Equipment

The muscle action created by rubberized equipment is virtually the same regardless of the environment. Any muscle action away from the anchored point is resisted and concentric. Any muscle action toward the anchored point is assisted and eccentric. The position of the anchor determines the muscle group being worked.

Muscle Actions for Common Exercises Using Rubberized Equipment		
Exercise	Anchor	Anchor
Biceps Curl Flexion of the forearm Extension of the forearm	**High** Eccentric Triceps brachii Concentric Triceps brachii	**Low** Concentric Biceps brachii Eccentric Biceps brachii
Leg Curl Flexion of the lower leg Extension of the lower leg	**Front** Concentric Hamstrings Eccentric Hamstrings	**Back** Eccentric Quadriceps Concentric Quadriceps
Lateral Arm Raise Abduction of the arm Adduction of the arm	**High** Eccentric Latissimus Concentric Latissimus	**Low** Concentric Deltoid Eccentric Deltoid
Lateral Leg Raise Abduction of the leg Adduction of the leg	**Medial** Concentric Abductor Eccentric Abductor	**Lateral** Eccentric Adductor Concentric Adductor
Transverse Arm Adduction and Abduction Transverse Adduction Transverse Abduction**	**Front** Eccentric P. Deltoid/ Infraspinatus/ Teres Minor Concentric P. Deltoid Infraspinatus/ Teres Minor	**Back** Concentric Pectoralis/ A. Deltoid Eccentric Pectoralis/ A. Deltoid

** Squeeze the shoulder blades together on Transverse Abduction to contract the Middle Trapezius.

Exercise	Anchor	Anchor
Front Arm Raise Flexion of the arm Extension of the arm	**Front** Eccentric P. Deltoid/ Latissimus/ Triceps Concentric P. Deltoid/ Latissimus/ Triceps	**Back** Concentric A. Deltoid/ Pectoralis/ Biceps brachii Eccentric A. Deltoid/ Pectoralis/ Biceps brachii
Front Kick Flexion of the leg Extension of the leg	**Front** Eccentric Gluteus Maximus/ Hamstrings Concentric Gluteus Maximus/ Hamstrings	**Back** Concentric Iliopsoas/ Rectus femoris Eccentric Iliopsoas/ Rectus femoris

Appendix E:
Answers to Chapter Review Questions

Chapter 1
Review Questions:
1. The rib cage is _____ to the pelvic girdle. (Use an anatomical reference term.)
   Answer: superior
2. The humerus is classified as a _____ bone.
   Answer: long
3. Which characteristic of muscle allows it to shorten and thicken?
   Answer: contractility
4. The _____ muscle group flexes the leg at the knee.
   Answer: hamstrings
5. What is a motor neuron?
   Answer: A specialized nerve cell that innervates muscle fibers.
6. Describe the Valsalva maneuver.
   Answer: Closing the glottis and bearing down to create pressure in the chest resulting in a drop in blood pressure and diminished blood flow to the heart.

Chapter 2
Review Questions:
1. _____ states that you only train that part of the system or body which is overloaded.
   Answer: Specificity
2. Name three muscle pairs in the body.
   Answer: Biceps and triceps; anterior deltoid and posterior deltoid; pectoralis and trapezius/ latissimus dorsi; rectus abdominis and erector spinae; iliopsoas and gluteus maximus; hip abductors and adductors; quadriceps and hamstrings; tibialis anterior and gastrocnemius/soleus
3. Which metabolic system yields the highest amount of ATP for the working muscle?
   Answer: Oxidative system
4. Protein is broken down into _____.
   Answer: amino acids
5. Define the "all or none" principle.
   Answer: All of the muscle fibers in a motor unit contract, or none contract.
6. Which type of muscle tissue is best suited for endurance activities?
   Answer: Slow twitch

7. Concentric and eccentric muscle actions are part of an _____ muscle contraction.
   Answer: isotonic
8. When initiating exercise, the time of inadequate oxygen supply is called _____.
   Answer: oxygen deficit

Chapter 3
Review Questions:
1. _____ is moving away from the midline of the body.
   Answer: Abduction
2. Flexion and extension are performed primarily in the _____ plane.
   Answer: sagittal
3. In a third class lever, the _____ is between the _____ and _____.
   Answer: effort, fulcrum, resistance
4. What type of joint is the elbow?
   Answer: Hinge
5. Name the three normal curves in the spine.
   Answer: Cervical, thoracic, and lumbar
6. In deep water, you primarily manipulate your center of _____.
   Answer: buoyancy

Chapter 4
Review Questions:
1. _____ is defined as the maximum force that can be exerted by a muscle or muscle group against a resistance.
   Answer: Muscular strength
2. Which proprioceptor is found in the tendons of your muscles and measures muscle tension?
   Answer: Golgi tendon organ
3. Name the 6 skill-related components of fitness.
   Answer: Balance, coordination, speed, power, agility, reaction time
4. What is the difference between maximal heart rate and heart rate reserve?
   Answer: Maximal heart rate is the highest heart rate a person can achieve. It is measured with a max test or estimated with 220 minus your age. Heart rate reserve is your maximal heart rate minus your resting heart rate.

5. How does compression lower your heart rate in the water?

   Answer: The water is thought to act like a compressor on all body systems including the vascular system, causing a smaller venous load to the heart reducing heart rate.

6. What are the recommended guidelines for duration of training?

   Answer: 20-60 minutes of continuous training

7. Describe circuit training.

   Answer: A class format of strength or cardio-respiratory stations, or a combination of the two; usually equipment is utilized.

8. List 5 benefits of regular exercise.

   Answer: Improve physical appearance; increases functional capacity; heart becomes stronger; strengthens the walls of the blood vessels; improves strength and endurance; improves the efficiency of the nervous, lymph, and endocrine systems; improves psychological function.

Chapter 5

Review Questions:

1. How is radiation different than convection in heat dissipation?

   Answer: Radiation is heat lost through vasodilation of surface vessels, and convection is the transfer of heat by the movement of a liquid or gas between areas of different temperatures.

2. What are the possible pitfalls of doing vertical exercise in water under 80 degrees (27 C)?

   Answer: Physiological responses will be altered; it will take longer to warm up; participants may chill.

3. What is an ideal water temperature range for a typical cardiorespiratory aquatic fitness class?

   Answer: 83-86 degrees F (28-30 degrees C)

4. What is ideal water depth range for a pool to conduct a shallow water aquatic fitness program?

   Answer: 3.5-4.5 feet (1-1.4 meters)

5. What is usually the primary irritator in the aquatic environment in a chlorinated pool?

   Answer: Chloramines

Chapter 6

Review Questions:

1. By adding the element of travel in aquatic choreography, you are increasing intensity using the law of _____.

   Answer: inertia

2. What is the difference between linear and rotational movement?

   Answer: Linear movement is motion of the entire body forward/ back or right/left. Rotational movement is motion at a joint.

3. Friction between the molecules of a liquid or gas is referred to as _____.

   Answer: viscosity

4. Which movement is more intense based on frontal resistance: an alternating side leg lift traveling forward, or an alternating side leg lift traveling to the side?

   Answer: An alternating side leg lift traveling forward.

5. True or False? Increasing speed in the water considerably reduces range of motion for most movements.

   Answer: True

6. Would pushing the arms forward while jogging forward in the water increase or decrease intensity?

   Answer: Increase – impeding arms

7. Will you sink or float if you weigh more than the water you displace.

   Answer: Sink

8. What is the primary force that causes resistance in the aquatic environment: buoyancy, gravity, or the water's viscosity/drag?

   Answer: The water's viscosity/drag

Chapter 7

Review Questions:

1. List five factors to consider when selecting and purchasing aquatic equipment.

   Answer: Usability, population appropriate, storage and transportation, durability and maintenance, works in your pool, brings in additional participants

2. When the movement is facilitated by the properties of the equipment, it is considered to be _____ movement.

   Answer: assisted

3. When performing a standing leg curl on land, knee flexion is a(n) _____ action of the hamstring muscles, and extension is a(n) _____ action of the hamstring muscles.

   Answer: concentric, eccentric

4. When performing a front kick in the water, hip flexion is a(n) _____ action of the iliopsoas muscles, and extension is a(n) _____ action of the gluteus maximus muscles.

   Answer: concentric, concentric

5. With drag equipment, a lateral arm raise is (resisted or assisted) up and (assisted or resisted) down.
   Answer: resisted, resisted
6. Describe how the anchor point affects muscle use when working with rubberized equipment.
   Answer: Any movement away from the anchored point is resisted; any movement toward the anchored point is facilitated by the equipment or assisted.

Chapter 8
Review Questions:
1. What is the difference between beats and tempo?
   Answer: Beats are regular pulsations having an even rhythm. Tempo is the rate of speed at which the beats occur.
2. Which choreography style replaces moves with other moves one at a time in the original pattern or sequence?
   Answer: Layered
3. What tempo does the following chart represent?
   Answer: Water Tempo

Chapter 9
Review Questions
1. Name three primary options available for the endurance component of an aquatic work out.
   Answer: Cardiorespiratory endurance training; muscular fitness training; muscular flexibility/ ROM training
2. What is the difference between aquatic dance exercise and striding?
   Answer: Dance exercise has more highly developed choreography sequences and may incorporate dance-oriented moves. Striding is water walking or jogging.
3. Give an example of a footwork cue.
   Answer: Knee lift 3, and bounce center- right, left, right, bounce center, left, right, left, bounce center.
4. Which type of cueing (verbal, visual, or tactile) is best to use at all times?
   Answer: Visual- most people are visual learners.
5. Which type of transition requires the greatest degree of core strength and coordination to safely execute?
   Answer: Advanced

6. Name three options for demonstrating or teaching movements from deck.
   Answer: High impact, low impact, non-impact
7. Why are prone flutter kicks considered a high risk movement for most class populations?
   Answer: They may lead to cervical and lumbar hyperextension.
8. List four qualifications employers may look for in an aquatic instructor.
   Answer: Education and knowledge; experience; energy and enthusiasm; motivation; good interpersonal skills; adaptability; responsible; sincere.

Chapter 10
Review Questions
1. What are the 7 positive risk factors for cardiovascular disease?
   Answer: Family history; smoking; hypertension; hypercholesterolemia; impaired fasting glucose; obesity; physical inactivity
2. A heart rate taken three mornings in a row, after you wake and before you rise is a _____ heart rate.
   a. true resting
   b. sitting
   c. sub maximal exercise
   d. maximum
   Answer: true resting
3. Is the Rockport Walking test considered a laboratory or field test for cardiorespiratory fitness?
   Answer: Field test
4. Name three assessments commonly used for measuring muscular endurance.
   Answer: Push-ups, curl-ups, and pull-ups

Chapter 11
Review Questions
1. Which chronic condition is due to excessive, prolonged pressure or from repetitive movement?
   Answer: Bursitis
2. What do the letters in RICE represent for basic first aid treatment?
   Answer: Rest, Ice, Compression, and Elevation
3. You should remove a victim who is having an epileptic seizure from the water immediately.   True or False.
   Answer: False

Chart for Review Question 3

Beat → 8 LAND Tempo Beats	1	2	3	4	5	6	7	8
Front Kick	R		L		R		L	

4. You should always remove a victim from the water before administering CPR. True or False.
Answer: True

5. List three common markers indicating cardio-respiratory overtraining.
Answer: Decreased performance; decreased percentage of body fat; decreased maximal oxygen uptake; altered blood pressure; increased muscle soreness; decreased muscle glycogen; altered resting heart rate; increased submaximal exercise heart rate; altered cortisol concentration; decreased total testosterone concentration; aecreased sympathetic tone (decreased nocturnal and resting catecholamines); increased sympathetic stress response

6. List 3 tips to avoid vocal abuse and injury.
Answer: Keep your throat moist; avoid overuse; renew your breath frequently; use a microphone; if using music, keep it at a moderate level; check ventilation and chemical fume levels in the pool area; project your voice with proper posture and body alignment; minimize background noise; limit talking when you have an upper respiratory infection; substitute a swallow for excessive throat clearing

7. Before using the AED machine, it is <u>not</u> necessary to dry the victim. True or False
Answer: False

8. Obtain a copy of your facility's emergency action plan and see if it adequately addresses all of the emergencies discussed here.

Chapter 12
Review Questions
1. Name the 4 primary categories for changes that occur as the body matures.
Answer: Sensory, physical, heart, psychological
2. Cardiorespiratory exercise in water temperatures above 90 degrees F (32 degrees C) is safe and prudent for larger adults. (True or False)
Answer: False
3. Which cardiovascular disease is caused by blockage to arteries in the brain?
   a. Coronary artery disease
   b. High blood cholesterol
   c. Stroke
   d. Myocardial infarction
Answer: Stroke
4. Which neurological disease is characterized by a loss in muscle function due to the deterioration of the myelin sheaths around the nerves?
   a. Muscular Dystrophy
   b. Multiple Sclerosis
   c. Cerebral palsy
   d. Epilepsy
Answer: Multiple Sclerosis

Chapter 13
Review Questions
1. What function do nutrients perform in the body?
Answer: Provide energy, serve as building material, help maintain or repair body parts, promote or sustain growth, and regulate or assist in body processes.
2. How many calories are found in one gram of carbohydrate, fat and protein?
   a. Carbohydrate 6, Fat 7, and protein 4.
   b. Carbohydrate 4, Fat 4, and protein 9.
   c. Carbohydrate 2, Fat 9, and protein 4.
   d. Carbohydrate 4, Fat 9, and protein 4.
Answer: Carbohydrate 4, Fat 9, and protein 4.
3. Which type of cholesterol is considered to be good cholesterol because it helps lower the risk of plaque sticking in the arteries?
   a. Low Density Lipoprotein (LDL)
   b. High Density Lipoprotein (HDL)
   c. Triglycerides
   d. Fiber
Answer: High Density Lipoprotein (HDL).
4. It is prudent practice for an exercise professional to recommend supplements to their clients. (True or False)
Answer: False
5. Which condition is characterized by starvation and weight loss to alleviate fear of gaining weight?
   a. Anorexia
   b. Bulimia
   c. Binge Eating Disorder
Answer: Anorexia
6. Which type of exercise is commonly prescribed and effective for weight loss efforts?
   a. Resistance training only.
   b. High intensity, short duration aerobic activity with moderate resistance training.
   c. Moderate intensity, long duration aerobic activity with moderate resistance training.
   d. Moderate, short duration aerobic exercise only.
Answer: Moderate intensity, long duration aerobic activity with moderate resistance training.

Chapter 14
Review Questions
1. Exercise drop out after the first year averages about _____ percent.
   a. 20
   b. 30
   c. 40
   d. 50
Answer: 50

2. Which is the most prevalent indicator of exercise dropout?
   a. Smoking
   b. Depression
   c. Exercising alone
   d. Poor exercise leadership

   Answer: Smoking

3. Which psychological concept promotes the premise that internal thoughts are the cause of every effect or result?
   a. The Law of Attraction
   b. The Law of Cause and Effect
   c. The Transtheoretical Model
   d. Self-Efficacy

   Answer: The Law of Cause and Effect

4. List three common motivators that may serve as factors for <u>initiating</u> an exercise program.

   Answer: A desire for improved physical appearance (weight reduction, weight gain, toned muscles, muscle mass); a doctor's recommendation or the desire to improve health; prompting from a significant other or parent; the desire to feel better and have more energy; stress reduction; rehabilitation from surgery, injury or disease; seeing a friend or spouse participating; a desire to do something for oneself, or have time for oneself; improve one's quality of life.

Chapter 15
Review Questions

1. A(n) _____ is legally responsible for covering your liability insurance and paying federal and state taxes on your behalf based upon compensation paid to you.

   Answer: employer

2. Define negligence.

   Answer: Committing an act that a person exercising ordinary care would not do under similar circumstances.

3. Duty is my _____ and moral obligation to my students and facility.

   Answer: responsibility

4. _____ is defined as the process of measuring or assessing risk and then developing strategies to manage the risk.

   Answer: Risk management

5. The 1976 U.S. Copyright Act provides protection for _____.

   Answer: the copyright owners of music

6. The Americans with Disabilities Act was established in _____ to protect the rights of _____.

   Answer: 1990; people with disabilities

Chapter 16
Review Questions

1. _____ is greater in deep water because of depth of immersion.
   a. Frontal resistance
   b. Music tempo
   c. Lever length
   d. Air temperature

   Answer: Frontal resistance

2. A _____ in deep water exercise is when you insert a move to regain vertical alignment.
   a. basic transition
   b. transition move
   c. tempo transition

   Answer: transition move

3. Deep water is beneficial for clients with back conditions because of:
   a. the hydrostatic properties of the water.
   b. increased tempo of movement.
   c. reduced compression load on the spine.
   d. reduced stress entering and exiting the pool.

   Answer: reduced compression load on the spine.

4. Shoes are mandatory for deep water exercise. (True or False)

   Answer: False

5. Applying more force against the resistance of the water with the arms and legs to increase intensity in deep water exercise is an example of _____.

   Answer: acceleration

Glossary

1/2 Water Tempo
Performing water tempo movements with a bounce every other water beat. There are options for placement of the bounce – "doubles" and "bounce center."

A

Abduction
Moving a limb away from the midline of the body.

Acceleration
The reaction of a body as measured by its acceleration is proportional to the force applied, in the same direction as the applied force, and inversely proportional to its mass.

Action / Reaction
For every action there is an equal and opposite reaction.

Acute Injury
An injury with sudden onset and short duration.

Adaptation
The ability of a system or organ to adjust to additional stress or overload over time by increasing in strength or function.

Adduction
Moving a limb toward the midline of the body.

Adenosine Triphosphate (ATP)
A chemical compound that is the most immediate chemical source of energy for a cell.

Afferent
Part of the peripheral nervous system. An afferent neuron carries an impulse toward the central nervous system; also known as a sensory neuron.

Agility
The ability to rapidly and fluently change body positioning during movement.

Agonist
The muscle in a muscle pair that is actively contracting at any given time to move the bone. It is also called the prime mover.

Alignment
Proper posture.

Alveoli
Small balloon-like air sacs in the lungs where oxygen and carbon dioxide are exchanged.

Amenorrhea
The absence of menstruation.

Amino Acids
Strands of carbons, hydrogen, oxygen, and nitrogen. Proteins are comprised of amino acids.

Anatomical Position
The body is in an upright, erect position with the forearms supinated, and all joints in neutral position.

Angina
A feeling of pressure or tightness in the chest. This cardiac pain can radiate to the arm, shoulder, upper back, or jaw.

Anorexia Nervosa
A psychological condition manifested by a refusal to eat to achieve an abnormally thin appearance.

Antagonist
The muscle in a muscle pair that is relaxed or stretched when the other muscle is contracting.

Antioxidants
Protect the cell membrane, lipids, proteins, DNA, or cholesterol molecules by being destroyed themselves.

Anterior
A term used in exercise to describe one body part's position in relation to another. Anterior means "in front of."

Anterior Tilt
Anterior tilt of the head means flexion (flatting) of the cervical spine. With the pelvis, the lumbar spine goes into extension and the top part of the pelvis moves forward.

Aorta
A large artery stemming from the left ventricle of the heart through which blood travels on its way to the body.

Appendicular Skeleton
Refers to the bones associated with the "appendages" and includes the bones in the arms, shoulders, legs, and hips.

Archimedes' Principle
The loss of weight of a submerged body equals the weight of the fluid displaced by the body.

Arteries
Vessels which carry oxygenated blood from the heart muscle to all parts of the body.

Arterioles
A small arterial branch that delivers blood to a capillary.

Arteriosclerosis
An arterial disease in which the blood vessel walls become thickened and hardened.

Arthritis
Inflammation of a joint.

Assisted Movement
Assisted movement refers to any part in the range of motion of an exercise that is facilitated by the forces of gravity or buoyancy, or the properties or mechanics of an apparatus or particular piece of equipment.

Asthma
Constriction of the airway passages.

Atherosclerosis
A form of arteriosclerosis in which fatty deposits of cholesterol and calcium develop on the blood vessel walls.

ATP-PCr System
A metabolic anaerobic system providing immediate fuel from stored phosphocreatine.

Atrophy
Loss or wasting of muscle tissue or function through lack of use or disease.

Autonomic Nervous System
Part of the efferent nervous system and consists efferent neurons that transmit impulses to involuntary muscles and glands.

Axial Skeleton
Consists of the bones found around the "axis" or imaginary midline of the body including the skull, vertebral column, sternum, and the ribs.

B

Balance
Controlling the position of the body's center of gravity, or maintenance of equilibrium while stationary (static balance) or moving (dynamic balance).

Ballistic Stretching
Bouncing, tugging, or overstretching a muscle which can actually cause the muscle to tighten instead of relax. Elicits the stretch reflex arc.

Basal Metabolism
The amount of energy needed by the body for maintenance of life when the person is at digestive, physical, and emotional rest.

Beats
Regular pulsations having an even rhythm.

Binge Eating Disorder
A condition characterized by eating unusually large amounts of food and often feeling guilty or secretive about it.

Biomechanics
The area of kinesiology that deals more specifically with analysis of movement.

Body Composition
The body's relative percentage of fat as compared to lean tissue (bones, muscles, and organs).

Bromide
An alternative sanitizer used in pool disinfecting systems that has much of the same effect as chlorine, with slightly different results. It is used to eliminate pathogens such as bacteria.

Bronchial Tubes
Smaller branches of the bronchi in the lungs.

Bulimia
A condition characterized by an abnormal increase in hunger along with a binge-purge syndrome.

Buoyancy
The force that is exerted on an object by the fluid in which it is submerged; mathematically, this force equals the volume of the fluid displaced time its density.

Bursitis
An inflammation of the bursa, which is a synovial-lined sac of fluid that helps reduce friction between tendon and bone or tendon and ligament.

C

Calories
A measurement of energy or units of heat.

Capillaries
Where the arteries and veins meet. Very thin membranes that readily allow the exchange of oxygen and nutrients for carbon dioxide and waste products through their walls.

Carbohydrates
An essential nutrient. Compounds composed of simple sugars or multiples of them. Carbohydrates are made by green plants in a process called photosynthesis.

Cardiac Muscle
Muscle found in the heart.

Cardiorespiratory Cool Down
To gradually decrease the heart rate and respiration rate before continuing with isolated muscular conditioning and/or stretching.

Cardiorespiratory Endurance
The capacity of the cardiovascular and respiratory systems to deliver oxygen to the working muscles for sustained periods of energy production.

Cardiorespiratory Warm Up
This segment of class is designed to gradually overload the cardiovascular and respiratory systems in preparation for the aerobic training segment. Movements progressively become more vigorous to increase the workload.

Cardiovascular Disease
Diseases of the heart and blood vessels.

Cardiovascular System
Comprised of the heart, blood vessels, and blood. It distributes oxygen and nutrients to the cells, removes carbon dioxide and wastes from the cells, and maintains the acid-base balance of the body.

Center of Buoyancy
The center of the volume of the body displacing the water.

Center of Gravity
The center of a body's mass. In the human body, the position of the body parts determines where the center of gravity will be at any one time.

Central Nervous System
The brain and spinal cord.

Cervical Spine
The part of the vertebral column found in the neck which contains 7 smaller vertebrae.

Chloramines
Combined available chlorine formed when the free chlorine in water combines with other elements such as ammonia.

Chlorine
A popular disinfecting agent used in swimming pool systems. Its purpose is to eliminate dangerous pathogens such as bacteria which thrive in water making the pool safe for bathing.

Chondromalacia
A gradual degenerative process in the knee.

Choreography
The arrangement or written notation of a series of movements.

Choreography Styles
Different ways of linking together moves or patterns either in sequencing, number of repetitions, or both.

Chronic Bronchitis
Inflammation and increased mucous production of the bronchi and bronchial tubes.

Chronic Injury
An injury with a long onset and long duration.

Chronic Obstructive Pulmonary Disease (COPD)
An obstruction of air flow from chronic asthma, bronchitis, or emphysema.

Chronological Age
Physical age as measured in years.

Circumduction
A movement at a joint where the proximal end of the bone remains relatively stable and the distal end of the bone inscribes a circle. It is a combination of flexion, extension, hyperextension, abduction, and adduction.

Circuit Training
A station formatted workout. Stations can train an individual aerobically or for muscular strength and endurance, or a mixture of the two. Usually equipment is utilized.

Coccyx
The tailbone in the spine that is made up of 4 vertebrae fused into one or two bones.

Component
The smallest part or segment in choreography. A knee lift, kick, or jumping jack would be considered a "move" or basic component of choreography.

Concentric Muscle Action
A muscle action in which the muscle creates tension while shortening or contracting.

Conduction
The transfer of heat to a substance or object in contact with the body.

Contractility
The property of muscle that allows it to shorten and thicken or to contract when it is stimulated to do so.

Continuous Training
Resembles a bell curve. After warming up, a steady state level of training is maintained in the target training zone for a prescribed length of time.

Convection
The transfer of heat by the movement of a liquid or gas between areas of different temperatures.

Coordination
The integration of many separate motor skills or movements into one efficient movement pattern.

Coronary Arteries
The blood vessels in the heart.

Coronary Artery Thrombosis
An obstruction or a blood clot in the coronary artery.

Coronary Heart Disease (CHD)
Also know as coronary artery disease (CAD) in which atherosclerosis develops in the arteries of the heart.

D

Deep Water Exercise
Exercise performed in water depths that allow the participant to remain vertical and yet not touch the pool bottom providing a truly non-impact workout. Flotation equipment is typically utilized to maintain correct alignment.

Depression
Moving a body part toward the feet, e.g., pressing your shoulders downward.

Diabetes
A blood sugar disorder characterized by chronically elevated blood glucose levels in the body.

Diaphragm
A dome-shaped skeletal muscle between the thoracic and abdominal cavities.

Directional Cue
Transitional cue to explain the desired direction you want your students to travel or move their bodies.

Diastasis Recti
A separation of the abdominal muscle that may occur during pregnancy.

Dopamine
A neurotransmitter responsible for increased alertness.

Dorsal
The back surface of the body and also the top part of the foot (the instep).

Drag
The fluid-dynamic resistance that acts upon an object that is moving through a particular fluid.

Drag Coefficient
Experimentally determined value that represents the relative effect of an object's frontal profile on its fluid drag.

Duration of Training
The length of time an individual exercises.

Duty
The responsibility and moral obligation of the professional to perform the services following industry standards and guidelines.

Dynamic Stabilization
The body's ability to maintain neutral, or near neutral postural alignment (a stable position) while moving.

Dyspnea
Difficult or labored breathing.

E

Eccentric Muscle Action
Retaining tension in a muscle as it lengthens.

Eddies
Rotary movements of a fluid.

Efferent
Part of the peripheral nervous system. The efferent neurons, also known as motor neurons, relay "outgoing" information from the central nervous system to the muscle cells.

Elasticity
A property which allows a muscle to return to its original shape after it is contracted or extended.

Elevation
Moving a body part towards the head, e.g. shrugging the shoulders upward.

Ellipsoidal or Condyloid Joint
This joint is formed by an oval convex surface placed near an elliptical concave surface. Example: Radiocarpal (wrist) joint.

Embolism
A sudden obstruction of a blood vessel, usually caused by a clot carried in the blood stream.

Emphysema
A lung disease causing thinning and loss of elasticity of the lung tissue.

Employee
A person who is hired to provide services to a company on a regular basis in exchange for compensation, and who does not provide these services as part of an independent business.

Enzymes
Proteins that are produced in living cells that accelerate metabolic reactions.

Erythrocytes
Red blood cells that contain the protein hemoglobin, which is the site where oxygen is carried in the blood.

Evaporation
Loss of body heat through the sweating mechanism. The evaporation of sweat from the skin cools the body.

Eversion
Turning the sole of the foot outward or laterally.

Excitability
A property of muscle that allows the muscle to receive and respond to stimuli.

Exercise Adherence
An individual's commitment to participating in a regular exercise program.

Exercise Behavior
Behaviors that motivate an individual to initiate and maintain regular exercise. It also dictates how a person chooses to exercise.

Exercise Compliance
An individual participating in an exercise program following the recommended parameters for mode, intensity, duration, and frequency.

Extensibility
A property in muscle that allows the muscle to stretch.

Extension
Increasing the angle at a joint or returning to anatomical position.

Extrinsic Reinforcement
External incentives and rewards that provide motivation.

F

Fascia
A connective tissue covering found on the muscle.

Fascicules
Bundles of fibers in the muscle that are actually bundles of muscle cells bound by connective tissue.

Fast-Twitch Muscle Fiber
A "white" muscle fiber characterized by its fast speed of contraction and a high capacity for anaerobic glycolysis.

Fats
An essential nutrient. Lipids as a whole are referred to as fats. Lipids are a family of compounds that are soluble in organic solvents but not in water.

Flat Bone
A flat bone is thin and generally flat as the term implies. Examples would include the cranial bones and the scapula.

Flexibility
The ability of limbs to move at the joints through a normal range of motion.

Flexion
Decreasing the angle at a joint or moving out of anatomical position.

Fiber
The part of the plant that the human body cannot typically digest. There are two forms of dietary fiber, soluble (can absorb water) and insoluble (cannot absorb water) and each has important health benefits.

Footwork Cue
A transitional cue that provides detailed movement cues specific to the lower body, usually expressed as left or right.

Form Cue
A signal to participants to take note of body alignment and technique.

Forward Head
The mastoid process landmark is anterior to the lateral line of gravity.

Free Radicals
Highly reactive molecules often containing oxygen, produced by normal body processes.

Frequency of Training
How often you should exercise or train.

Frontal Axis
The axis that extends horizontally from one side of the body to the other side at about waist height.

Frontal Plane
An imaginary longitudinal plane that divides the body into anterior and posterior halves.

Frontal Resistance
Results from the horizontal forces of the water.

Functional Age
Age as measured by the ability of the individual to maintain daily activities related to independent living.

G

Genu Recurvatum
Knee hyperextension. The knee landmark is posterior to the lateral line of gravity.

Gluconeogenesis
The formation of glucose from something other than carbohydrate.

Glucose
The simple sugar made by the body from carbohydrates.

Glycogen
Sometimes called animal starch, is the storage from of glucose found in animals.

Glycogenolysis
The breakdown of glycogen.

Glycolytic System
An anaerobic metabolic system providing an intermediate source of ATP and the by-product lactic acid.

Golgi Tendon Organ
A sensory organ in the tendon that recognizes changes in tension in the muscle.

H

Health History
A process conducted using a questionnaire or interview to collect information about a client and determine any health risks.

Heart Attack
Medically known as myocardial infarction in which a section of the heart dies due to lack of blood supply.

Heart Rate Reserve (HRR)
Maximal heart rate minus resting heart rate.

Heat Cramps
Overexposure to heat combined with inadequate rehydration can cause muscle cramping (calf cramping is common).

Heat Exhaustion
Overexposure to heat combined with inadequate rehydration can cause heat exhaustion. The symptoms are pale, clammy skin; profuse sweating; dizziness; weak, rapid pulse; shallow breathing; nausea; headache; and loss of consciousness.

Heat Stroke
Overexposure to heat combined with inadequate rehydration can cause heat stroke which is a medial emergency. The symptoms are hot, dry, very red skin; generally no perspiration; rapid and strong pulse; labored breathing; loss of consciousness.

Hemoglobin
Protein in the blood where oxygen is carried. Iron is an essential component of hemoglobin and bonds with oxygen.

Hinge or Ginglymus Joint
Involves two articular surfaces that restrict movement primarily to one axis. Example: elbow, knee, ankle.

High Density Lipoproteins (HDL)
HDL act as scavengers and pick up excess cholesterol and phospholipids from the tissues and return them to the liver for disposal. HDL have earned themselves the labels of being "good cholesterol."

Hydrostatic Pressure
The pressure exerted by molecules of a fluid upon an immersed body.

Hyperextension
Going beyond neutral extension.

Hyperglycemia
An imbalance of glucose levels (elevated level) due to various factors. Signs and symptoms include fatigue, extreme thirst, frequent urination, hunger, blurred vision and sudden weight loss.

Hypertension
High blood pressure.

Hypertrophy
A term used to describe an increase in the size, girth, or function of muscle tissue.

Hypoglycemia
An imbalance of glucose levels (low level) due to various factors. Signs and symptoms include sweaty/clammy skin, hunger, feeling confused, dizziness, rapid heart rate, feeling nervous/shaky, and mood changes.

I

Independent Contractor
A person or business that provides goods or services to another entity under terms specified in a contract

Indirect Reinforcement
Motivation resulting from one or more factors in the participant's surroundings.

Inertia
An object remains at rest or in motion with constant velocity unless acted on by a net external force.

Inferior
A term used in exercise to describe one body part's position in relation to another. Inferior means "below."

Informed Consent Form
A signed form documenting that the client has been fully informed of the risks and possible discomforts involved in a physical fitness program.

Insertion
Most muscles have at least two tendons, each one attaching to a bone. The one which tends to be more mobile is called the insertion.

Insulin
A hormone that stimulates the movement of glucose and amino acids into most cells and stimulates the syntheses of protein, fat, and glycogen.

Intensity of Training
An objective or subjective measure of how hard an individual is exercising.

Interval Training
Consists of "harder" bouts of exercise (work cycles) interspersed with "easier" bouts of exercise (recovery cycles).

Intrinsic Reinforcement
Motivation resulting from the activity itself being the reward.

Inversion
Turning the sole of the foot inward or medially.

Irregular Bone
A bone with a complex shape such as a vertebra.

Isokinetic
A type of muscular action where movement occurs at the joint as in an isotonic action, however, the tension remains constant as in an isometric action.

Isometric
Muscle actions that occur when tension is developed in the muscle without movement at the joint or a change in the muscle length. The tension remains constant because the length of the muscle does not change.

Isotonic
Muscle actions where the muscle shortens and lengthens and movement occurs at the joint.

J

Joint
The mechanisms by which bones are held together. The point where two bones meet allowing some degree of movement. There are three basic categories of joints – immovable, slightly moveable and freely moveable (synovial).

K

Karvonen's Formula
A mathematical equation which figures in heart rate reserve for determining a target heart rate range. Personalizes heart rate measurement by factoring in a person's resting heart rate.

Ketosis
A condition in which ketones, or abnormal products of fat metabolism, accumulate in the blood.

Kilocalorie
The amount of heat required to raise the temperature of a kilogram (a liter) of water 1 degree Celsius.

Kinesiology
The study of human movement.

Kyphosis
Abnormal curvature of the spine. Kyphosis (humped back) refers to an exaggerated curve in the thoracic region. The head is often too far forward with rounded shoulders and sunken chest.

L

Land Tempo (LT)
Movement at the same speed used on land. Movement occurs at each beat.

Lateral
A term used in exercise to describe one body part's position in relation to another. Lateral means "away from the midline."

Lateral (External) Rotation
Also called outward rotation and occurs primarily at the hip and shoulder joints. Rotation refers to movement around the long axis of the limb.

Layer Technique
A pattern in choreography that can be repeated; the pattern first can be taught via pure repetition, add-on, or pyramid choreography.

Left Atrium
A receiving chamber of the heart where the oxygenated blood arrives from the alveoli in the lunges.

Left Ventricle
A sending chamber of the heart that pumps the oxygenated blood out of the heart.

Leukocytes
White blood cells that protect the body from infectious diseases and provide immunity.

Level I
Standing in an upright position and rebounding, or pushing off, from the pool bottom.

Level II
Flexing at the hips and knees to lower the body to a position where the shoulders are at the water's surface. The feet will still contact the pool bottom but without the rebounding or jumping forces.

Level III
Flexing at the hips and knees to lower the body to a position where the shoulders are at the water's surface while keeping the feet elevated from the pool bottom for several repetitions.

Lever
Rigid bars that turn about an axis. The axis or fulcrum can be visualized as a pivot point. In the body the bones represent the rigid bars and the joints are the axis (fulcrum).

Lifeguard Lung Disease
An asthma-like condition resulting from bacteria in indoor aquatic facilities that have water spray features.

Ligament
A band of tissue, usually dense, white, and fibrous, which attaches bone to bone.

Linear Progression or Freestyle Choreography
A style of choreography where a series of moves are performed without a predictable pattern (hence the term "Freestyle").

Lipids
A family of compounds that are soluble in organic solvents but not in water.

Long Bone
A bone that is longer than it is wide. Long bones include the femur, tibia, and humerus.

Longitudinal Axis
A line from the top of the head running vertically to the feet through the center of the body.

Lordosis
Abnormal curvature of the spine. Lordosis (bent backward) is an increased concave curve in the lumbar region of the spine. Lordosis is often accompanied by an increased anterior pelvic tilt. The abdomen and the buttocks will protrude and the arms hang further back.

Low Density Lipoproteins (LDL)
LDL carry cholesterol and triglycerides from the liver to the tissues. It is the cholesterol in LDL that finds its way into the plaques of atherosclerosis, and LDL cholesterol has been named the "bad cholesterol."

Lumbar Spine
The low back area of the vertebral column that consists of 5 large vertebrae.

M

Maximal Heart Rate (HRmax)
The highest heart rate an individual can achieve during an exercise session. A commonly accepted estimate of maximal heart rate is 220- age.

Medial
A term used in exercise to describe one body part's position in relation to another. Medial means "toward the midline."

Medial (Internal) Rotation
Also called inward rotation and occurs primarily at the hip and shoulder joints. Rotation refers to movement around the long axis of the limb.

MET Level
Metabolic equivalent. Term used to describe exercise intensity. A single MET equals the energy expended during 1 minute of rest.

Metabolic Respiration
The conversion of chemical energy to mechanical energy needed for muscular contractions.

Metabolism
The sum of all chemical processes occurring within a living cell or organism.

Minerals
An essential nutrient. Naturally occurring, inorganic homogeneous substances.

Mitochondria
Specialized sub cellular compartment in the muscle cell. The powerhouse of the cell, capable of producing mass quantities of ATP to fuel muscular contractions.

Mode of Training
The type of exercise being done.

Monounsaturated
When there is only one point of unsaturation in the chain of fatty acids.

Motion
Motion occurs when a person changes his or her location in space.

Motivational Cue
A verbal of nonverbal signal used for encouragement and reinforcement.

Motor Neurons
Specialized nerve cells that innervate muscle fibers.

Motor Unit
Consists of one motor neuron and all of the myofibrils it stimulates.

Movement or Step Cue
A transitional cue that expresses the basic movement that is being performed.

Muscle Balance
Balance in strength and flexibility in muscle pairs allowing for proper posture and stability in the body.

Muscle Spindle
A sensory organ in the muscle that relays information about length and speed of stretch to the central nervous system.

Muscular Conditioning
A segment of class designed to isolated specific muscle groups in order to promote strength and/ or endurance through resistance training.

Muscular Endurance
The capacity of a muscle to exert force repeatedly or to hold a fixed or static contraction over time.

Muscular Strength
The maximum force that can be exerted by a muscle or muscle group against a resistance.

Muscular System
Comprised of skeletal, visceral, and cardiac muscle tissue. There are more than 600 muscles in the human body.

Musculoskeletal Disorders
Any problem dealing the muscles, tendons, ligaments, bones, and/ or joints.

Myofibrils
Protein filaments that bundled together make the fibers that bundled together make muscles.

N

Nervous System
Is comprised of the brain, spinal cord, nerves, and the sense organs, It serves as the control center and communication network within the body.

Neutral Buoyancy
The gravity-versus-buoyancy relationship that results from the force of weight being equal to the force of buoyancy (causing the object to remain suspended at some intermediate point within the fluid).

Numerical Cue
A transitional cue that communicates the desired repetitions of each movement.

Nutrients
Components of food that help to nourish the body by performing any of the following functions: provide energy, serve as building material, help maintain or repair body parts, promote or sustain growth, and regulate or assist body processes.

Nutrition
The study of nutrients in foods and their functions in the body.

O

Obesity
A condition where there is "an excess of body fat frequently resulting in a significant impairment of health," a level of 20% or more above ideal body weight.

Origin
Most muscles have at least two tendons, each one attaching to a bone. One of these attachments tends to be more stationary or immobile and is referred to as the muscle's origin.

Ossification
The process by which bone grows in the body.

Osteoarthritis

A form of arthritis in which degenerative changes occur in the joint causing pain, swelling, and loss of normal mobility.

Overload

A greater than normal stress or demand placed upon a physiological system or organ typically resulting in an increase in strength or function.

Overtraining

Excessive exercise resulting in various physical symptoms such as chronic fatigue or insomnia.

Overuse Injuries

Repetitive injury caused by repetitive activities, i.e., tendonitis, bursitis.

Overweight

A condition where an individual's weight exceeds the population norm or average, which is determined by height-weight tables based on gender, height, and frame size.

Oxidative System

An aerobic metabolic system in the body that yields large amounts of ATP and the by-products carbon dioxide, water and heat.

Oxygen Debt or EPOC

The volume of oxygen required to oxidize the lactic acid produced by exercise.

Oxygen Deficit

The time when commencing exercise where there is an inadequate oxygen supply.

P

Pattern

A pattern or combination is two or more moves linked together to form some type of repeatable sequence in choreography.

Peripheral Nervous System

(PNS) Connects the brain and spinal cord with receptors, muscles, and glands.

Physical Fitness

The ability of the body's physical parts to function, measured by the level at which these physical parts are capable of functioning.

Physician's Consent Form

A written medical clearance by a physician.

Pivot or Trochoid Joint

Formed by a central bony pivot surrounded by osteoligamentous ring. Rotation is the only movement possible. Example: Superior radioulnar joint.

Plane or Gliding Joint

These joints are formed by the proximity of two relatively flat surfaces. This allows gliding movements to occur. Example: Intertarsal joints (in the foot).

Plantar

Refers to the bottom surface or the sole of the foot.

Plantar Fasciitis

A chronic condition that affects the bottom or heel of the foot.

Platelets

Blood cells which function to prevent blood loss, including the clotting mechanism.

Polyunsaturated

Refers to a triglyceride in which two or more carbons have double bonds.

Posterior

A term used in exercise to describe one body part's position in relation to another. Posterior means "in back of" or "behind."

Posterior Tilt

Movement used to describe movement of the head or pelvis. With the head, it will result in extension of the cervical spine (chin up), with the pelvis, it will be opposite, with the lumbar spine flexing or flattening.

Post-stretch

Part of the cool down, consisting of stretching exercises to return muscles to pre-exercise length.

Power

A function of strength and speed. The ability to transfer energy into force at a quick rate.

Pre-stretch

Static stretching exercises performed after the thermal warm up and before the cardio respiratory warm up.

Preventive Nutrition

The concept of eating well in order to stave off certain disease conditions.

Progression

Gradually increasing intensity, duration, and frequency over time to reduce the risk of injury and improve exercise compliance.

Progressive Overload
A gradual and systematic increase in the stress or demand placed upon a physiological system or organ to avoid the risk of chronic fatigue or injury.

Projected Area
The surface area of a piece of equipment that will determine the amount of drag force.

Pronation
Rotating or turning the forearm inward, so the palm of the hand is facing behind in anatomical position.

Prone
Refers to the body lying in a "face-down" position.

Proteins
An essential nutrient. Proteins are compounds of carbons, hydrogen, oxygen, and nitrogen arranged into strands called amino acids.

Protraction
Forward movement of the shoulder girdle away from the spine. Abduction of the scapula.

Proximate
To physically hold the separated abdominal muscle together while performing an exercise.

Pulmonary Disease
Limits the body's ability to provide oxygen to the body's tissues.

Pure Movement
Muscle action void of gravity, water, or equipment.

Pyramid Choreography
The number of repetitions for each move in a combination is gradually decreased and/or increased.

Radiation
Loss of body heat through vasodilatation of surface blood vessels. Heat radiates from the body into the surrounding environment.

Rating of Perceived Exertion (RPE)
A subjective assessment, including all of the body's responses, of how hard one is working. There is a 6-20 scale or a 1-10 scale which can be used to determine level of perceived exertion.

Reaction Time
The amount of time elapsed between stimulation and acting upon the stimulus.

Relative Velocity
The speed to one object as measured in respect to the speed of another object.

Resisted Movement
Resisted movement refers to any part in the range of motion of an exercise movement where additional resistive force is created by moving a load against the forces of gravity or buoyancy. The additional resistance force can also be created by the properties or mechanics of an apparatus or particular piece of equipment.

Respiratory System
Made up of the lungs and a series of passageways leading into and out of the lungs.

Resting Heart Rate (HRrest)
The heart rate after being at rest for an extended period of time. A "true" resting heart rate is found by taking the heart rate for 60 seconds, three mornings before rising, and averaging the three.

Retraction
Backward movement of the shoulder girdle toward the spine. Adduction of the scapula.

Reversibility
This principle states that the body will gradually revert to pre-training status when you do not exercise.

Rhythmical Stretching
Moving body parts through a full range of motion in a slow controlled manner.

Rhythmic Cue
Transitional cue that expresses the musical counts used during movement. Tempo changes and complex counts are considered rhythm cues.

RICE
Basic first aid for injuries. RICE stands for rest, ice, compression, and elevation.

Right Atrium
A receiving chamber of the heart where blood first arrives from the body.

Right Ventricle
A sending or pumping chamber which sends blood from the right atrium through the pulmonary artery to the capillaries at the alveoli in the lungs.

Risk Management
The process of measuring or assessing risk, and then developing strategies to manage that risk.

Rotation

Rotation refers to movement around the long axis of the limb.

S

Sacrum

The bone below the lumbar area of the spine which is made up of 5 fused sacral vertebrae.

Saddle Joint

Each joint surface has a convexity at right angles to a concave surface. All movements except rotation are possible at this joint. Example: First carpometacarpal joint (thumb).

Sagittal Axis

A line from the front to the back of the body at about waist height.

Sagittal Plane

An imaginary vertical plane extending from front to back, dividing the body into right and left halves.

Saturated

A triglyceride which has hydrogen attached to every available bond on the carbons.

Scoliosis

Abnormal "S" shaped curve of the spine. Scoliosis refers to a lateral bending of the spine. The shoulders and pelvis will appear uneven and the rib cage may be twisted.

Septum

A wall between the right and left sides of the heart.

Shallow Water Exercise

Exercises typically performed in a vertical position in a water depth of waist to chest level. Lower impact than land-based training, but joint loading does occur.

Shin Splints

Pain and irritation in the shin region of the lower leg.

Short Bone

A short bone is basically cube shaped and is about as wide as it is long. Examples of short bones include the tarsals and carpals.

Skeletal Muscle

The skeletal muscles are voluntary muscles under conscious control, which attach to the bones and allow the skeleton to move.

Skeletal System

All of the bones of the body, associated cartilage, and joints.

Slow-Twitch Muscle Fiber

A red muscle fiber characterized by its slow speed of contraction and a high capacity for aerobic glycolysis.

Somatic Nervous System

A part of the peripheral nervous system made up of efferent somatic fibers that run between the central nervous system and the skeletal muscles.

Specificity

A principle which states that you only train that part of the system or body which is overloaded.

Speed

The rate at which a movement or activity can be performed.

Spheroidal or Ball-and-Socket Joint

A ball-shaped surface articulates with a cup-shaped surface. Example: Hip, Shoulder.

Standard of Care

The degree of care a reasonable person would take to prevent an injury to another.

Static Stretching

Stretching to the point of pain, backing off slightly, and holding the elongated position. Elicits the inverse stretch reflex arc and facilitates muscle relaxation.

Steady State

An exercise state where the body is able to supply the oxygen needed for exercise and oxygen supply meets oxygen demand.

Streamlined Flow

Continuous, steady movement of a fluid.

Stroke

An obstruction of an artery in the brain.

Superior

A term used in exercise to describe one body part's position in relation to another. Superior means "above."

Supination

Rotating the palm outward so it faces forward in anatomical position.

Supine

Refers to the body lying in a "face-up" position.

Swimmer's Ear

Is caused by a bacterial infection resulting from failure to dry the ear adequately following swimming. Symptoms of this condition include itching, a greenish-colored discharge, pain when chewing, and a blocked feeling of the ear.

Synovial Joint
A fully movable joint in which a synovial cavity is present between the two articulating bones.

T

Tempo
The rate of speed at which the beats occur.

Tendonitis
Is a chronic condition that involves inflammation of the tendon or musculotendinous junction.

Tendons
Strong fibrous connective tissue that connects the fascia of a muscle to bones or muscles to muscles.

Thermal Warm up
The purpose is to elevate the core temperature of the body, increase oxygen delivery to the working muscles of the body and release synovial fluid within the joints.

Thermogenesis
The process by which the body produces extra heat, usually by stepping up metabolism or shivering.

Thoracic Spine
The part of the vertebral column found behind the rib cage which consists of 12 midsized vertebrae.

Thrombosis
A clot in a blood vessel.

Tilt
Movements of the head, scapula, and pelvis. The head and pelvis have anterior and posterior tilts.

Trachea
The tube that connects the nasal passages to the lungs.

Transition
A transition occurs when there is a change from one move to another move; changing from a knee lift to a jog would be a transition.

Transitional Cue
A verbal or nonverbal instruction to make a change in activity or direction.

Transverse Plane
The imaginary horizontal plane that divides the body into upper and lower halves.

Triglycerides
The storage form of fat. It consists of free fatty acids and glycerol.

Turbulence
Disturbed or disrupted water flow.

Turbulent Flow
Irregular movement of a fluid with movement varying at any fixed point.

V

Valsalva Maneuver
Closing the glottis and bearing down to create pressure in the chest resulting in a drop in blood pressure and diminished blood flow to the heart.

Valves
Membranous folds which open to allow blood to flow into the heart's chambers, then close to prevent backflow.

Variability
The varying of intensity, duration, or mode (cross training) of exercise sessions to obtain better muscle balance and overall fitness.

Veins
Small vessels that carry deoxygenated blood back through the body to the heart.

Vena Cava
Two large veins that carry blood from the body to the right atrium.

Ventral
The front surface of the body.

Visceral Muscle
The smooth or involuntary muscle in the body over which we have no control.

Viscosity
Refers to the friction between molecules of a liquid or gas, causing the molecules to tend to adhere to each other (cohesion) and in water, to a submerged body (adhesion).

Vitamins
An essential nutrient. Noncaloric organic nutrients needed in tiny amounts in the diet.

Vocal Cords
Pair of membrane covered muscles and ligaments located in the mid-throat. They vibrate to produce sound.

Vocal Injury
Abuse of the vocal cords causing an alteration in the normal manner of speaking such as hoarseness and lowered pitch.

Vocal Nodules

Small, callused growths formed on the vocal cords due to overuse and abuse of one's voice.

W

Waiver of Liability

An agreement between the club and the client that if the club permits the client to exercise in its facility, the client agrees not to sue the club should the client become injured.

Water

Essential nutrient class needed by the body.

Water Specific Movements

Movements that can be performed safely in water, but are impossible to perform on land or considered high risk.

Water Tempo

An appropriate rate of speed used in the aquatic environment to allow for slower reaction time and full range of motion in water choreography.

Manual Contributors

SUSAN ALLEN
B.S. Nutritional/Medical Dietetics
Susan Allen, a registered dietitian and the president of HealthWise, is accomplished as a nationally known nutrition education speaker and consultant for the American Heart Association's weight management program as well as for several health, fitness, and medical facilities.

JUNE M. ANDRUS
June Andrus is a choreographer, seasoned trainer and instructor holding American Red Cross certifications in all aspects of aquatics, a national and international conference presenter at venues including IDEA, AEA, USWFA, and the International School of Aerobic Training.

DEBORAH ASHLIE
Registered Nurse
B.A.
Deborah Ashlie has over 29 years experience as a Registered Nurse in Cardiology as well as Obstetrical Care. She is a water fitness instructor with AEA and is well known for her work with seniors and special populations, in particular her Aqua Hearts © program for Cardiac Rehabilitation patients.

STEPHANIE BARRERA
M.S. Nutrition and Food Sciences
R.D.
Stephanie Barrera holds bachelors and masters degrees in Nutrition and Food Sciences, is a Registered Dietitian, and has ten years experience teaching undergraduate nutrition courses. She currently works in the Cancer Prevention Division at the University of Texas M.D. Anderson Cancer Center in Houston, Texas.

PAULA BRIGGS
M.S. Exercise Physiologist
B.S. Physical Education
Paula Briggs is an expert in water safety and has developed in and outpatient therapeutic aquatic programs, as well as community group aquatic classes for special populations. As an educator Paula shares her expertise in areas of aquatic therapy principles and practice as an instructor to college interns.

JUNE M. (LINDLE) CHEWNING - Editor
M.A. Exercise Physiology
B.S. Physical Education / Co-major Biological Sciences
June (Lindle) Chewning is the owner and manager of Harrison Health and Fitness Center. She is an AEA Aquatic Training Specialist, Chairperson of the AEA Aquatic Research Council and recipient of AEA's 1995 Achievement Award and 2001 Contribution to the Industry Award. June has developed curriculum and serves as adjunct faculty for the Health and Fitness Technologies degree program at Cincinnati State Technical and Community College. June is also the owner of Fitness Learning Systems.

CHRISTINE CRUTCHER
B.A.
Christine Crutcher, an Aquatic Supervisor for Willamalane Park and Recreation District in Springfield, Oregon, has actively been training water exercise instructors in deep and shallow techniques for 26 years. She serves on the AEA Advisory Council and has presented training courses on a national level.

LINDA DELZEIT
M.A. Physical Education emphasis Exercise Physiology
B.A. Physical Education / Health Education Minor
Linda Delzeit has been a junior college instructor in health and physical education, has received honors in World Who's Who of Women, Who's Who in the West, Who's Who in American Education, and from The French Embassy in Washington, D.C.

PATRICIA FOSSELLA
B.S. Physical Education
Patricia Fossella, Operations Manager of the Cranford Pools & Fitness Center in New Jersey, is a member of the AEA Board of Directors and a former member of the AEA Advisory Council. She is a Red Cross Certified Instructor for CPR, First Aid, WSI and Lifeguarding and is a Certified Pool Operator (CPO).

GARY GLASSMAN, M.D.
Gary Glassman, an Emergency Physician from Bucks County, Pennsylvania, is a member of the AEA Board of Directors, writes the Medical Update column for *AKWA* magazine and has presented at IAFC. His goal is that instructors, therapists, and lifeguards be able to recognize, react and respond to emergencies immediately.

SARA KOOPERMAN, J.D.
Sara Kooperman is the director of Sara's City Workout and MANIA Fitness Conventions and was a proud recipient of the AEA Global Award for Contribution to the Aquatic Fitness Industry. She was an adjunct faculty member for the IAR, a lecturer/trainer for ACSM, and a former AEA Advisory Board Member.

PAULINE IVENS

M.S. Adapted Physical Education
B.Ed. Education & Physical Education
Secondary Teaching Certificate in Arts &
   Science of Movement

Pauline Ivens, recipient of the 1997 AEA Global Award for education excellence, owner of Aqua Aerobics Unlimited, has been a movement specialist since 1973, with expertise in dance, aquatics, and exercise for special populations facilitating workshops nationally and internationally.

MICHAEL W. LENK

B.S. Mechanical and Aerospace Engineering

Michael Lenk is a former mechanical/aerospace engineer and aerobic fitness studio owner working as an independent international fitness consultant. He is on staff at the Engineering Department of the Delaware Technical & Community College and is a contributing author for *AKWA* magazine.

RITA MONASTERIO

M.S. Dance
B.S. General Studies

Rita Monasterio is a Dance Scientist of Human Motor Control & Neuromechanisms and movement specialist with expertise in dance and fitness. Rita is a published author and specialist in wellness curriculum development who runs a successful personal trainng business in Eugene, Oregon.

CHARLOTTE NORTON

B.S. Physical Education
M.S. Exercise and Sports Psychology
D.P.T. Doctorate of Physical Therapy

Charlotte Norton received her Doctorate of Physical Therapy at Creighton University and is a national presenter with extensive experience in aquatic therapy. She is a past member of the AEA Research Committee and a contributing author to the *AKWA* magazine.

ANGIE T. PROCTOR

Angie Proctor, Executive Director of AEA and President of Personal Body Trainers, Inc., is a leading international presenter on topics of aquatic fitness, personal training, management and marketing. Angie has produced over 58 aquatic fitness videos and has contributed numerous articles in fitness and health publications worldwide.

JULIE L. SEE

Julie See is the President of AEA, Editor of *AKWA* magazine and Founder of Innovative Aquatics. Active in the industry in a variety of capacities, Julie is a global fitness leader. She has produced numerous fitness videos for instructors and consumers and co-authored a book.

MARSHA STRAHL

Marsha Strahl, Owner of Networking Educational Workshops, is the Fitness Consultant for The Club for Women Only in Chapel Hill, NC. Marsha has guest lectured at many colleges in the Triad area, produced audio cassettes, lectured frequently at Fitness Conferences, and author of Become a Vocal Athlete.

TERESA L. TRIPLETT

B.S. Athletic Training / Sports Medicine
M.S. Exercise Science

Teresa Triplett is a certified Athletic Trainer with experience in commercial fitness, academic health and fitness, and medical fitness. She shares her skills as an instructor, presenter, advisor for ACE, and Director of the Dance Medicine program at the Orthopedic Specialty Hospital in Salt Lake City.

CHRISTINE VEGA, R.D.

B.S. Physical Education
B.A. Biology M.P.H.

Christine Vega is a registered dietitian, physical education teacher on the U.S. Naval Station in South Korea, co-director of Aerobic Training International and author of numerous articles on nutrition and fitness. She serves as an International Aquatic Training Specialist for AEA.

JACK F. WASSERMAN, PH.D.

B.S. Aerospace Engineering
M.S. Mechanical Engineering
Ph.D. Mechanical Engineering – Biomedical Option
Associate of Science Physician's Assistant

Jack F. Wasserman is a professor of Mechanical & Aerospace Engineering and Engineering Science at the University of Tennessee and is the coordinator for the Biomedical Engineering degree program in the department. He has received numerous teaching awards and serves on the AEA Aquatic Research Council.

SUSAN H. WOLFORD

B.A. Physical Education

Susan Wolford, owner of Sun Valley Aquatics in Ketchum, Idaho, teaches water fitness at her own pool and at Sun Valley Athletic Club. She is a former member of the AEA advisory board and a contributing author for *AWKA* magazine. Susan is recognized for prenatal aquatic programs and parent-child exercise.

Manual Reviewers

PAUL BARAN
B.S.Ed., Russian Language & Physical Education
Paul Baran, AEA's *AKWA* Shop Coordinator, is an AEA certified Aquatic Fitness Professional and active in a variety of fitness activities including running, triathlons, kayaking, and drumming.

KELLY DENOMME
Certified Human Resource
Professional Graduate
Kelly Denomme is an AEA certified Aquatic Fitness Professional, Canadian Red Cross Authorized Provider and certified First Aid, CPR & AED Instructor for the Canadian Red Cross and Ontario Heart & Stroke Foundation.

BERYL MICHAELS
B.A.
M.A.
LSW
Beryl Michaels, an AEA Certified Aquatic Fitness Instructor teaching for California Family Fitness Health Clubs, is Principle and Owner of Jaybee Consultants and is the editor of a published collection of short stories.

SHANA SIMMONS
Shana Simmons is AFAA certified (personal trainer, group exercise instructor, youth fitness instructor and aquatics instructor) as well as an AFPA certified nutrition consultant.

RISE STEIN
M.S. Exercise Physiology
Rise Stein has been involved in aquatics for more than twenty-five years and has developed, implemented and coordinated programs for diverse groups ranging from children through seniors.

Index

C

F

fats 31, 209, 228, 230-232, 236-237, 239-240, 337

fatty acids 31, 33-34, 230, 237, 240

feedback cues 141

femoral nerve 19

fetus 203-206

fiber 18, 35-36, 229-230, 233, 237, 239-240, 252, 337

fibrocartilaginous membranes 50

Fibromyalgia Syndrome (FMS) 222

field testing 167-172

filtration system 82

fine motor skills 58, 139, 199

first-class lever 48-49

fitness assessment 158, 163-172, 269

fitness pool 79

fixation 56

flat bones 3

flexibility 12, 28, 30, 59-61, 65-67, 72-75, 89, 134-139, 151-152, 163, 166, 171, 185, 187, 195, 200-201, 209-210, 212, 214-216, 218-219, 222, 224, 277, 293, 337

flexion 8-14, 16-17, 42-47, 51-56, 59, 61-62, 88, 90, 107-109, 111-112, 117, 120, 152-153, 170-172, 186, 283, 286, 337

flotation belt 111, 117, 278, 280-282, 284-285, 295, 310

flotation cuffs 280, 282

flotation device 179, 276, 281-282

flotation equipment 108, 111, 137-138, 153, 220, 276, 280-282, 284, 293

flotation vests 282

fluid density 100

fluid replacement guidelines 241-242

fluoride 234

foam hand bars 104, 108, 111, 277

foam logs 282

folate 234

Food and Drug Administration (FDA) 242

food diaries 250

food safety 237

footwork cue 140, 143

form 45, 116, 140, 200-201, 213-214

form and technique 72, 186

form cues 140

forms, consent 269-271

forward head 60, 166, 203, 337

fractures 176, 183, 188, 215

Framingham Study 68

free radicals 233, 337

free weights 66, 170

freely moveable (synovial joints) 50

freestyle choreography 118-119, 340, *see also linear progression*

frequency 28, 69, 72, 75, 212, 218, 249-250, 260, 277

frequency of training 69, 337

friction 89-92, 186

frontal axis 47, 53, 286, 337

frontal plane 44, 46-47, 123, 286-287, 289, 337

frontal resistance 89, 91-93, 98, 290, 337

frontal surface area 92-93, 98, 100-101, 109, 291

fuel sources 33-34

fulcrum (F) 48

full (high) impact 147

full range of motion 55, 67, 91, 93, 109, 116, 121, 126-127, 138, 217, 286, 290-291, 294

functional capacity 58, 65-66, 69, 73, 189, 221, 225, 283, 285, 327

functional performance 218

functional training 68

G

gait 218-219

games 199- 203

gases 22

gastrocnemius 9, 16, 30, 56, 185, 306-307, 314, 316

genu recurvatum 166, 337

gestational diabetes 206, 216

glandular secretions 17

glenohumeral joint 52, 59

gluconeogenesis 33, 249

glucose 31-34, 159, 179-180, 216, 229, 249, 337

glucose intolerance 216

gluteus maximus 9, 14-15, 29, 44, 56, 113, 214, 307, 313, 324

gluteus medius 9, 15, 56

gluteus minimus 15

glycogen 31-34, 38, 189, 229, 249, 337

Q

R

regular physical activity 74, 194, 236, 256

relative risk 221

relative velocity 91, 109-110, 343

relaxation 137, 139-140, 203, 219-220, 222, 251, 262

relaxation cues 140

relaxin 203

repetitions 66, 72, 98, 116, 118-119, 121, 136, 139-140, 143, 147-148, 152, 170, 172, 200, 289, 292

reproductive system 2

research 29-30, 36, 66, 68-71, 73-74, 89, 122, 166-167, 171-172, 188, 194, 198, 204, 206, 209-210, 214-215, 217, 220-221, 228, 230, 240-241, 244, 249-250, 256, 276-277, 290

resistance (R) 48-50

resistance arm 49, 97

resistance training 28, 36, 61, 72-73, 79, 103-104, 121, 132, 188, 195, 211, 215-218, 222, 224, 250, 292

resisted movement 106, 108, 343

respiratory system 2, 19-20, 37, 66, 73, 178, 195, 343

resting heart rate (HRrest) 69, 73-74, 163-164, 166, 189, 278, 343

retain members 261

retraction 8, 10, 42-43, 45, 58-59, 63, *see also scapular retraction*

reversibility 29, 343

rewards 258-260, 262

rheumatic heart disease 207

rheumatoid arthritis 186, 213-214

rhythmic cue 140, 143

rhythmic movements 134

rhythmical stretching 67, 314, 343, *see also dynamic stretching*

riboflavin 233-234

RICE 175-176, 184, 191, 229, 231, 328, 343

right atrium 21, 23, 343

right ventricle 21, 23, 343

ring buoy 178-179

risk assessment 158-159, 161, 163, 173, 269

risk factors 159, 161, 166, 207, 214, 216, 218-219, 221, 240

risk management 268, 343

rotation 8-10, 14, 42-48, 51-56, 58-59, 61-62, 88, 98, 116-117, 153, 281, 286, 306, 343

rotational motion 88-89

rubberized equipment 30, 36, 106, 110-112, 321, 324

runner's high 260

S

sacral plexus 19

sacrum 5, 19, 50, 171, 343

saddle joint 51, 53, 343

safe transitions 127, 145, 286

safety 81, 83-84, 93, 97, 108, 116-117, 122-125, 135, 139-140, 142, 146-147, 149-153, 176-179, 183-184, 191, 195, 205, 215, 217, 242, 261-262, 265, 268-269, 279-282, 292-293, 295

sagittal axis 47, 53, 286, 343

sagittal plane 41, 46-47, 123, 144, 286-289, 343

saphenous nerve 19

sarcomere 34, 106

saturated 230-231, 236-237, 240, 343

scapula 3-4, 8, 10, 43, 45-47, 52, 56, 58-59, 106, *see also shoulder blade*

scapular retraction 8, 206, *see also retraction*

sciatic nerve 19

scoliosis 60, 166, 344

second-class lever 48-49

sedentary lifestyle 68, 159

seizures 177, 181-182, 218

selenium 235, 240

self-confidence 196, 203

self-efficacy 258

self-rescue techniques 279

self-starvation 245

self-talk 262

semimembranosus 9, 16, *see also hamstrings*

semitendinosus 9, 16, *see also hamstrings*

sensory change 194

septum 21, 344

set-point theory 244

shallow water exercise 69, 78, 80-81, 207, 213, 216, 276, 279, 297-308

shallow water running test 171

shin splints 185, 271, 344

shoes 81, 84, 147-148, 150, 154, 180, 185, 197, 204, 217, 276, 280, *see also water shoes*

Y

Z